THE PEDIATRIC PROCEDURAL SEDATION HANDBOOK

The Pediatric Procedural Sedation Handbook

EDITED BY

Cheryl K. Gooden, MD
Associate Professor of Anesthesiology and Pediatrics
Division of Pediatric Anesthesia
Yale University School of Medicine
Yale-New Haven Hospital
New Haven, CT

Lia H. Lowrie, MD
Director, Division of Pediatric Critical Care Medicine and Procedural Sedation
Professor of Pediatrics
St. Louis University School of Medicine at SSM Health Cardinal Glennon Children's Hospital
St. Louis, MO

Benjamin F. Jackson, MD
Associate Professor of Pediatrics
Pediatric Emergency Medicine
PEM Director of Procedural Sedation
Medical University of South Carolina
Charleston, SC

SPS
SOCIETY FOR PEDIATRIC SEDATION
SAFE AND SOUND

OXFORD
UNIVERSITY PRESS

OXFORD
UNIVERSITY PRESS

Oxford University Press is a department of the University of Oxford. It furthers the University's objective of excellence in research, scholarship, and education by publishing worldwide. Oxford is a registered trade mark of Oxford University Press in the UK and certain other countries.

Published in the United States of America by Oxford University Press
198 Madison Avenue, New York, NY 10016, United States of America.

CIP data is on file at the Library of Congress
ISBN 978–0–19–065911–0

9 8 7 6 5 4 3

Printed by Webcom, Inc., Canada

Contents

Contributors

David Banks, MD
Pediatric Emergency Medicine Associates, LLC
Children's Healthcare of Atlanta, Scottish Rite

Judson Barber, MD
Department of Pediatrics
Division of Pediatric Emergency Medicine
University of Alabama at Birmingham
Birmingham, AL

John Berkenbosch, MD
Professor of Pediatrics
Pediatric Critical Care
University of Louisville
Louisville, KY

Maala Bhatt, MD, MSc
Assistant Professor of Pediatrics
University of Ottawa
Ottawa, ON

Jennifer Biber, MD
Pediatric Intensivist
Akron Children's Hospital
Akron, OH

Laura Bredbenner, CCLS
Child Life Specialist
Children's Hospital of San Antonio
San Antonio, TX

Eileen Briening, MSN, DNP
Pediatric Nurse Practitioner
A.I. Dupont Hospital for Children
Wilmington, DE

Mark A. Buckmaster, MD
Associate Professor of Pediatrics and Anesthesiology
University of Alabama School of Medicine
Director, Simon Sedation Service
Children's of Alabama
Birmingham, AL

Rebecca K. Burger, MD
Department of Pediatrics
Division of Pediatric Emergency Medicine
Emory University School of Medicine
Children's Healthcare of Atlanta
Atlanta, GA

Laurie J. Burton, MD
Assistant Professor
Department of Pediatrics
Emory University
Vice-Chief
Children's Sedation Services, CHOA
Atlanta, GA

Tracy Campbell, MSN
Nemours A.I. duPont Hospital for Children

Andrea R. Carberry, MD
University of Wisconsin—American Family Children's Hospital
Madison, WI

Peter A. Chin, MBBS, MMHC
Associate Professor of Clinical Anesthesiology
Vanderbilt University Medical Center
Nashville, TN

Jill Chorney, PhD
Dalhousie University and IWK Health Centre
Halifax, NS

Corrie E. Chumpitazi, MD, MS
Associate Professor of Pediatrics
Section of Emergency Medicine
Baylor College of Medicine
Houston, TX

Lowell Clark, MD
Associate Professor of Pediatrics
Pediatric Critical Care Medicine
Mercer University School of Medicine
Macon, GA

Jerard (Mick) Connors, MD
Pediatric Emergency Medicine
Anytime Telehealth Inc.
CEO/Founder
Nashville, TN

Jacinta Cooper, MD, PhD
Department of Pediatrics
Division of Pediatric Emergency Medicine
University of Alabama at Birmingham
Birmingham, AL

Kevin G. Couloures, DO, MPH
Yale School of Medicine
New Haven, CT

Joseph P. Cravero, MD
Associate Professor of Anesthesiology
Harvard Medical School
Senior Clinical Associate
Boston Children's Hospital
Boston, MA

Nancy Crego, PhD
Assistant Professor
Duke University
School of Nursing
Durham, NC

Barbara Dilos, DO
Clinical Assistant Professor
Icahn School of Medicine
Director of Anesthesia
Elmhurst Hospital Center
Elmhurst, NY

Rebecca H. Evans, MD
Department of Anesthesiology
University of Vermont Medical Center Children's Hospital
Burlington, VT

David Fagin, MD
Pediatric Emergency Medicine Associates, LLC
Children's Healthcare of Atlanta, Scottish Rite
Atlanta, GA

MaryKay Farrell, RN-BC
Children's Minnesota—Sedation and Procedural Services
St. Paul, MN

Debra J. Faulk, MD
University of Colorado
Children's Hospital Colorado
Aurora, CO

Jenna Fine, DO
Assistant Professor of Pediatrics
Eastern Virginia Medical School
Children's Hospital of the King's Daughters
Norfolk, VA

Kimberly Fugok, DO
Pediatric Emergency Medicine
Lehigh Valley Physician Group
Allentown, PA

Gordon Gale, MD
Professor of Pediatrics
Saint Louis University School of Medicine
SSM Health Cardinal Glennon Children's Hospital
St. Louis, MO

Jennifer K. Gillen, MD
Assistant Professor of Pediatrics
Pediatric Intensive Care
Mount Sinai Kravis Children's Hospital
New York, NY

Cheryl K. Gooden, MD
Associate Professor of Anesthesiology and Pediatrics
Pediatric Anesthesia Division
Yale University School of Medicine
Yale New Haven Hospital
New Haven, CT

Sarah Greenaway, MBBS
Clinical Research Fellow
Great Ormond Street and Royal London Hospitals
London, UK

Jeana E. Havidich, MD, MS
Department of Anesthesiology
Children's Hospital at Dartmouth
Lebanon, NH

Mary A. Hegenbarth, MD
Section of Emergency Medicine
Children's Mercy Kansas City
Department of Pediatrics
University of Missouri-Kansas City School of Medicine
Kansas City, MO

James H. Hertzog, MD
Department of Pediatrics
Division of Critical Care Medicine
Nemours/Alfred I. duPont Hospital for Children
Wilmington, DE
Professor of Pediatrics
Sidney Kimmel Medical College at Thomas Jefferson University
Philadelphia, PA

Joanne M. Hojsak, MD
Associate Professor of Pediatrics and Medical Education
Pediatric Intensive Care
Mount Sinai Kravis Children's Hospital
New York, NY

Gregory A. Hollman, MD
Professor of Pediatrics
Medical Director, Diagnostic and Therapy Center
University of Wisconsin—American Family Children's Hospital
Madison, WI

Constance S. Houck, MD, MPH
Associate Professor
Department of Anesthesiology, Perioperative and Pain Medicine
Boston Children's Hospital
Harvard Medical School
Boston, MA

Melissa Howlett, BSc
Department of Psychology & Neuroscience
Dalhousie University
Halifax, NS

Benjamin F. Jackson, MD
Associate Professor of Pediatrics
Pediatric Emergency Medicine
PEM Director of Procedural Sedation
Medical University of South Carolina
Charleston, SC

Shobhit Jain, MD
Division of Emergency Medicine
Department of Pediatrics
Children's Mercy Kansas City
University of Missouri-Kansas City
Kansas City, MO

Nicole M. Johnson, MD
Pediatric Critical Care Medicine
Rainbow Babies & Children's Hospital
University Hospitals Cleveland Medical Center
Cleveland, OH

Pradip P. Kamat, MD, MBA
Associate Professor of Pediatrics
Pediatric Critical Care Medicine
Emory University School of Medicine
Director of Children's Sedation Services
Children's Healthcare of Atlanta, Egleston
Atlanta, GA

John S. Kopec, MD
Pediatric Intensivist, Pediatric Intensive Care Unit
Director of Pediatric Sedation Service
Helen DeVos Children's Hospital at Spectrum Health
Grand Rapids, MI

Susanne Kost, MD
Sedation Service
Children's Hospital of Philadelphia
Philadelphia, PA

Ashwin Krishna, MD
Department of Pediatrics
University of Kentucky
Heinrich A Werner Division of Pediatric Critical Care
Lexington, KY

Cheri Landers, MD
Department of Pediatrics
University of Kentucky
Heinrich A Werner Division of Pediatric Critical Care
Lexington, KY

Mary Landrigan-Ossar, MD, PhD
Senior Associate in Perioperative Anesthesia
Boston Children's Hospital
Assistant Professor of Anaesthesia
Harvard Medical School
Boston, MA

Melissa Langhan, MD, MHS
Department of Pediatrics and Emergency Medicine
Section of Pediatric Emergency Medicine
Yale University School of Medicine
New Haven, CT

Deborah LaViolette, BSN
Children's National Medical Center
Washington, DC

Storm Liebling, MD
Department of Pediatrics
Section of Pediatric Emergency Medicine
Yale University School of Medicine
New Haven, CT

Jeffrey Linzer Sr., MD
Professor of Pediatrics and Emergency Medicine
Emory University— Children's Healthcare of Atlanta
Atlanta, GA

Lia H. Lowrie, MD
Director
Division of Pediatric Critical Care Medicine and Procedural Sedation
Professor of Pediatrics
St. Louis University School of Medicine at
SSM Health Cardinal Glennon Children's Hospital
St. Louis, MO

Elizabeth Mack, MD, MS
Division of Pediatric Critical Care
Medical University of South Carolina
Charleston, SC

Christina Mannix, MD
Assistant Professor
Pediatrics
St. Louis University School of Medicine
St. Louis, MO
St. Louis University School of Medicine at
SSM Cardinal Glennon Children's Hospital
St. Louis, MO

Bryan P. McKee, MD
Pediatric Intensivist
Akron Children's Hospital
Akron, OH

Laura Mitchell, CCLS
Certified Child Life Specialist III
Nemours/A.I. du Pont Hospital for Children
Wilmington, DE

Ndidi Nwokorie, MBBS
Pediatric Emergency Medicine
Assistant Professor of Clinical Pediatrics
Georgetown University
Washington, DC

Kimberly Paula-Santos, BSN
Radiology/Sedation Nurse
Connecticut Children's Medical Center
Hartford, CT

Janey Phelps, MD
Associate Professor of Anesthesiology and Pediatrics
Medical Director of the Pediatric Sedation Service
University of North Carolina at Chapel Hill
Chapel Hill, NC

Elysha Pifko, MD
Division of Pediatric Emergency Medicine
Department of Pediatrics
Nemours/A.I. du Pont Hospital for Children
Wilmington, DE

Chris A. Rees, MD, MPH
Fellow
Division of Pediatric Emergency Medicine
Boston Children's Hospital and Harvard Medical School
Boston, MA

Lorie Reilly, MSN
Sedation/Radiology Nurse Practitioner
The Children's Hospital of Philadelphia
Philadelphia, PA

Jason Reynolds, MD
Pediatric Palliative Care
Cook Children's Hospital

Michelle M. Rhoads, MSN
Nemours A.I. duPont Hospital for Children

Mark G. Roback, MD
Professor of Pediatrics and Emergency Medicine
Division Director, Pediatric Emergency Medicine
University of Minnesota Medical School
Minneapolis, MN

Amber Rogers, MD
Texas Children's Hospital
Baylor College of Medicine
Houston, TX

Patricia Scherrer, MD
Sedation Physician – Sedation Services
Children's Healthcare of Atlanta
Atlanta, GA

Daniel J. Sedillo, MD, MBA
Associate Professor
Chief, Section of Pediatric Sedation Medicine
The Children's Hospital of San Antonio
Baylor College of Medicine
Houston, TX

Paul G. Smith, DO
Pediatric Intensivist/
Pulmonologist
Community Medical Center
Pediatric Intensive Care Unit
and Pediatric Speciality Clinic
Missoula, Montana

Anne Stormorken, MD
Associate Professor of Pediatrics
Case Western Reserve
University School of Medicine
Medical Director,
Pediatric Pain Service
UH Rainbow Babies and
Children's Hospital
Cleveland, OH

Jesse J. Sturm, MD, MPH
Associate Professor
Chief of the Division of
Sedation Services
Connecticut Children's
Medical Center
Hartford, CT

Michael Sury, MBBS, PhD
Consultant Anaesthetist
Department of Anaesthesia
Great Ormond Street Hospital
NHS Trust
Portex Unit of Anaesthesia
Institute of Child Health
University College London
London, UK

Christine Tatem, MEd, CCLS
Lead Child Life Specialist
Connecticut Children's Medical
Center
Hartford, Connecticut

Urmila Tirodker, MD
Visiting Clinical Associate
Professor
University of Pittsburgh
Sedation Service
Division of Anesthesiology
Children's Hospital of
Pittsburgh, UPMC
Pittsburgh, PA

Joseph D. Tobias, MD
Chairman, Department of
Anesthesiology and Pain
Medicine
Professor of Anesthesiology and
Pediatrics
Nationwide Children's Hospital
The Ohio State University
College of Medicine
Columbus, OH

Stephen Tomek, MD
Clinical Assistant Professor of
Pediatrics
Mercer University School of
Medicine
Macon, GA

Daniel S. Tsze, MD, MPH
Assistant Professor of Pediatrics in Emergency Medicine
Department of Emergency Medicine
Columbia University Vagelos College of Physicians & Surgeons
NewYork-Presbyterian Morgan Stanley Children's Hospital
New York, NY

Michael Turmelle, MD
Associate Professor of Pediatrics
Division Co-Chief of Hospital Medicine
Medical Director of St. Louis Children's Hospital Children's Direct
Washington University School of Medicine
St. Louis, MO

John H. Unkel, DDS, MD, MPA
Residency Director and Medical Director
Pediatric Dentistry
St. Mary's Hospital of Richmond
Bon Secours Health System Inc.

Élise W. van der Jagt, MD, MPH
Professor of Pediatrics and Critical Care
Division of Pediatric Critical Care
Department of Pediatrics
Golisano Children's Hospital/ University of Rochester School of Medicine/Dentistry
Rochester, NY

Samuel Vanderhoek, MD
Assistant Professor
Anesthesiology and Critical Care Medicine
Johns Hopkins University School of Medicine
Baltimore, MD

Rhea Vidrine, MD
Division of Critical Care Medicine
Cincinnati Children's Hospital Medical Center
Cincinnati, OH

Amy E. Vinson, MD
Assistant Professor
Department of Anesthesiology, Perioperative and Pain Medicine
Boston Children's Hospital
Harvard Medical School
Boston, MA

Sara Walls, MD
Staff Anesthesiologist
Greenville Health Systems
Greenville, SC

Sally Webb, MD
Professor of Pediatrics
Pediatric Critical Care Medicine
Medical University of South Carolina
Charleston, SC

David Werner, MD
Pediatric Emergency Medicine Associates, LLC
Children's Healthcare of Atlanta, Scottish Rite

Jenna Wheeler, MD
Clinical Assistant Professor
Florida State University College of Medicine
Pediatric Critical Care
Arnold Palmer Hospital for Children
Orlando, FL

Don Wiest, PharmD
Associate Professor
Clinical Pharmacy and Outcome Sciences
Medical University of South Carolina, College of Pharmacy
Charleston, SC

Feifei Z. Williams, MD
Division of Pediatric Critical Care Medicine
Division of Pediatric Cardiology
Emory University of School of Medicine
Children's Healthcare of Atlanta
Atlanta, GA

Michael J. Wolf, MD
Division of Pediatric Critical Care Medicine
Division of Pediatric Cardiology
Emory University of School of Medicine
Children's Healthcare of Atlanta
Sibley Heart Center
Atlanta, GA

Seth Wolf, MD
Department of Pediatrics
Section of Pediatric Emergency Medicine
Yale University School of Medicine
New Haven, CT

Judith L. Zier, MD
Children's Minnesota—Pediatric Critical Care
Minneapolis, MN

Samuel L. Zuckerman, MD
Associate Professor
Chief, Division of Pediatric Critical Care Medicine
Department of Pediatrics
School of Medicine at Amarillo
Texas Tech University Health Sciences Center
Amarillo, TX

PART 1

FUNDAMENTALS OF SEDATION

1

Pediatric Sedation

Evolution of a Medical Discipline During a Professional Lifetime

LIA H. LOWRIE

The unique psychological and physical needs of children during anesthesia have been recognized since the earliest reports of creating a state of unawareness during surgery. Indeed. the third reported ether anesthesia procedure by Dr. Crawford Long in 1849 was for a 7-year-old boy undergoing toe amputation. By 1900 tonsillectomy and orthopedic procedures were common in children using ether, and attention to a child's anxiety level preanesthesia was remarked upon in 1907 when it was recommended to "add a few drops of the mother's cologne to the ether mask and induce the child in the mother's arms."[1] Modern medicine after World War II was characterized by an explosion of technological advances in equipment and techniques. Advanced care for infants and children was provided in a few medical centers with often jerry-rigged equipment with inadequate patient/technology interface because of the engineering challenge inherent in smaller-sized equipment (endotracheal tubes, vascular access), limitations of surgical field in infants, and lack of understanding of infant physiology. Indeed, it was not until the late 1980s that a widely held tenet that infants did not require anesthesia during surgery or analgesia afterwards was finally put to rest by Anand and Hickey.[2]

The author's medical training started in the mid-1980s at a respected full-service children's hospital. Training in that era stressed local anesthesia and physical patient immobilization techniques for common procedures such as lumbar puncture or tube thoracostomy. More elaborate or prolonged invasive procedures such as endoscopy or dental care were regularly performed with the proceduralist administering a "cocktail" of meperidine, promethazine, and chlorpromazine, often intramuscular. Barbiturates with relatively long half-lives were a mainstay of sedation in radiologic testing or electroencephalography requiring primarily immobility in children. Parents were routinely instructed to administer chloral hydrate at home before bringing the child in (without a car seat, of course) for a scheduled procedure. The decade of the 1980s represented an awakening of interest in the safety of pediatric sedation care in the United States—extending the dramatic success demonstrated by anesthesiologists in reducing morbidity and mortality from anesthesia in the operating suite. The Society for Pediatric Anesthesia was formed in 1986 in the United States. The American Academy of Pediatrics (AAP) and the American Academy of Pediatric Dentistry (AAPD) published in 1985 their first of a series of guidelines for the monitoring and management of children during elective administration of sedation for tests and procedures outside the operating room.[3] The terms *conscious sedation, deep sedation,* and *general anesthesia* were defined; minimal monitoring recommended consisted of a precordial stethoscope and blood pressure cuff; and the concept of a clinician monitoring the child without being involved in the procedure was introduced.

The decade of the 1990s brought about rapid and often politically charged discussion about which medical professionals were best equipped to provide procedural sedation care for children. Use of medications outside the operating room such as fentanyl, midazolam, and ketamine and the introduction of propofol in intensive care settings allowed proceduralists access to medications for which they may have had little training. Anesthesiologists (who did have the appropriate training) were unable to provide the services needed to meet the demand represented by the rapidly evolving technology appropriate for infant and child diagnosis and treatment. Pulse oximetry was the "fifth vital sign" as it moved out of the operating room and intensive care setting, becoming ubiquitous in pediatric hospital care. The AAP and AAPD revised their guidelines to include much more specific requirements for monitoring, preprocedural patient assessment, and postprocedure care.[3] Reports of creation of pediatric sedation services or units separate from anesthesiology control began to surface. Case series of tens or hundreds of procedures performed with certain regimens of sedation were touted as evidence of safety and efficacy despite being inappropriately statistically powered to support the claims.[4]

The early 2000s were marked by continued reports of pediatric permanent morbidity and deaths after sedation care in children marred by poor presedation risk assessment, medication delivery errors, and failure to rescue children from known sedation medication risks (airway obstruction, apnea, hypoxemia, etc.). In the United States, the Centers for Medicare and Medicaid Services (CMS) and The Joint Commission (TJC) joined the national conversation about sedation safety by mandating oversight of all care in the hospital involved in the continuum of sedation—moderate, deep, and general—by the department of anesthesiology. Revision of the language of the AAP guidelines eliminated the use of the term *conscious sedation*; the definition of that patient state is likely unachievable in infants and young children. CMS revised the definition of the sedation continuum to be more applicable to pediatrics, also removing the term *conscious sedation*, acknowledged in particular the amount of sedation occurring in dental practices, and laid out directives about standards for sedation care needing to be consistent across hospital and nonhospital settings. Reimbursement was denied to systems and practitioners that could not meet these new standards. Recognizing the evolving multiprofessional approach to pediatric procedural sedation, a group of diverse practitioners met for a conference supported by a National Patient Safety Foundation grant in 2000 about pediatric procedural sedation organized by Drs. Cravero and Blike at the Dartmouth-Hitchcock Medical Center.[5] This conference contributed impetus toward the formation in 2003 of a multi-institutional Pediatric Sedation Research Consortium (PSRC) that focused on gathering data about pediatric procedural sedation care across the United States, eventually becoming the research tool of the Society for Pediatric Sedation (SPS), formed in 2007. Several multicenter research studies have been produced from the PSRC database with sufficient power to produce early benchmarks about the skills and techniques associated with safe pediatric procedural sedation delivery.[6]

The decade beginning in 2010 sharpened the focus on skills and techniques of providing care rather than solely on the credentials of the clinician needed to hold hospital privileges to provide the care. Recognition of the need for specific procedural sedation services for children has grown to the extent that individual clinicians from a variety of background training—anesthesiology, critical care, emergency services, hospitalists, advanced practice nursing—are considered sedationists with pathways to hospital privileging. Fueled in part by an SPS-sponsored forum about quality as it relates to this new professional field in 2011,[7] we are beginning to move beyond safety as a single determinant of quality to include assessing the patient state attained during sedation beyond whether the procedure could be completed, the efficiencies of care represented by sedation service line creation, and creating specific patient-centered approaches to sedation rather than procedure-specific protocols. New medications such as dexmedetomidine and a focus on less invasive administrative techniques have allowed tailoring of sedative approaches and more integration with distraction techniques so skillfully applied by child life specialists. Assessment of the efficacy of new and old medications has resulted in appropriately questioning the "continuum" of sedation as a useful paradigm; widespread use of hypnotics such as ketamine and dexmedetomidine mandates new ways of assessing how much physiologic risk is actually occurring during the sedation process. Technology has also continued to evolve to allow shorter, quieter MRI scanning, and for sedation care, many practitioners would tout noninvasive end-tidal carbon dioxide measurement as now the "sixth vital sign." The concept of safety and benefit of anesthetics and sedatives is being reexamined after young animal research data have raised significant concerns about neuronal apoptosis during exposure to commonly used medications. Only very recently have we seen the publication of the first human studies attempting to assess risk to the developing human brain from exposure to agents such as midazolam, fentanyl, ketamine, and inhaled general anesthetics.[8]

The author has several more years of a productive career in which to look forward to even more attention to achieving high-quality healthcare for children and infants focusing on not only their physiologic state but also their psychological health and resiliency. It is exciting to imagine how much farther we can go in another professional lifetime of shared multidisciplinary quality and research work toward perhaps non-painful sedative and procedural techniques and new technology interfaces that eliminate the need for pharmacologic sedation at all.

References

1. Rockoff MA. History of pediatric anesthesia. In: Davis PJ, Cladis FP, eds. *Smith's Anesthesia for Infants and Children.* 9th ed. Philadelphia: Elsevier, 2017:1332–1345.
2. Anand KJS, Hickey PR. Pain and its effects in the human neonate and fetus. *N Engl J Med.* 1987;317:1321.
3. Coté CJ, Wilson S. Guidelines for monitoring and management of pediatric patients before, during and after sedation for diagnostic and therapeutic procedures: update 2016. *Pediatrics.* 2016;138(1):20161212.
4. Havidich JE, Cravero JP. The current status of procedural sedation for pediatric patients in out-of-operating room locations. *Curr Opin Anesthesiol.* 2012;25:453–460.
5. Blike GT, Cravero JP. Pride, prejudice and pediatric sedation: a multispecialty evaluation of the state of the art: report from a Dartmouth summit on pediatric sedation. National Patient Safety Foundation; 2001. Available at http://www.npsf.org/pdf/r/PediatricSedation.pdf. Accessed November 9, 2010.
6. http://www.pedsedation.org/resources/research/articles/

7. Connor JM, Cravero JP, Kost S, et al. Great expectations—defining quality in pediatric sedation: outcomes of a multidisciplinary consensus conference. *J Healthcare Quality.* 2015;37(2):139–154.
8. www.smarttots.org/research-and-grants/
9. Mason KP. Challenges in paediatric procedural sedation: political, economic, and clinical aspects. *Br J Anaesth.* 2014;113(S2):ii48–ii62.
10. Willams MR, Ward DS, Carlson D, et al. Evaluating patient-centered outcomes in clinical trials of procedural sedation. Part 1, efficacy: sedation consortium on endpoints and procedures for treatment, education, and research recommendations. *Anesth Analg.* 2017;124:821–830.

2

The Impacts of Procedural Stress

JILL CHORNEY AND MELISSA HOWLETT

Children undergo stressful medical procedures as part of routine (e.g., immunizations) and specialty care (e.g., lumbar puncture). The stress experienced by children around these procedures is produced by a combination of factors:[1]

- The degree of pain associated with the procedure
- The child's behavioral and emotional response (e.g., fear, lack of control, temperament)
- How much attention is focused on the procedure.

Interactions among the child, parent, and healthcare provider and the physical environment are also important contributors to procedural stress.[2] Procedural stress is often family-wide, with parents experiencing fear and anxiety about the procedures; parent anxiety accounts for approximately 50% of the variance in child procedural distress.[3]

Being aware of the factors that contribute to procedural stress can help healthcare providers identify children who may be at risk. Research on children having frequent medical procedures (e.g., immunizations, blood draws, dental work) suggests that procedural stress can be predicted by factors such as the following:

- Difficult, fearful, or shy child temperament (e.g., increased inhibition, withdrawal, high activity)

- Child psychopathology (e.g., preexisting anxiety)
- Parent anxiety (children can often recognize when their parent is anxious, which can influence their own anxiety and thus contribute to children's procedural stress)
- Prior negative medical experiences (i.e., high frequency of procedures, intense pain, distress, or procedural complications)

Although these factors cannot be changed at the time of the procedure, identifying these factors can alert healthcare providers that the child and family may require more support.

High procedural stress is associated with the following:

- Less use of effective coping during the procedure
- Prolonged completion time and decreased ease with which the procedure is completed, and thus increased costs associated with the procedure
- Poor behavioral compliance and cooperation leading to negative interactions between healthcare providers, children, and/or parents, including the need for child restraint

Procedural stress can exert both immediate and long-term impacts following procedure completion, influencing pain, recovery, postprocedure behavior, and emotions. For example, children who are more anxious before surgery have more of the following:

- Postoperative pain, negative postsurgical behavioral disturbances (e.g., separation anxiety, eating and sleep challenges), and general anxiety during the recovery period[4]
- Postoperative emergence delirium, a higher need for analgesia, and a prolonged recovery period[4]

The impacts of procedural stress during childhood have even been shown to translate into adulthood: reports of fear around medical events and even total avoidance of preventive, diagnostic, and/or necessary medical care have been documented.[5]

Managing Anticipatory Distress

Anticipatory distress refers to fear and anxiety experienced before the procedure even begins. Even if a child will be sedated for a procedure, anticipatory distress may be present and should be assessed and managed by doing the following:

- Providing information about the procedure and effective use of coping behaviors (e.g., distraction, relaxation techniques)
- Teaching confidence and mastery of coping behaviors through preparation prior to the procedure. The content of preparation should include developmentally appropriate and specific procedural information:
    - How long the procedure will take
    - What tools will be used
    - Why the procedure is necessary
    - What the child will be asked to do (e.g., step-by-step expectations)
    - Sensory information (e.g., physical and emotional sensations that may be experienced during the procedure)
    - Planning for implementation of coping techniques (e.g., distraction, deep breathing, imagery, progressive muscle relaxation).

It is also important to address anticipated pain. If the procedure is going to be painful, children should be informed of this ahead of time and pain management strategies should be discussed proactively with children and parents.[6]

The timing of preparation delivery should be informed by the type of procedure (e.g., a few days prior to surgery; same day for injections) and the child's interpretation of the severity of the procedure. For example, preparation should be provided earlier to a child who perceives a needle to be a major procedure, as compared to a child who perceives a needle to be a minor procedure. If preparation is delivered too far in advance, the child may forget pertinent information or may actually experience increased anxiety if he or she dwells on the information provided. Alternatively, preparation delivered too close to the procedure may not allow the child enough time to process the information, thereby heightening stress and anxiety. The overall goal of preparation is to do the following:

- Reduce children's fear of the unknown
- Allow children to feel they have as much control and choice as possible
- Ensure children have the skills they need to facilitate effective coping throughout the procedure

Given the important role that parent factors play in maintaining and predicting child procedural distress, parents must be included in the preparation process. Preparation should target parents' anxiety directly and provide training as to how to effectively support their child during the procedure, such as coaching the child to use learned coping strategies (e.g., relaxation techniques) and lead distraction. Parents should also be informed of unhelpful behaviors consistently shown to influence child distress during medical procedures and coached in how to engage with their child in a way that promotes coping during the procedure.

Managing Distress During the Procedure

Distraction, which involves directing attention away from the undesirable (e.g., procedure) and toward something more pleasant and engaging, is consistently shown to be effective in managing child distress and improving behavioral cooperation during medical procedures. There are many different ways in which distraction can be implemented (Table 2.1). Distraction appears to be effective whether or not the child independently chooses what to use as a distraction, whether technology is used passively (e.g., video clips) or

TABLE 2.1 Examples of age-appropriate distraction techniques

	Distraction Techniques
Toddlers	• Introducing toys • Bubbles (if child blowing, could also be relaxation) • Books • Singing songs • Directing child's attention to something in the room • Watching a video on an iPad or tablet
School-aged Children	• Actively playing with age-appropriate toys • Books • Telling stories • Watching a video on an iPad or tablet • Playing a game on an iPad or tablet • Listening to music • Nonprocedural talk (e.g., school, pets, favorite movie, hobbies) • Actively playing age-appropriate games. • Blowing on a pinwheel or party blower (also serves to facilitate deep breathing) • Counting forward/backward • Puzzles • Drawing or coloring
Adolescents	• Watching a video on an iPad or tablet • Playing a game on an iPad or tablet • Listening to music • Nonprocedural talk (e.g., school, vacation, hobbies) • Listening to music • Virtual reality (interactive video equipment, goggles) • Mental imagery • Telling jokes • Solving problems

interactively (e.g., playing games on a smartphone), and whether or not an adult is involved.

Parent and healthcare provider behaviors during procedures are strongly related to child anxiety and behavioral distress. Behaviors that promote distress in children and should be avoided during the procedure include criticism, reassurance, apologizing, and empathic statements. Although many of these behaviors, especially empathic statements ("I know this is hard") and reassurance ("It will be OK"), are well intentioned, they actually direct the child's attention to his or her own distress and pain, and suggest fear in the adult.[7] Healthcare providers and parents are encouraged to engage in behaviors that promote coping during procedures, such as distracting talk about things other than the procedure, humor, prompting children to engage in coping behaviors (e.g., distraction, relaxation techniques), and medical reinterpretation (i.e., reframing medical equipment as less threatening). It is also important that healthcare providers and parents limit questions that suggest children have control over aspects of the procedure that they actually cannot control (e.g., start of the medical procedure, "are you ready for the needle?"); rather, they should offer choices over aspects children can control (e.g., "which arm would you like the needle in?"). Examples of both unhelpful and helpful adult behaviors are summarized in Table 2.2.

Research has shown high correlations between healthcare provider and parent behaviors, suggesting that parents likely take cues from healthcare providers and follow their behaviors.[7] As such, it is important for healthcare providers to model behaviors that promote coping during procedures.

Preventing Future Procedural Stress

Children who experience higher procedural stress and pain frequently develop negatively exaggerated and less accurate memories, which then translate into higher stress toward subsequent procedures.[8] Fortunately, children's memory of medical procedures

TABLE 2.2 Unhelpful/helpful parent and healthcare provider behaviors during pediatric medical procedures

Unhelpful		*Helpful*	
Label	***What Not to Say***	***Label***	***What to Say***
Reassurance	*"There is nothing to worry about."* *"You're going to be okay."*	Distraction (nonprocedural talk)	*"Tell me about your favorite movie."* *"What did you do in school today?"*
Criticism	*"Stop acting like a baby and sit still."*	Praise	*"You did a great job staying still."* *"I'm proud of you."*
Too much control	*"Tell me when you're ready to begin."*	Limited control	*"Which arm would you like the needle in?"*
Apologizing	*"I'm so sorry you have to go through this."* *"I'm sorry for hurting you."*	Encouragement	*"You're being very brave."*
Lying	*"This won't hurt at all."*	Sensory information	*"You might feel a pinch, but it will be very quick,"*
Empathic statements	*"I know this is hard."* *"I know this is painful."*	Coping skills coaching	*"On the count of three take a big breath and blow as many bubbles as you can."* *"Look around the room and tell me how many black objects you can see."*
		Medical reinterpretation	During mask anesthesia induction: *"Let's see how big you can blow up this balloon!"* *"Let's play the astronaut game."*

is malleable and the language used to discuss pain memories with children can influence the content of procedural memories.[9] For example, when children's memories are reframed in a positive light (e.g., highlighting how the child effectively coped during the procedure), less pain and distress is noted at subsequent procedures. Therefore, it can be helpful to talk to the child and family about the child's success, highlighting his or her ability to cope, as well as the parent's ability to coach and support the child during the procedure.

Table 2.3 provides a guide for healthcare providers outlining what should be done before, during, and after procedures to manage procedural stress and pain.

TABLE 2.3 Guide for healthcare providers to manage procedural stress at each stage of procedure completion with children

What to Do . . .	*Recommendations*
Before the Procedure	• Assess the presence of predictors of high procedural stress among patient and family (e.g., temperamental factors, child anxiety, parent anxiety, prior negative medical experiences, child response/coping during previous medical procedures). • Encourage parents and children to prepare for the procedure ahead of time. • For procedures requiring an injection, encourage the use of topical anesthetics. • Provide clear, detailed, honest, and age-appropriate procedural and sensory information. • Teach parent and child positive coping strategies (e.g., distraction, diaphragmatic breathing, imagery, progressive muscle relaxation). • Educate parents on how to effectively support their child during the procedure (e.g., coach through mastered coping strategies, lead distraction). • Educate parents on the importance of adult behaviors during the procedure and what they should/should not say. • Plan for implementation of coping strategies (e.g., select distraction stimuli).

TABLE 2.3 Continued

What to Do . . .	*Recommendations*
During the Procedure	* **Manage procedural stress and pain through the use of evidence-based strategies.** • Ensure child is in the most comfortable position for the given procedure (e.g., for injections, children should be sitting upright, held by parent, or on chair/bed). • Prompt child to take slow deep breaths. Deep breathing can be facilitated using bubbles or pinwheels, which also act as distraction techniques. • Encourage the use of distraction. Redirect child's attention to the distraction stimuli if his or her focus switches to the procedure. • Model helpful adult behaviors for the parent. • Manage pain during painful procedures (e.g., for injections, rub/stroke the skin near the injection site with moderate intensity prior to and during the injection).
After the Procedure	• Praise child for his or her efforts and for engaging in positive coping strategies. • Highlight how effectively the child coped during the procedure. • Continue distraction as necessary until the child is calm.

References

1. Baxter AL. Best practices for outpatient procedural sedation. *Pediatr Annals.* 2012;41:471–475.
2. Racine NM, Pillai Riddell RR, Khan M, et al. Systematic review: predisposing, precipitating, perpetuating, and present factors predicting anticipatory distress to painful medical procedures in children. *J Pediatr Psychol.* 2016;41:159–181.
3. Cohen LL, Blount RL, Cohen RJ, Johnson VC. Dimensions of pediatric procedural distress: children's anxiety and pain during immunizations. *J Clin Psychol Med.* 2004;11:41–47.
4. Kain ZN, Caldwell-Andrews AA, Mayes LC, et al. Family-centered preparation for surgery improves perioperative outcomes in children: a randomized controlled trial. *Anesthesiology.* 2007;106:65–74.

5. Pate JT, Blount RL, Cohen LL, Smith AJ. Childhood medical experience and temperament as predictors of adult functioning in medical situations. *Child Health Care.* 1996;25:281–298.
6. Taddio A, Appleton M, Bortolussi R, et al. Reducing the pain of childhood vaccination: an evidence-based clinical practice guideline. *CMAJ.* 2010;182:1989–1995.
7. Chorney JM, Torrey C, Blount R, et al. Healthcare provider and parent behavior and children's coping and distress at anesthesia induction. *Anesthesiology.* 2009;111:1290–1296.
8. Martin SR, Chorney JM, Tan ET, et al. Changing healthcare providers' behavior during pediatric inductions with an empirically based intervention. *Anesthesiology.* 2011; 115:18–27.
9. Noel M, McMurtry CM, Chambers CT, McGrath PJ. Children's memory for painful procedures: the relationship of pain intensity, anxiety, and adult behaviors to subsequent recall. *J Pediatr Psychol.* 2010;35:626–636.

3

Sedation as a Continuum

3.1

The Sedation Continuum

Minimal, Moderate, Deep and Other Sedation States

ÉLISE W. VAN DER JAGT

Sedationists must understand not only the specific levels of sedation that have been formally defined by professional and regulatory bodies, but also the concept of a sedation continuum, with its implications for sedation care. Just as there are various depths of sleep, there are various depths of sedation which can be induced by both nonpharmacologic (e.g., hypnosis) and/or pharmacologic means. And like sleep, these levels cannot be compartmentalized neatly into phases with well-delineated beginnings and ends but must be thought of in the context of a dynamic process that is influenced by both internal and external stimuli.

Definitions of Sedation

Initially defined by the American Society of Anesthesiologists in 1999[1] and subsequently adopted by multiple other societies and regulatory bodies, including the Society of Pediatric Sedation, the American Academy of Pediatrics, the American College of Emergency Physicians, and the Centers for Medicaid/Medicare Services, the classic definitions for specific levels of sedation are shown in Table 3.1.1. All levels of sedation are described in terms of changes that occur in neurologic (level of consciousness), respiratory (airway and ventilation), and/or cardiovascular function, including what might be anticipated when verbal, tactile, and/or painful stimuli are applied.

Not included in these classic definitions is the amnesia that may occur at each level of sedation depending on the particular agents used to induce that state. This amnesia is especially important to attain for children when management of an illness or injury requires multiple painful and/or anxiety-provoking procedures (e.g., repeated lumbar punctures in patients with childhood leukemia). In addition, no mention is made of the dissociative sedation state, which has been associated specifically with ketamine, a common agent used in procedural sedation/analgesia, particularly in the pediatric emergency department setting, and defined by the American College of Emergency Medicine as indicated in Table 3.1.1.[2]

TABLE 3.1.1 Levels of sedation

Minimal Sedation/Anxiolysis
A drug-induced state during which patients respond normally to verbal commands. • Cognitive function and coordination may be impaired. • Ventilatory and cardiovascular functions are unaffected.
Moderate Sedation/Analgesia
A drug-induced depression of consciousness during which patients respond purposefully* to verbal commands either alone or accompanied by light tactile stimulation. • No interventions are required to maintain a patent airway, and spontaneous ventilation is adequate. • Cardiovascular function is usually maintained.

(Continued)

TABLE 3.1.1 Continued

Deep Sedation/Analgesia
A drug-induced depression of consciousness during which patients respond purposefully* following repeated or painful stimulation. • The ability to independently maintain ventilatory function may be impaired. • Patients may require assistance in maintaining a patent airway and spontaneous ventilation may be inadequate. • Cardiovascular function is usually maintained.
General Anesthesia
A drug-induced loss of consciousness during which patients are not arousable even by painful stimulation. • The ability to maintain ventilation independently is often impaired. • Patients often require assistance in maintaining a patent airway and positive-pressure ventilation may be required because of depressed spontaneous ventilation or drug-induced depression of neuromuscular function. • Cardiovascular function may be impaired.
*Reflex withdrawal from a painful stimulus is NOT considered a purposeful response.
Dissociative Sedation
A trancelike cataleptic state characterized by profound amnesia and relative unawareness of surroundings • Protective airway reflexes, spontaneous respirations, and cardiopulmonary stability are usually retained.

Finally, although general anesthesia is included in the formal definitions as the deepest level of sedation, the term *procedural sedation/analgesia* generally refers only to minimal, moderate, and deep sedation states, not to the general anesthetic state.

Minimal sedation or anxiolysis is associated with few significant adverse effects and much benefit for the child who is anxious about a procedure. In this state, the child should not fall asleep but will:

- Maintain awareness of the surroundings
- Be able to understand and respond to speech appropriately
- Obey commands without tactile stimulation.

Many times a child who can speak becomes significantly loquacious, uninhibited, and "happy" appearing (thus the term "happy-juice" for agents such as midazolam, commonly used for anxiolysis). Usually, the agents that provide minimal sedation/anxiolysis also produce significant amnesia.

Moderate sedation still requires that the patient is able to obey verbal commands, although there may be light sleep/dozing off and on, but with easy awakening by speaking to the patient either alone or with some light touching. If the patient is not able to be awakened easily and/or is not able to follow verbal commands, the patient has passed into a state of deep sedation requiring more monitoring.

Deep sedation occurs when the patient:

- is asleep
- does not respond to verbal commands
- still responds purposefully to repeated or painful stimulation (e.g., reaching for the location of a painful stimulus).

It is important to note that if only reflex withdrawal is present, the patient has entered a general anesthetic plane and is at a much higher risk for an adverse respiratory or cardiovascular event.

Dissociative sedation is a term that is relatively new and was coined because this state does not fall neatly into the other three. This state is often observed when using ketamine and appears to result in a disconnection between cortical and limbic system processes. The patient usually:

- is not aware of surroundings, although eyes may be open in a trancelike state

- can partly obey verbal commands and speak
- is expected to have excellent amnesia
- has preservation of respiratory and cardiovascular function.

As defined, the risk of an adverse event increases as the depth of sedation increases, with the greatest risk of adverse events occurring during deep sedation and general anesthesia. Monitoring intensity and personnel skillset should be determined by the intended level of sedation, with preparation for managing at least one level deeper. Airway and respiratory drive–related events are by far the most common[3] and the most serious. (See Chapter 9 for an in-depth discussion of adverse events.)

Sedation Continuum

It is important to recognize that the process whereby a patient attains or leaves a given level of sedation is very fluid. Intermediate states between levels are the norm, and assessment of these states is often difficult since they are influenced by:

- types and blood or tissue levels of specific sedation agents
- the variable nature and timing of stimuli occurring during the procedure
- the innate physiology and individualized responses of the patient to the procedure, the environment, and/or the medications used.

Given the dynamic nature of the levels of sedation with many intermediate states, some pediatric sedation scales have incorporated ranges of sedation levels rather than sharply defined levels.[4] An example of this type of scale is the Wisconsin Sedation Scale, where levels are designated as conscious-moderate, moderate-deep, deep responsive to painful stimuli, and deep unresponsive to pain. More detail on how to assess the various states of sedation is provided in Chapter 3.2.

References

1. American Society of Anesthesiologists Task Force on Sedation and Analgesia by Non-Anesthesiologists. Practice guidelines for sedation and analgesia by non-anesthesiologists. *Anesthesiology.* 2002;96:1004–1017.
2. Green SM, Roback MG, Kennedy RM. Clinical practice guideline for emergency department ketamine dissociative sedation: 2011 update. *Ann Emerg Med.* 2011;57:449–461.
3. Cravero JP, Beach ML, Blike GT, et al., Pediatric Sedation Research Consortium. The incidence and nature of adverse events during pediatric sedation/anesthesia with propofol for procedures outside the operating room: a report from the Pediatric Sedation Research Consortium. *Anesth Analg.* 2009;108(3):795–804.
4. http://www.asahq.org/quality-and-practice-management/standards-and-guidelines/search?q=sedation. Continuum of depth of sedation: definition of general anesthesia and levels of sedation/analgesia. May 25, 2016.

3.2

Assessing Patient State and Efficacy

JOSEPH P. CRAVERO

The provider of pediatric procedural sedation should strive to produce a "state" wherein the patient is not moving and is not experiencing stress or pain (so he or she has no adverse recall of the procedure), and there should be control of the sympathetic or parasympathetic nervous system response to the procedure. In short, the patient should be in an optimized condition for the procedure, both from the perspective of the patient and the person performing the procedure—this is the desired "patient state." This state will represent a balance between the need to alter consciousness to make a procedure tolerable and the need to maintain a stable physiologic condition. These goals are generally accomplished through the induction of a state of sedation (varying depths) that may be combined with analgesia (local or systemic) for those procedures that involve painful stimuli. On the other hand, behavioral interventions such as games or movies may suffice for some children to produce a similar (acceptable) state for a minor procedure. The very fact that pediatric procedural sedation involves children implies that sedation and behavioral control will be required to produce an optimal state for procedures in which this could be achieved without intervention on more mature, developmentally appropriate, patients.

If one accepts the concepts outlined above, the simple cataloging of the depth of sedation for a given patient is not adequate to describe the appropriateness of the patient state for a procedural intervention. For instance, a child may be deeply sedated with a pure sedative such as midazolam or propofol but will move wildly when a painful stimulus (e.g., the pain of needle insertion for a lumbar puncture) is applied. On the other hand, a patient could be fully awake yet be comforted or distracted (with a favorite movie or game) to an extent that all of the goals of an adequate procedural state may be accomplished. In light of these issues, when evaluating the adequacy of any procedural sedation intervention, some measure of patient state should accompany (or replace) the measure of sedation level.

The safety of a patient during sedation must remain the primary concern for everyone involved in the practice of pediatric sedation. Any measure of patient state should include an appreciation of the patient's physiologic state. For instance, if the patient is sedated and movement is controlled but the patient's breathing is impaired and therefore he is hypoxic, that state is not appropriate. Likewise, evaluation of the patient's cardiovascular status should be included. Hypotension due to excessive sedative effect or hypertension due to undersedation should both be avoided. Any scale that attempts to catalog the patient state should include a measure of physiologic safety.

Attempts to assess the quality and safety of sedation practice have suffered from the lack of an objective scale that specifically allows the comparison of the *effectiveness* as well as the safety of sedation provided by various strategies and systems. Scales are available that specifically measure the level of sedation of children during procedures, including the following:

- Observer's Assessment of Alertness and Sedation (and modifications)
- University of Michigan Sedation Scale
- Ramsay Scale (and modifications).

In addition, pain scales (intended for the intensive care unit or perioperative environment) that measure the "comfort and stress" of pediatric patients have also been utilized to measure the effectiveness of procedural sedation, including the following:

- COMFORT score
- Children's Hospital of Eastern Ontario Pain Scale (CHEOPS)
- Faces, Legs, Activity, Cry, Consolability (FLACC) scale
- Critical-Care Pain Observation Tool.

These scales (described more completely in Chapter 7.4) do not account for specific features that are relevant to providing the best possible patient "state" during procedures. The ideal scale would measure a variety of factors outlined above, such as control of movement, stress, and pain, while at the same time allowing for categorization of respiratory depression or other effects related to sedation. Importantly, this scale should be simple enough to be applied in a timeframe that is appropriate for clinical procedural sedation.

One attempt at a scale that addresses the specific issues related to describing patient state is the Dartmouth Operative Conditions Scale (DOCS). This scale uses four separate categories (or dimensions) of patient behaviors: pain/stress, movement, consciousness, and sedation side effects. Numeric values are assigned to signify the balance desired between increasing activity associated with reaction to the procedure that is being performed (increasingly positive), and effects of interventions (usually medications) aimed at ameliorating pain and stress (increasingly negative) (Table 3.2.1). The overall score is derived by summing the levels in all four categories to yield one numeric value describing the patient state. It is important to recognize that there is no connotation of adverse behavior associated with negative numbers in this scale. Rather, the scale was designed to reflect the desire to balance patient activity with intervention to yield neutral (acceptable) states for procedures. DOCS scores can be divided into three general categories of patient states during procedures: (1) under-controlled states with DOCS score of greater than 2, correlating with patient behaviors such as crying, thrashing, and severe agitation; (2) safe states with DOCS scores of 2 through –2, correlating

TABLE 3.2.1 Dartmouth Operative Conditions Scale (DOCS)

Patient State	*Observed Behaviors*			
Pain/Stress	(0) eyes closed or calm expression	(1) grimace or frown	(2) crying, sobbing, screaming	
Movement	(0) still	(1) random little movement	(2) major purposeful movement	(3) thrashing, kicking, biting
Consciousness	(0) eyes open	(−1) ptosis, uncoordinated, "drowsy"	(−2) eyes closed	
Sedation side effects	(−1) $SpO_2 < 92\%$	(−1) noise with respiration	(−1) respiratory pauses >10 seconds	(−1) BP decrease of >50% from baseline

with patient behaviors that lacked any evidence of pain, stress, or side effects from sedation medications; and (3) oversedated states where the total DOCS score was less than −2, correlating with states in which the sedative effects and respiratory compromise associated with sedation medications were not adequately treated.

A simpler scale that has recently been developed to help categorize patient state during procedures is the Pediatric Sedation State Scale (PSSS) (Table 3.2.2). This scale is a simple linear (ordinal) description of patient conditions that varies from distressed patients requiring restraint due to lack of effective sedation (level 5) to those experiencing dangerous physiologic disturbance associated with excessive sedative effect (level 0). The scale is designed to be used clinically to measure the appropriateness of patient "state" and adjust interventions based on outcome.

TABLE 3.2.2 Pediatric Sedation State Scale (PSSS)

State	*Observed Behaviors*
5	Patient is moving (purposefully or nonpurposefully) in a manner that impedes the proceduralist and requires forceful immobilization. Patient may be partially sedated or awake. This includes crying or shouting during the procedure, but vocalization is not required—score based on movement.
4	Moving during the procedure (awake or sedated) that requires gentle immobilization for positioning. May verbalize some discomfort or stress, but there is no crying or shouting that expresses stress or objection.
3	Expression of pain or anxiety on face (may verbalize discomfort) but *not* moving or impeding completion of the procedure. May require help positioning (as with a lumbar puncture) but does not require restraint to stop movement during the procedure.
2	Quiet (asleep or awake) not moving during procedure, no frown (or brow furrow) indicating pain or anxiety. No verbalization of any complaint.
1	Quiet (asleep or awake) not moving during procedure, no frown (or brow furrow) indicating pain or anxiety. No verbalization of any complaint.
0	Sedation associated with ABNORMAL physiological parameters that require ACUTE intervention (i.e., oxygen saturation less than 90%, blood pressure is 30% lower than baseline, bradycardia receiving therapy)

Suggested Reading

Ambuel B, Hamlett KW, Marx CM, et al. Assessing distress in pediatric intensive care environments—the COMFORT scale. *J Pediatr Psychol.* 1992;17(1):95–109.

Barker R, Nisbet HI. The objective measurement of sedation in children: a modified scoring system. *Can Anaesth Soc J.* 1973;20:599–606.

Chernik DA, Gillings D, Laine H, et al. Validity and reliability of the Observers Assessment of Alertness/Sedation Scale: study with intravenous midazolam. *J Clin Psychopharmacol.* 1990;10:244–251.

Cravero JP, Askins N, Sriswasdi P, et al. Validation of the Pediatric Sedation State Scale. *Pediatrics.* 2017;139(5):e20162897.

Cravero JP, Blike GT, Surgenor SD, Jensen J. Development and validation of the Dartmouth Operative Conditions Scale. *Anesth Analg.* 2005;100(6):1614–1621.

Malviya S, Voepel-Lewis T, Tait AR, et al. Depth of sedation in children undergoing computed tomography: validity and reliability of the University of Michigan Sedation Scale (UMSS). *Fr J Anaesth.* 2002;88:241–245.

Marx CM, Smith PG, Lowrie LH, et al. Optimal sedation of mechanically ventilated pediatric critical care patients. *Crit Care Med.* 1994;22(1):163–170.

Williams MR, Ward DS, Carlson D, et al. Evaluating patient-centered outcomes in clinical trials of procedural sedation, part 1, efficacy: Sedation Consortium on Endpoints and Procedures for Treatment, Education, and Research Recommendations. *Anesth Analg.* 2017;124(3):821–830.

4

Pediatric Airway and Respiration

4.1

The Pediatric Airway

LOWELL CLARK AND STEPHEN TOMEK

The practice of procedural sedation involves the use of medications that alter upper airway function and patency because of myoneural suppression of anatomic airway elements. It is the specific responsibility of the sedationist to ensure upper airway patency during conditions induced by pharmaceuticals in which the airway is almost certain to be threatened, if not totally obstructed. A sedationist's knowledge of the anatomy and physiology of the upper airway[1] (Figures 4.1.1, 4.1.2) and proficiency in clinical application of airway supportive principles is of utmost importance.

The upper airway serves several physiologic functions:

- Air access to the lungs for O_2 delivery and CO_2 removal
- Humidification and warming of inspired air
- Heat preservation from exhaled air
- Ingestion, mastication, and initial digestion of foodstuffs
- Olfaction
- Phonation and speech.

Airway stability is dependent on several factors:

- Anatomic structure
- Neuromuscular tone
- Central ventilatory control
- Level of consciousness

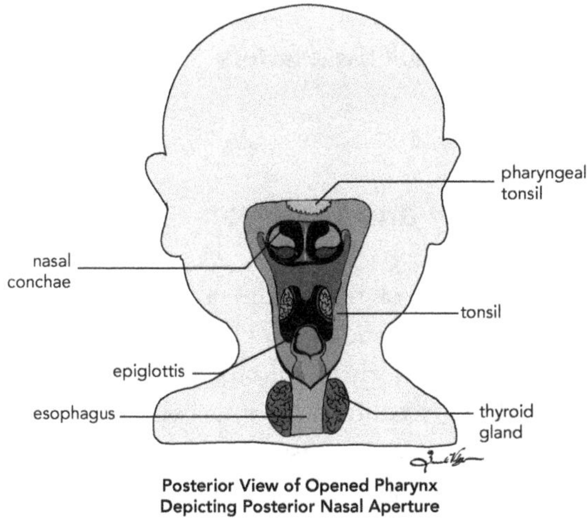

FIGURE 4.1.1.

Coronal section of airway at posterior nasal aperture

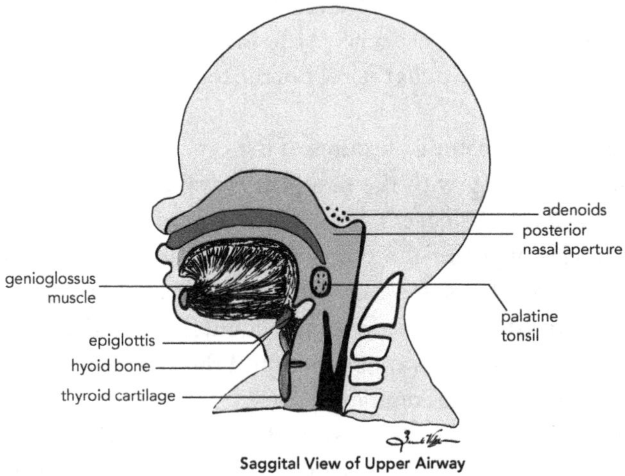

FIGURE 4.1.2.

Midline sagittal section of upper airway

- Upper airway reflexes
- Craniofacial and soft tissue factors
- Body position.

Airway Anatomy and Function

The **nose** is the organ of respiration and smell. Ambient air is humidified by a mechanism in which arterial blood to mucosal surfaces is directed anteriorly in countercurrent flow to posteriorly directed inspired air. Nasal inspiration accounts for ~50% of total airway resistance. Resistance exists during exhalation as well, reflecting back to the alveolar level providing a degree of positive end-expiratory pressure to minimize alveolar collapse.

The **tongue** is a large mass within the oral cavity with the potential to become a major force for obstruction. However, the mass of the tongue is subject to myoneural forces opening the oropharyngeal airway.[2] The genioglossus muscle originates at the anterior-most reach of the mandible and attaches to the body of the tongue. During consciousness, especially with inspiration, the genioglossus is tonically active and pulls the base of the tongue anteriorly, opening the airway.

Other major anatomic features of the oral cavity are the palatine tonsils, which along with the nasopharyngeal adenoids and lingual tonsils make up Waldeyer's ring. When hypertrophied these lymphatic tissues augment the potential for upper airway obstruction during sedation. The soft palate also contributes to upper airway dynamics, serving to direct air, food, and liquid flows. In deep sleep and sedated states, upper airway obstruction at the level of the soft palate, tonsils, and adenoids is common.[3]

Suspended from the skull base by digastric and stylohyoid muscle and ligament, the mandible, tongue, hyoid, and larynx form an interconnected working complex in which movement of one element induces change throughout the complex (Figure 4.1.3). The mandible moves through the temporomandibular joint, which functions

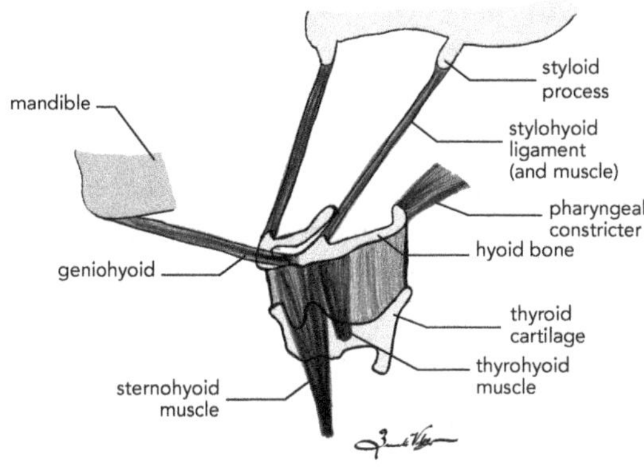

FIGURE 4.1.3.

Suspension of larynx from genu of mandible and styloid process

as a gliding joint and hinge, allowing for one of the most useful airway maneuvers, the jaw thrust.[3]

The **pharynx** consists of three anatomic divisions: nasopharynx, oropharynx, and laryngopharynx. The roof of the nasopharynx is lined by pharyngeal tonsil (adenoids), immediately behind the posterior nasal aperture. The oropharynx is bound superiorly by the soft palate and inferiorly by the base of the tongue and epiglottis. The laryngopharynx contains the larynx. Importantly, the pharynx is ensheathed circumferentially by the paired superior, middle, and inferior pharyngeal constrictor muscles, overlapping with the superior muscle innermost. The superior constrictor attaches to the pterygoid plate anteriorly, the middle to the hyoid bone, and the inferior to the larynx. The pharyngeal airway is best depicted by the concept of a Starling resistor. A Starling resistor exists when a collapsible tube (the pharyngeal airway) is positioned and enclosed (by surrounding tissue) between two noncollapsible tubes (nose and larynx). In such an arrangement, collapse of the airway is dependent on the interplay among the proximal/nasal airway, intraluminal, surrounding tissue, and distal/laryngeal pressures. The pressure surrounding the pharyngeal airway is subject to the dilatory influence of the genioglossus and geniohyoid muscles, to pharyngeal constrictor tone, and, less obviously, to surface tension phenomena and factors such as obesity. Distal laryngeal pressures fluctuate with normal inspiration (–2 to 4 cm H_2O) and expiration and can be dramatically increased (by cough) or decreased (by forceful inspiration).

Neuromotor Control

Afferent sensation of the pharynx is provided via the trigeminal nerve (V) superiorly and the glossopharyngeal nerve (IX). Central integration with cranial nerves IX, X (vagus), and XII (hypoglossal) allows exquisite myoneural control of the pharyngeal airway. Hence, neurologic or neuromuscular conditions that involve spasticity or brainstem pathology can have a major impact on airway control.

Little is known about neuromotor control of the upper airway, but ventilatory muscle tone and sequential activation are coordinated by central respiratory drive from the pons and medulla and effected through the glossopharyngeal, vagus, hypoglossal, and phrenic nerves. This drive is affected by sleep state, chemical control (pH, CO_2, and O_2), and airway mechanoreceptors. Dilating forces on the airway are due to activities of the pharyngeal dilatory muscles, primarily the genioglossus and geniohyoid and less so the tensor and levator palatine, sternothyroid, and thyrohyoid muscles. Neuromotor control of the upper airway musculature is tightly connected and coordinated by the brainstem with the muscles of breathing. During the respiratory cycle, upper airway dilators act sequentially and synergistically with the diaphragm to optimize the rate and extent of inspiratory lung expansion and expiratory flow resistance. A significant factor in stabilizing the pharyngeal airway is the "tracheal tug": tracheal traction generated along the raphe during inspiration alters pharyngeal collapsibility by increasing longitudinal tension on the posterior pharyngeal wall, functionally "stiffening" the pharynx.

The anatomy and pathophysiology of dynamic upper airway obstruction during sedation is highly influenced by aberrations in neuromotor control resulting in:

- Relaxation of the soft palate
- Posterior and inferior displacement of the mandibuloglossal hyoid complex due to gravity and loss of pharyngeal dilator control, resulting in narrowing throughout the oro- and laryngopharynx[3]
- Loss of sequential activation of coordination between various muscles of respiration
- Loss of swallow.

Airway Protective Reflexes

Airway protective reflexes are primitively evolved to continuously protect the upper airway during consciousness and sleep. The pharmaceuticals used in sedation practice may profoundly affect or abolish these protective reflexes. Afferent arms occur primarily through the trigeminal, glossopharyngeal, and vagus nerves, whereas efferent control is expressed primarily through the vagus and phrenic nerves. These reflexes include the following:

- Sneeze
- Gag
- Swallow
- Cough
- Laryngospasm.

Sneezing serves to expel foreign materials from the nose. The gag serves to clear the supraglottic airway, beginning with the afferent signal via the glossopharyngeal nerve and efferent response via the vagus resulting in forceful pharyngeal constrictors expelling foreign material. Swallowing is considerably more complex and requires exquisite coordination between oral, pharyngeal, and laryngeal neuromuscular function. In relation to sedation practice, cessation of swallowing may lead to pooling of secretions in the hypopharynx, increasing risks for aspiration, laryngospasm, and apnea. The cough reflex protects the lower airways and forcefully expels either aspirated foreign or native materials from the trachea and larger bronchial airways. Laryngospasm is a protective reflex that consists of sustained, tight closure of the laryngeal inlet and vocal cords stimulated by direct laryngeal irritation with food, a foreign object, or saliva. The tendency to laryngospasm is increased by hyperventilation, hypocapnia, and light levels of sedation. The ultimate purpose of these reflexes is to protect the delicate alveolar-capillary unit from exposure to foreign substances that would prevent O_2 and CO_2 exchange.

References

1. Motoyama EK, Finder JD. Respiratory physiology in infants and children. In: Motoyama EK, Davis PJ, eds. *Smith's Anesthesia for Infants and Children.* 8th ed. Philadelphia: Elsevier Mosby, 2011:22–79.
2. Hammer J, Reber A, Trachsel D, Frei FJ. Effect of jaw-thrust and continuous positive airway pressure on tidal breathing in deeply sedated infants. *J Pediatrics.* 2001;138(6): 826–830.
3. Marcus CL, Smith JH, Mankarious LA, et al. Developmental aspects of the upper airway. *Proc Am Thorac Soc.* 2009;6:513–520.

4.2

Sedation Effects

MARY LANDRIGAN-OSSAR AND

SAMUEL VANDERHOEK

While the medications used for sedation have many advantageous effects in terms of providing anxiolysis, hypnosis, and analgesia, they possess some disadvantageous properties that must be understood by anyone providing sedation. Data from the Pediatric Sedation Research Consortium demonstrate that adverse events involving the airway and respiratory system are among the most commonly reported, with up to 1 in 200 sedations requiring airway and ventilation interventions. Sedationists administering medications inducing sedation should have an understanding of their deleterious consequences so that they can prepare appropriately to mitigate these effects. The deleterious effects of sedative drugs can be divided into central effects on the respiratory drive and peripheral effects on airway musculature.

Respiratory Drive

The control of ventilation is highly complex and involves multiple behavioral and chemical systems. The chemical control system depends on chemosensors in cerebrospinal fluid and arterial blood that send signals to the brainstem in response to changes in pH, pCO_2, and pO_2. This allows the brainstem to maintain homeostasis by directing upregulation and downregulation of ventilation. Receptors on respiratory neurons can be activated or inhibited by medications used in procedural sedation.

Most sedatives lead to a dose-dependent decrease in respiratory rate, sometimes to the point of apnea:

- Activation of opioid receptors in the brainstem results in depression of the ventilatory response to hypercapnia and hypoxia, resulting in decreases in respiratory rate and volume.
- Propofol has a depressant effect on respiratory rate and volume.
- Benzodiazepines have a minimal depressant effect on respirations, but when they are given in conjunction with opioids they have an additive effect on respiratory depression.

Two sedative medications, dexmedetomidine and ketamine, are used commonly precisely because they do preserve the normal respiratory drive. In the case of alpha-2 agonists such as dexmedetomidine, there is no effect on the response to pCO_2. Ketamine similarly maintains respiratory drive, although larger doses administered rapidly will result in transient respiratory depression.

Airway Musculature

Medication effects on airway muscular tone and coordination are seen much more commonly during pediatric procedural sedation than the depressant effects on respiratory drive. Upper airway obstruction is quite common, and the resultant hypoventilation and desaturation must be promptly recognized and treated. Laryngeal or tracheal aspiration due to discoordination of pharyngeal musculature is fortunately more rare but is also a concern.

Most sedative medications, including opioids, benzodiazepines, propofol, and to a lesser extent dexmedetomidine cause a reduction in pharyngeal muscle tone and decreased airway patency.

Ketamine is the major exception to this rule, acting instead to maintain airway muscle tone and airway reflexes. Whether this maintenance of airway reflexes helps explain the increased rate of laryngospasm seen with ketamine sedation is unclear but plausible.

A final effect on respiratory musculature is opioid-induced chest wall rigidity. This phenomenon may be related to the rate of administration and is most commonly seen with high doses but has been reported in sedative or even analgesic doses. This will impede spontaneous ventilation and is treated with supportive respiratory maneuvers and ultimately with opioid reversal.

Special Considerations

Several patient conditions increase the risk of airway obstruction under sedation. Obesity and tonsillar hypertrophy can predispose patients to airway obstruction, either by extra soft tissue compressing the airway externally or with tonsils obstructing the airway from within. A careful history of snoring or sleep apnea should be elicited, and the risk-versus-benefit ratio should be considered before proceeding in concerning cases.

Trisomy 21 patients present particular airway challenges. They possess a constellation of macroglossia, narrow nasopharynx, and hypotonia that strongly predisposes them to airway collapse and obstruction with sedative medications. The potential for atlantoaxial instability should also be borne in mind, which may limit one's ability to reposition the head to relieve obstruction.

The cornucopia of sedative agents available, as well as the suite of their attendant side effects, demands a rational and judicious approach to selecting an appropriate sedative regimen. A thorough understanding of the procedure or diagnostic study being performed (e.g., duration, depth of sedation required, likelihood of hemodynamic instability, positioning required), together with the patient's own medical condition (including chronic comorbidities and acute exacerbations), is necessary in order to create a safe and effective experience for the pediatric patient.

Suggested Reading

Chatterjee D, Friedman N, Shott S, Mahmoud M. Anesthetic dilemmas for dynamic evaluation of the pediatric upper airway. *Semin Cardiothorac Vasc Anesth.* 2014;18(4):371–378.

Coruh B, Tonelli MR, Park DR. Fentanyl-induced chest wall rigidity. *Chest.* 2013;143(4):1145–1146.

Cravero JP, Blike GT, Beach M, et al. Incidence and nature of adverse events during pediatric sedation/anesthesia for procedures outside the operating room: report from the Pediatric Sedation Research Consortium. *Pediatrics.* 2006;118(3):1087–1096.

Haas DA, Harper DG. Ketamine: a review of its pharmacologic properties and use in ambulatory anesthesia. *Anesthesia Progress.* 1992;39(3):61–68.

Jacobs IN, Gray RF, Todd NW. Upper airway obstruction in children with Down syndrome. *Arch Otolaryngol Head Neck Surg.* 1996;122(9):945–950.

Scherrer PD, Mallory MD, Cravero JP, et al. The impact of obesity on pediatric procedural sedation-related outcomes: results from the Pediatric Sedation Research Consortium. *Paediatr Anaesth.* 2015;25(7):689–697.

Simons JC, Pierce E, Diaz-Gil D, et al. Effects of depth of propofol and sevoflurane anesthesia on upper airway collapsibility, respiratory genioglossus activation, and breathing in healthy volunteers. *Anesthesiology.* 2016;125(3):525–534.

4.3

Techniques for Managing the Airway

MARY LANDRIGAN-OSSAR AND

SAMUEL VANDERHOEK

Deciding which technique to use during a pediatric procedural sedation can be overwhelming when the options are considered. A variety of devices are shown in Figure 4.3.1. The decision of which to choose involves determining the level of sedation required for the procedure, the anticipated duration of the procedure, the remoteness of the patient from the provider, the child's medical condition, and any airway conditions the child may have. The overarching goal is to maximize the child's safety and mitigate the risks to the airway that sedation may pose.

The least invasive form of airway management in a sedated patient is to maintain the natural airway with effective positioning while providing supplemental oxygen. The rationale behind providing supplemental oxygen is that sedation can depress minute ventilation as well as decrease functional residual capacity, predisposing the patient to both hypercapnia and hypoxia. Supplemental oxygen increases the partial pressure of oxygen in the alveoli and buffers the hypoxic risk.

In a spontaneously breathing patient, supplemental oxygen can be provided in various forms. A nasal cannula consists of two prongs that sit in the nares, whereas a face mask provides an enriched oxygen environment to both the mouth and nose. Noninvasive monitoring of expired carbon dioxide can be performed with either of these delivery sources and can provide an early indication of inadequate ventilation or loss of airway patency. Signs of inadequate ventilation should be

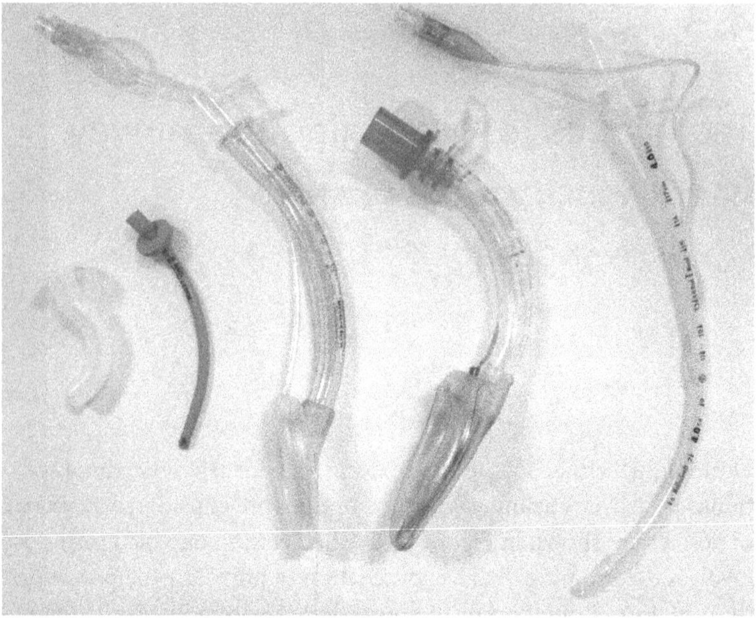

FIGURE 4.3.1.

Devices for airway management. From left to right, oropharyngeal airway, nasopharyngeal airway, laryngeal mask airway (LMA Unique, Teleflex), Air-Q supraglottic device (Mercury Medical), endotracheal tube.

evaluated and acted upon promptly to avoid further deterioration of a patient's cardiopulmonary status.

In sedated, supine children, the posterior displacement of the tongue against the pharyngeal wall and soft palate can lead to airway obstruction. Several maneuvers can be employed to relieve this obstruction and restore airway patency. Initially, a simple chin lift can be applied. If this is insufficient, one can perform a jaw thrust by lifting both angles of the mandible and displacing it anteriorly. These maneuvers are often successful in relieving pharyngeal obstruction. Turning the head from a neutral position to one side will often relieve mild obstruction, but this may not be possible depending on the procedure (e.g., MRI of the brain).

Oropharyngeal and nasopharyngeal airways are essential adjuncts in managing the pediatric airway due to the relatively larger tongue size in children and its tendency to obstruct the airway under sedation (see Figure 4.3.2). These airways must be carefully sized. An oropharyngeal airway that is too large can cause laryngeal damage, complete airway obstruction, and impaired venous drainage from the tongue and uvula, leading to swelling of these structures. Conversely, an undersized oropharyngeal airway can displace the base of the tongue inferiorly, thereby worsening the obstruction. Nasopharyngeal airways are often better tolerated in children than oropharyngeal airways but should be well lubricated prior to their insertion to avoid traumatic placement and subsequent bleeding into the nasopharynx.

A laryngeal mask airway (LMA) is another option for supraglottic airway management. Typically, it can be inserted only in patients who are deeply sedated or anesthetized. The mask portion of the LMA, when inserted correctly, will face the laryngeal inlet, and the tip will sit against the upper esophageal sphincter. It is important to note,

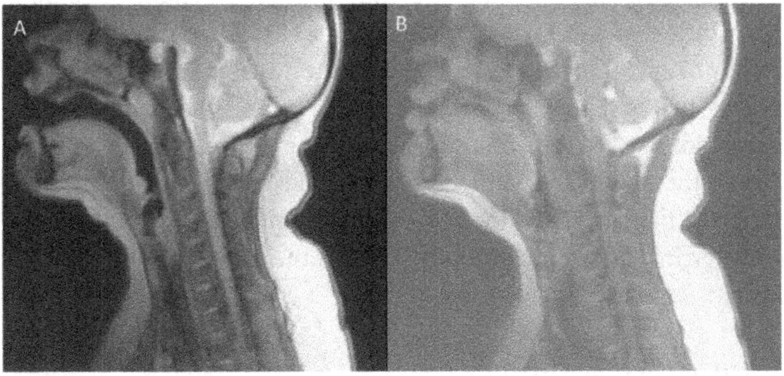

FIGURE 4.3.2.

MRI demonstrating effect of oral airway in creating patent passage for air movement. (A) Sagittal image with oral airway in place. (B) Sagittal image of same patient with no oral airway.

From Chatterjee et al. *Semin Cardiothorac Vasc Anesth.* 2014 Dec;18(4):371–8. Used with permission.

however, that the LMA is not a secure airway device, nor is it designed to deliver controlled ventilation. Additionally, it poses the risk of gastric insufflation during positive-pressure ventilation and possible aspiration. Nevertheless, the LMA has emerged as a useful temporary airway management device in patients with known difficult airways. Many versions of supraglottic devices are now available on the market, with a host of features designed to improve on the LMA. Some are intended as a conduit for easier intubation (Air-Q, Mercury Medical), and some are intended to provide easier placement (i-gel, Intersurgical).

An endotracheal tube provides the most definitive form of airway management in a pediatric patient. It is traditionally placed using direct laryngoscopy, a technique in which the glottic opening is visualized and the endotracheal tube is subsequently passed into the trachea. Due to the short distance between the vocal cords and carina in children, care must be taken ensure placement in the trachea and not into the right mainstem bronchus. A variety of endotracheal tubes are available for use, including ones for nasal intubation.

Management of a difficult airway in a child requires planning, preparation, and teamwork, often in consultation with a pediatric anesthesiologist. Often, the best intervention may be no intervention at all—that is, allowing the child to breathe spontaneously. There are other times, however, when the airway must be definitively secured. While the specifics of difficult airway management are beyond the scope of this chapter, various tools can be utilized to care for these children in a safe, thoughtful, and vigilant manner.

Suggested Reading

Holzman RS. Airway management. In: Cladis FP, Davis PJ, eds. *Smith's Anesthesia for Infants and Children*. Philadelphia: Elsevier, 2017:349–369.

McNiece WL, Dierdorf SF. The pediatric airway. *Semin Pediatr Surg.* 2004;13(3):152–165.

5

Cardiovascular System

5.1

Sedation Effects

JEFFREY LINZER SR.

Medications commonly used in sedation care include benzodiazepines, barbiturates, opioids, and less well-categorized agents: ketamine, dexmedetomidine, etomidate, and propofol. While much attention is paid to respiratory depressive effects, all these medications can exert effects on vascular resistance, cardiac contractility, and heart rate that the sedationist must understand and manage, particularly with respect to specific patient pathophysiologic states (Table 5.1.1).

Benzodiazepines may be used as an adjunct with other medications or as a primary sedative agent. Their most common hemodynamic affect is a modest decrease in arterial blood pressure resulting from a decrease in systemic vascular resistance. Occasionally heart rate may increase, although cardiac output is generally not affected. While homeostatic reflex mechanisms are preserved, the baroreceptor reflex may be diminished. These effects are dose-dependent. Midazolam tends to produce a greater effect on blood pressure than diazepam. Cardiovascular depressant effects may be unmasked when given with opioids.

Barbiturates typically produce modest decreases in blood pressure. Depression of the medullary vasomotor center and decreased sympathetic portion of the central nervous system outflow leads to peripheral vasodilation, resulting in pooling of blood and decreased venous return. There can be a transitory blunting of the baroreceptor reflex, especially in hypovolemic patients, which can lead to a significant drop

TABLE 5.1.1 Cardiovascular effects of commonly used sedation agents

Medication/Effect	*Heart Rate*	*Systemic Vascular Resistance*	*Systemic Blood Pressure*
Midazolam	Unchanged	Unchanged to decreased	Unchanged to decreased
Methohexital	Increased	Decreased	Decreased
Ketamine	Increased	Increased	Increased
Dexmedetomidine	Decreased	Decreased	Decreased
Etomidate	Unchanged to increased	Unchanged to decreased	Unchanged to decreased
Propofol	Unchanged to decreased	Decreased	Decreased
Morphine/Fentanyl	Unchanged to decreased	Decreased	Decreased

in cardiac output and arterial blood pressure. An increase in heart rate is due to changes in blood pressure and a central vagolytic effect. This increase in heart rate maintains cardiac output. Larger doses and rapid administration can make the hemodynamic effects more pronounced. Making sure the patient is well hydrated and using a slow rate of administration tends to reduce the cardiovascular effects.

Opioids are sedating at large doses but are used for pain control during and after procedures and may exert additive cardiovascular effects on patient reactions to other sedatives. Opioids decrease sympathetic tone and increase parasympathetic tone, resulting in bradycardia, although this is generally more pronounced with large doses. Dose-dependent peripheral vasodilation also occurs likely mediated by nitric oxide, so hypotension may occur, particularly in dehydrated patients or in patients who are already vasodilated (sepsis). Opioids can have a direct depressive action on the myocardium, particularly if contractility is already compromised. Morphine stimulates mast cells to release histamine, causing vasodilation and hypotension. Fentanyl and remifentanil are not associated with histamine release.

Ketamine transiently increases heart rate, systemic vascular resistance, and blood pressure principally due to CNS stimulation. It increases the release of systemic catecholamines as well as depressing the reuptake of norepinephrine. This also results in increased cardiac output with a consequential increase in myocardial oxygen consumption. These actions allow maintenance of cardiac stability in children with marginal cardiac reserve. However, direct myocardial depressant activity can be seen in catecholamine-depleted patients. While there are no significant changes in shunt directions or fraction in those with congenital heart disease, patients who have increased pulmonary artery pressure may have a more pronounced increase in pulmonary vascular resistance than that seen systemically. Effects such as tachycardia and systemic hypertension can be blunted by giving a benzodiazepine prior to ketamine administration or by using a continuous infusion. High total doses of ketamine may amplify the side effects.

Dexmedetomidine is a selective α_2-adrenergic agonist. It causes decreases in heart rate and systemic vascular resistance resulting in a decrease in mean arterial blood pressure. Paradoxical hypertension associated with systemic vasoconstriction can occur with rapid infusion due to peripheral α_2-receptor stimulation. Bolus dosing has been associated with bradycardia, hypotension, and sinus arrest and may be due to unopposed vagal activity. These effects can be countered with anticholinergic medications.

Etomidate is an imidazole derivative that has minimal cardiovascular effect. There may be a small increase in heart rate. A decrease in systemic vascular resistance may cause a minimal decrease in blood pressure. This effect can become more prominent in patients with hypovolemia. There is minimal direct effect on the myocardium.

Propofol, of all the sedation medications used outside of the operating room, is most likely to cause hypotension. A decrease in systemic vascular resistance, due to impairment of normal baroreceptor reflex response to hypotension, leads to vasodilation and dropping of the blood pressure. There can be a slight increase in heart rate however not enough to make up for the transient reduction in preload and afterload. There is minimal direct effect on the myocardium. Hypotension can be exacerbated with rapid medication administration and in very young children. Propofol should be used with caution in patients who cannot tolerate systemic afterload reduction or have an ejection fraction of less than 50%. Premedication with anticholinergic agents does not appear to counter these effects.

Suggested Reading

Chapter 9, Intravenous Anesthetics. In: Butterworth JF, IV, Mackey DC, Wasnick JD. eds. *Morgan & Mikhail's Clinical Anesthesiology, 5e* New York, NY: McGraw-Hill; 2013.

Eilers H. Intravenous Anesthetics. In: Miller RD, Pardo Jr MC. eds. *Basics of Anesthesia, 6e* Philadelphia, PA: Elsevier Saunders, 2011.

Eilers H, Yost S. General Anesthetics. In: Katzung BG, Trevor AJ. eds. *Basic & Clinical Pharmacology, 13e* New York, NY: McGraw-Hill; 2015.

Gooding JM, Corssen G. Effect of etomidate on the cardiovascular system. *Anesth Analg.* 1977;56:717–771.

Schulte-Uentrop L, Goepfert MS. Anaesthesia or sedation for MRI in children. *Curr Opin Anaesthesiol.* 2010;23:513–517.

Simsek M, Bulut MO, Ozel D, Yucel IK, Aykac Z. Comparison of sedation method in pediatrics cardiac catheterization. *Eur Rev Med Pharmacol Sci.* 2016;20:1490–1494.

Vuyk J, Sitsen E, Reekers M. Intravenous Anesthetics. In: Miller RD. ed. *Miller's Anesthesia, 8e* Philadelphia, PA: Elsevier Saunders, 2015.

Wong J, Steil GM, Curtis M, et al. Cardiovascular effects of dexmedetomidine sedation in children. *Anesth Analg.* 2012;114:193–199.

5.2

Congenital Heart Disease Considerations

FEIFEI Z. WILLIAMS AND MICHAEL J. WOLF

Children with congenital heart disease (CHD) are at increased risk for sedation-related complications. The number of these patients with unrepaired or palliated disease requiring procedural sedation outside of the operating room continues to increase as staged surgeries and techniques are associated with better survival. The venues involved in follow-up care of CHD patients include the cardiac catheterization laboratory, interventional radiology, magnetic resonance imaging or computed tomography, and the emergency department. CHD patients may also require sedation for procedures or testing unrelated to their CHD. CHD patient characteristics associated with the highest risk of sedation-related complications include age under 2 years; single-ventricle physiology, including hypoplastic left heart syndrome (HLHS); left ventricular outflow tract obstruction; cardiomyopathy with impaired ventricular function; and pulmonary hypertension (Table 5.2.1).

Discussion

In preparing to sedate a child with CHD, the provider must understand the anatomic variations, surgical history, and physiologic

TABLE 5.2.1 When referral to cardiac anesthesia may be warranted

Consideration for Referral to a Pediatric Cardiac Anesthesiologist:
• Unrepaired cyanotic heart disease
• CHD and known history of a difficult airway
• Neonate with CHD
• Pulmonary hypertension
• Single-ventricle physiology
• Left ventricular outflow tract obstructive lesions
• Cardiomyopathy
• Prolonged procedure with complicated protocols for breath-holding

implications for each individual patient. There are three major anatomic variations of complex CHD:

1. Increased pulmonary blood flow (PBF) (e.g., left-to-right shunt lesions such as ventricular septal defect, atrial septal defect, and patent ductus arteriosus, which cause circulatory overload of the pulmonary vascular bed)
2. Decreased PBF (e.g., pulmonary valve stenosis/atresia, which leads to difficulties with oxygenation, resulting in hypoxemia)
3. Systemic outflow tract obstruction (e.g. aortic stenosis, coarctation of aorta), leading to increased ventricular work and reduced circulation distal to the obstruction.

These anatomic subsets are not exclusive and certain patients may fit into more than one of these categories.

There are 4 major consequences of either repaired or unrepaired CHD:

1. Congestive heart failure (CHF) caused by increased PBF from left-to-right shunting; left-sided obstructive lesions;

or impaired ventricular contractility. Impaired ventricular function can be the result of a primary cardiomyopathy (e.g., dilated cardiomyopathy), an acquired cardiomyopathy (e.g., myocarditis), or congenital heart disease. CHF can lead to increased pulmonary congestion, decreased effective cardiac output, and decreased oxygen delivery. Importantly, this can even occur in the setting of preserved ventricular function. Clinical features may include tachycardia, tachypnea, poor weight gain, gallop, and hepatomegaly.

2. Cyanosis can be present as a result of chronic hypoxia from decreased PBF and/or right-to-left shunting. It becomes apparent when the level of deoxyhemoglobin exceeds 2.5 g/dL. Thus, cyanosis is more noticeable when the patient's hemoglobin level is higher. Clinical features may include visible cyanosis, clubbing of extremities, exercise intolerance, and polycythemia.
3. Pulmonary hypertension (PH) can occur in longstanding unrepaired left-to-right shunts or mixing lesions (e.g., Eisenmenger syndrome) with increased PBF, prolonged pulmonary venous obstruction (e.g., total anomalous pulmonary venous drainage), and high left atrial pressure (e.g., HLHS with restrictive atrial septum or severe mitral valve regurgitation). Primary PH may also be present in the absence of any structural heart disease. Hypoxia, hypercarbia, acidosis, and hypothermia can precipitate a PH crisis.
4. CHD can be complicated by arrhythmias, which can require medication or pacemaker insertion. Patients with primary arrhythmias may require sedation as well. Monitoring of the ECG (QRS morphology) becomes mandatory in these patients rather than relying on monitoring of heart rate alone. The sedation provider must be aware of the presence of a pacemaker or implantable cardioverter-defibrillator and ensure they are functioning correctly and optimized prior to the administration of sedation.

There are a number of hemodynamic principles to keep in mind when managing shunts:

- Left-to-right shunts: Avoid increasing systemic vascular resistance (SVR), use inotropes, avoid fluid overload.
- Right-to-left shunts: Maintain high SVR, maintain adequate intravascular volume, avoid increase in pulmonary vascular resistance (PVR), minimize elevated intrathoracic pressure, remember that there is an increased risk for systemic embolic events.
- Left ventricular outflow tract obstructive lesions: Maintain SVR, maintain adequate intravascular volume, avoid medications that decrease SVR as this increases the outflow tract gradient.

In addition to understanding the cardiac pathophysiology and its hemodynamic consequences for each patient, it is important to remember that there are noncardiac consequences from CHD. Patients can have decreased lung compliance from increased PBF, airway compression by vascular structures, or phrenic/recurrent laryngeal nerve injury from previous surgeries. Phrenic nerve injury can lead to impaired respiratory mechanics from diaphragm dysfunction, and recurrent laryngeal nerve injury may result in chronic aspiration and lung disease from vocal cord dysfunction. Patients with chronic cyanosis can have polycythemia and resultant hyperviscosity syndrome. Older patients with unrepaired cyanotic CHD have an increased risk of paradoxical emboli or brain abscesses. There are several genetic syndromes that have strong associations with CHD as well (e.g., Down syndrome, DiGeorge syndrome, Noonan syndrome, mucopolysaccharidoses, tracheoesophageal fistula).

Presedation considerations are as follows:

- Minimize NPO time, specifically in shunt-dependent infants, who are very sensitive to small fluctuations in intravascular volumes. Allowing a clear liquid diet until 2 hours before

sedation and minimizing delays are both important in this population.
- Review cardiac medications (i.e., diuretics, antihypertensives, anticoagulants) and decide whether any of them need to be temporarily discontinued beforehand.
- Assess the need for endocarditis prophylaxis.
- Review the most recent echocardiogram, cardiac catheterization study (if applicable), and ECG.
- Review the most recent progress note from the cardiologist with sedation clearance.
- Obtain a baseline oxygen saturation value in room air.

Commonly used sedation medications in patients with CHD and their potential adverse effects are as follows:

- Ketamine provides sedation and profound analgesia with minimal negative side effects. It increases mean arterial pressure (MAP) but has minimal effect on SVR, PVR, or pulmonary artery pressure (PAP). It is also well tolerated in children with PH. Ketamine can act as a direct myocardial depressant in patients with catecholamine depletion.
- Propofol is a potent hypnotic drug with sedative and amnestic properties. It decreases MAP and SVR, while PVR and PAP remain unchanged. In patients with shunts, left-to-right flow decreases and right-to-left flow increases (thus reducing PBF and oxygenation). It should be used with caution in patients whose PBF is dependent on balancing their PVR and SVR and in those who cannot tolerate systemic afterload reduction. Propofol should be avoided in patients with impaired ventricular function as it also causes myocardial depression.
- Etomidate is a sedative–hypnotic agent with minimal hemodynamic effects in children. It is an excellent choice for patients with cardiomyopathy and impaired ventricular function.

Caution is advised in patients with suspected sepsis given the concern for adrenal suppression.

- Fentanyl is a potent analgesic with minimal hemodynamic effects. It is generally well tolerated in neonates, even in high doses (5–10 mcg/kg), although it may produce transient hypotension.
- Midazolam is an effective anxiolytic and amnestic medication, but it can lead to hemodynamic compromise (i.e., hypotension) and respiratory depression, particularly when used in conjunction with fentanyl.
- Dexmedetomidine has sedative, anxiolytic, and mild analgesic properties, with minimal risk of respiratory depression and relative lack of cardiovascular effects. The most commonly associated side effects include bradycardia and hypotension, usually relieved by discontinuation of the medication. It should be avoided in patients with preexisting bradyarrhythmias or atrioventricular block, as well as in patients receiving digoxin.

The following are postsedation considerations:

- Avoid hypovolemia.
- Maintain normothermia.
- Provide adequate analgesia if necessary.
- Ensure early hydration.

Summary

CHD is a common birth defect, with increasing numbers of patients requiring procedural sedation. This may be undertaken in many patients safely when adequate preparations are made. Understanding the often-complex physiology and the impact of sedation on that physiology is essential to ensure patient safety and appropriate referrals to a cardiac anesthesiologist when necessary.

Suggested Reading

Diaz LK, Jones L. Sedating the child with congenital heart disease. *Anesthesiol Clin.* 2009;27(2):301–319.

Thomas J. Anaesthesia for the child with congenital heart disease: pointers and pitfalls. *African Journals Online.* 2011;29(11):463–466.

6

The Pediatric Presedation Evaluation

6.1

Risk Assessment

MARK A. BUCKMASTER

Evaluation of patient risk is a critical aspect of the presedation phase of care. For scheduled procedures and tests, information obtained during the prescreening process is incorporated into the formal assessment of the patient at the time of the procedure. If the prescreening process has been sufficiently rigorous, the patient is likely to be appropriately prepared for sedation and the day-of-procedure evaluation (procedure screen) should be able to be done quickly and efficiently. These two processes (prescreening and procedure screening) determine the development of the sedation plan and allow for proper alignment of resources and skills to ensure as safe a conduct of sedation care as possible.

Prescreening for scheduled procedures is discussed fully in Chapter 6.2. Immediate preprocedural screening builds upon that information and for urgently performed procedures needs to incorporate prescreening considerations.

Preprocedural Screening

With review of the prescreening information, the sedation provider can make a preliminary assessment of the patient and begin to anticipate potential sedation pitfalls. Assessment of the patient at the time of procedure should be focused and easily done within a few minutes. Review of the presedation screening (if available) should give the provider a solid basis on which to plan his or her approach to sedation care. If unavailable, a quick assessment of past medical and surgical history and ongoing medical issues is made. A concentrated review of systems should be made in either situation and include information on last oral intake and the type of intake, any changes in care or status between the time of screening and the presentation for sedation, and other systems that sedation may impact (Box 6.1.1).

A directed physical exam should be performed prior to initiation of the sedation. The physical exam should assess overall body habitus, vital signs, overview of perfusion, pulses, auscultation of the chest, heart, and abdomen, and general assessment of neurologic function. A specific airway review should also be undertaken and can usually be done with little discomfort and distress to the child. Casual observation of the child while speaking with the parents can allow identification of abnormal neck positions, external masses, oral cavity size, and freedom of neck movement. Playful interaction and demonstration will often allow for inspection of teeth, tongue size, and ability to

BOX 6.1.1 Presedation Review

1. History of present illness
2. Medications
3. Oral intake
4. Anesthesia/sedation history
5. Perinatal history
6. Airway/respiratory
7. Cardiovascular
8. Gastrointestinal/hepatic
9. Neurologic
10. Renal

BOX 6.1.2 LEMON Airway Assessment Method

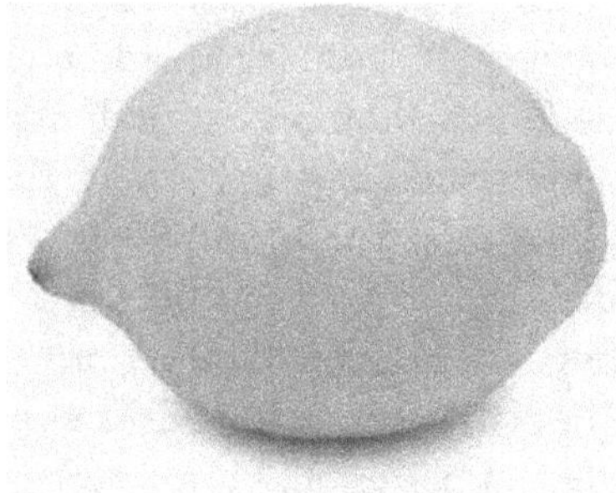

L = Look externally (facial trauma, large incisors, large tongue)

E = Evaluate the 3-3-2 rule (inter-incisor distance—3 child's fingerbreadths; hyoid-mental distance—3 child's finger-breadths; thyroid-hyoid distance—2 child's finger-breadths)

M = Mallampati (Mallampati score >3)

O = Obstruction (presence of any condition like epiglottitis, peritonsillar abscess, trauma)

N = Neck mobility (limited neck mobility)

visualize the uvula, which usually confirms the ability to successfully instrument the airway, if needed (Box 6.1.2).

Special Circumstances

Even with a comprehensive prescreening process, instances may arise that preclude proceeding with the sedation on the day of the procedure. This may occur due to changes in the condition of the patient or as the result of new information that has arisen since the initial prescreening evaluation was undertaken. In these situations you may be under outside pressure from parents, colleagues, or other personnel to proceed despite your best assessment of risk. In these circumstances, **safety** should always be the overriding aim. It is never wrong to say "no" if a given situation makes you as a sedationist uncomfortable. Alternative approaches are almost always available so that you can safely and successfully accomplish the procedure. With this in mind, there are certain conditions that do require a very measured review of the sedation circumstances before deciding how or whether to undertake the sedation.

Airway Procedures/Difficult Airways

When sharing the airway during a procedure such as a bronchoscopy, endoscopy, or dental or oral surgery cases, careful coordination between the sedationist and the proceduralist is necessary. Patient movement, coughing, desaturation, or other events must be anticipated. With sufficient practice and a close relationship between all involved, these types of cases can successfully be done under sedation.

Patients with known or expected difficult airways such as those with craniofacial abnormalities (Pierre-Robin sequence, Goldenhar syndrome), cervical spine abnormalities (Klippel-Feil syndrome), certain infiltrative metabolic processes (mucopolysaccharidoses such as Hurler's or Hunter's syndrome, Farber lipogranulomatosis, glycogen storage disorders such as Pompe's disease), or neck or oral pharyngeal masses that affect the airway present a different sort of problem. Ready access to a good pediatric syndrome reference book can be an invaluable source to assess the impact of the condition on the ability to manipulate the airway should this prove necessary. That is why prescreening should include review of prior sedation or anesthetic records as often problems relating to difficulty with the airway can be identified at this point and the patient funneled to the appropriate care provider. In any sedation situation, manipulation of the airway, while unlikely, is always a potential need for rescue from complications of sedation, and conditions that may make this difficult preclude the patient as a safe sedation risk.

Mediastinal Masses

Masses located in the mediastinum, particularly the anterior compartment, while not common often occur in conjunction with the need for sedation for related treatment and diagnostic procedures. The most common diagnoses associated with anterior mediastinal masses in children are Hodgkin's and non-Hodgkin's lymphoma, with germ cell tumors being the second most common. Symptomology is widely variable and may range from nothing to obvious positional dyspnea or cough, superior vena cava obstruction, or associated pericardial and pleural effusions. Careful review of all available imaging studies to evaluate the likelihood of possible airway collapse and compression or inability to secure the airway, if needed, is critical. Due to the potentially very tenuous nature of these patients and the absence of predictive symptoms even in the face of normal imaging studies, these patients should **never** be considered appropriate for routine sedation.

Obesity

Childhood obesity is a health problem currently approaching major proportions in the United States. As children with symptomatic obesity, defined as a body mass index (BMI) above 95% of predictive age norms, are increasingly common, their presentation and their need for sedation are becoming relatively routine. Obesity presents obvious potential problems for the sedationist related to airway management, including problems related to intubation, the establishment of adequate bag-mask ventilation, and decreased chest wall compliance. Secondarily associated conditions may also impact the conduct of sedation, such as breathing-related sleep disorders (obstructive sleep apnea), hypertension, diabetes, and cardiac issues. While the overall incidence of complications related to obesity during pediatric sedation is increased, the incidence of serious complications does not appear to change,[1] and the majority of these children are suitable for sedation with appropriate preparation and anticipatory care. Chapter 11.1 includes more information on obesity and pediatric sedation.

Age

Sedation risk increases with the increasingly younger age of the patient.[2] Patients less than 6 months of age are at higher potential risk than older children. Their increased basal metabolic rate and smaller physical size with decreased pulmonary reserve mean that potentially severe oxygen desaturations occur more quickly and are tolerated less well than in older patients. Infants with a history of prematurity also frequently have an increased degree of medical complexity, with associated problems such as bronchopulmonary dysplasia and chronic pulmonary issues that may further compromise their pulmonary safety margin. Considerations for the sedationist surrounding premature infants is discussed more completely in Chapter 11.4.

There is animal model evidence of the potential neurotoxicity of common sedative agents in younger children, although no specific guidelines for the restriction of or the approach to sedation in this population yet exists; it remains an active area of investigation. With these concerns in mind and appropriate sedation precautions, young children can be safely considered as sedation candidates.

Active Upper Respiratory Tract Infection

Upper respiratory tract infections in children are common and remain a difficult problem to easily resolve. The risk of sedation-related adverse events in the presence of an active upper respiratory infection is increased as compared with children without similar infections.[3] Distinguishing between upper respiratory infection and simple allergic rhinitis is often difficult. If the sedationist determines that an active infection is present, delaying the sedation is the prudent approach if the procedure is not urgently needed until symptoms have cleared and airway reactivity has returned to baseline (normally 3–4 weeks).

Summary

Careful prescreening will greatly aid in minimizing the inappropriate placement of patients and ensure that patients have access to the appropriate level of sedation care necessary to accomplish their procedures.[4] Despite best intentions, situations will arise where the sedationist is forced to make a judgment call as to the risk of complications in a particular patient at the time of the procedure. The degree of experience, the nature of the sedation system in which you operate, and alternative modalities will guide your decision, but overall patient safety should remain the prime directive.

References

1. Scherrer PD, Mallory MD, Cravero JP, et al. The impact of obesity on pediatric procedural sedation-related outcomes: results From the Pediatric Sedation Research Consortium. *Pediatr Anesth.* 2015;25(7):689–697.
2. Biber JL, Allareddy V, Gallagher SM, et al. Prevalence and predictors of adverse events during procedural sedation anesthesia outside the operating room for esophagogogastroduodenoscopy and colonoscopy in children: age is an independent predictor of outcomes. *Pediatric Critical Care Medicine.* 2015;16(8):e251–e259.
3. Tait AR, Shobha M. Anesthesia for the child with an upper respiratory tract infection: still a dilemma? *Anesthes Analges.* 2005;100(1):59–65.
4. Coté CJ, Wilson SW. Guidelines for monitoring and management of pediatric patients before, during, and after sedation for diagnostic and therapeutic procedures: update 2016. *Pediatrics.* 2016;138(1):e1–e31.

6.2

Prescreening

DEBORAH LAVIOLETTE

A successful pediatric procedural sedation program is dependent upon a structured and robust prescreening process. It is important that every patient be an appropriate candidate for elective, or even urgent, procedural sedation. Policies delineating which patients and procedures can be done with procedural sedation are set by each institution to conform to Center for Medicare and Medicaid Services (CMS) and Joint Commission guidelines depending upon the resources and skills available.

Prescreening is a process of checking for a match of the patient's medical and psychological risk and need factors with the available skills and equipment involved in achieving optimal sedation and procedure completion. For planned procedures, prescreening generally occurs days before the actual procedure date. The Institute of Medicine (IOM) defines six aims of quality in healthcare, and the prescreening process for procedural sedation has a direct impact on four of them:

Safety: Screening patient characteristics identifies those who are at high risk of physical or emotional harm during procedural sedation.

Efficiency and **Timeliness:** If a sedated procedure is scheduled, and the patient is deemed an inappropriate candidate for sedation *at the time of presentation* for the procedure, there is enormous preventable waste of patient and family time, clinician time and skills, and opportunity for other patients to receive care.

Patient- and family-centered care: Prescreening will ensure that the patient and family have all the information they need to be prepared physically and emotionally for the sedated procedure. By spending the time to go over what to expect, and listening to the family's questions and concerns, the sedation team can formulate a specific plan of care.

An effective prescreening process involves multiple touch points of contact among the patient, family, and sedation team members

Scheduling/Initial Screening

This is likely not done in person.

- A checklist of basic yes/no questions is often employed to ensure that the patient is appropriate for the institution's processes for procedural sedation.
  - Patient health-based questions may include:
    - Allergies
    - Previous surgeries or procedures and any adverse reactions
    - Family history of anesthesia reactions
    - Chronic pulmonary or cardiac disease
    - Obesity
    - Central or obstructive apnea
      - Sleep study documentation
      - Chronic snoring
      - Jaw or facial abnormality
    - Postgestational age of neonates
    - Swallowing dysfunction
    - Presence of fever or acute illness
    - Technology support (tracheostomy, ventriculoperitoneal shunt)
    - Epilepsy
    - Cerebral palsy

- Patient psychological factor screening questions may include:
  - Previous experience with sedation
  - General anxiety levels
  - Behavioral disorder diagnoses
  - Specific procedure-related phobias (needle, closed spaces)

These questions may be asked of the family by a nonclinically trained scheduler or answered electronically by referring providers. Any affirmative replies should prompt a more thorough review and follow-up with the family by a clinician member of the sedation team.

Secondary In-Depth Review

This review ideally is also performed before the actual procedure time (by phone).

- Elucidates details of the specific medical or psychological needs of the child to ensure the sedation team is adequately prepared with supplies, skills, and psychological supports (e.g., child life specialists)
- Results in referral to more appropriate sedation resources or gives an opportunity to inform the family of details of date, time, location, and preparation (e.g., NPO status) needs and allows an opportunity for them to ask questions. Discussion of family ideas about their presence during the procedure, for instance, allows better alignment of sedationist, proceduralist, and patient expectations.
- Allows discussion of travel concerns and potential needs for prolonged observation or even hospital admission after sedation
- Allows discussion of referral or insurance company authorization needs.

Preprocedural Follow-up

Many institutions then follow up by mailing a packet of information reviewing these same issues:

- NPO guidelines
- Physician referral or insurance prior authorization needs
- Date, time, and location of the procedure
- Importance of communication about cancellation or rescheduling needs (provide a specific phone number).

Another point of contact often employed is a reminder phone call or text message from the sedation team to the patient and family 24 to 48 hours before the scheduled procedure.

Day of Procedure

The day of the procedure represents a final point of review of the patient's pathophysiologic state (targeted history and physical) and a review with the family of concerns (which ideally were previously discussed) about the process of procedural sedation. A prepared sedation team can then meet the expectations of the patient and family, resulting in excellence in safety, efficiency, and patient satisfaction.

Suggested Reading

Connors JM, Cravero JP, Kost S, et al. Great expectations—defining quality in pediatric sedation: outcomes of a multidisciplinary consensus conference. *J Healthc Qual.* 2015;37(2):139–154.

Connors JM, Cravero JP, Lowrie L, et al. *Core Competencies for Providers who Deliver Deep Sedation.* Society for Pediatric Sedation (www.pedsedation.org).

6.3

Presedation Preparation

Equipment and Timeout/Checklists

ELIZABETH MACK AND RHEA VIDRINE

The American Academy of Pediatrics (AAP) and the American Academy of Pediatric Dentistry (AAPD) have published pediatric sedation guidelines with specific focus on appropriate monitoring during and after sedation.[1] The 2006 published guidelines also focus on the importance of a presedation safety culture using checklists to avoid preventable errors and promote availability of the necessary drugs, monitoring, and equipment in case of emergency. Several groups have published guidelines for appropriate sedation equipment, monitoring, and emergency equipment (see Chapter 17). Based on these guidelines, necessary sedation equipment can be divided into 3 main categories: vascular access equipment, monitoring equipment, and emergency equipment/medication (Figure 6.3.1).

Vascular Access Equipment

Even if the sedationist does not intend to use intravenous (IV) medications, IV supplies are necessary in case of complications. The following IV equipment should be standard in all pediatric sedation sites:

Intravenous Equipment	Monitoring Equipment	Emergency Equipment	Emergency Medications

• Gloves
• Tourniquets
• Alcohol wipes
• Sterile gauze
• IV catheters (18-24 gauge)
• Ped IV tubing (60drops/ml)
• IVF (NS, LR, D5 1/2NS)
• Syringes (1,3,5 10ml)
• Tape
• Sharps container
	• Cardiac:
	  • 3 lead EKG
	  • BP cuff
	• Respiratory
	  • Pulse ox
	  • Capnography
	• Temperature:
	  • Continuous monitoring for prolonged sedation
		• Cardiac defibrillator
		• Airway:
		  • Oral,nasal airways
		  • Ambu bag
		  • Suction apparatus
		  • Vacuum source
		  • Oxygen
		  • Nasal cannula, facemask
		  • Intubation equipment laryngoscope handles, blades, ETT, styles, LMA
			• Epinephrine (1:1000 and 1:10,000)
			• Atropine
			• Lidocaine
			• Glucose (25%, 50%)
			• Racemic epi
			• Diphenhydramine
			• Hydrocortisone
			• Albuterol
			• Midazolam
			• Ketamine
			• Etomidate
			• Vecuronium/ rocuronium
			• Succinylcholine
			• Naloxone
			• Flumazenil

FIGURE 6.3.1.

Equipment needs for pediatric sedation safety

- Gloves, tourniquets, alcohol wipes, sterile gauze, pediatric IV catheters (18–24 gauge), tape, syringes (1- to 10-mL assorted sizes), sharps disposal container.
- IV tubing, IV fluids (isotonic crystalloid and dextrose-containing fluids).
- Intraosseous needles are recommended for emergency access if IV access cannot be obtained promptly.

Monitoring Equipment

Multiple regulatory and professional society guidelines exist recommending monitoring practices in children before, during, and after pharmacologic sedation (Chapter 17). Monitoring during moderate or deep sedation should include the following:

- Assessment of depth of sedation: involves direct observation of the patient
- Blood pressure
- Oxygen saturation
- Heart rate and rhythm
- Capnography during moderate or deep sedation.

Patients undergoing sedation are at risk for hypothermia if exposed to cool room temperatures for a prolonged period of time. Attention to preventing exposure and temperature monitoring before, after, and in some cases continuously during moderate and deep sedation is recommended.[2] There are three primary subsets of monitoring equipment needed: cardiac monitoring, respiratory monitoring, and temperature monitoring. Cardiac monitoring equipment includes a 3-lead electrocardiogram, at minimum, to monitor heart rate and rhythm and repetitive blood pressure measurements during the sedation. Respiratory depression and airway obstruction are the most common significant adverse effects during sedation, and clinical observation may be unreliable in detecting these events in a timely manner. Respiratory monitoring should include continuous pulse oximetry monitoring (most modern machines will also record and sound heart rate) for all patients and capnography monitoring for patients under moderate to deep sedation. Many 3-lead electrocardiogram monitors will also monitor chest excursion plethysmography, which may be helpful for respiratory rate assessment. A precordial stethoscope will also provide the sedationist with assessment of heart rate in addition to assessment of quality and quantity of airflow. For more in-depth understanding of how to use these monitors during sedation, please see Chapter 7.

Emergency Equipment

In addition to preparing the appropriate monitors needed during sedation, it is important to have available appropriate pediatric emergency equipment and medications. Both equipment and medication should be checked and maintained on a regular basis to ensure proper function at time of emergency. As the most common adverse event associated with sedation is respiratory compromise, age- and size-appropriate emergency airway equipment should be immediately available. Emergency airway equipment includes oral and nasal airways, laryngeal mask airways, pediatric Ambu bag (either self-inflating or anesthesia/Mapleson) and appropriately sized mask, suction apparatus and vacuum source, oxygen, and nasal cannula and/or facemask. Intubation supplies include laryngoscope handles and blades (various types and sizes), end-tidal CO_2 monitoring, endotracheal tubes (various sizes, cuffed and uncuffed), and stylets. A cardiac defibrillator should always be readily available. Emergency medications must also be readily available for cardiac arrest, anaphylaxis, and/or emergent intubation. Emergency medications, at a minimum, should include epinephrine (1 mg/mL and 0.1 mg/mL concentrations), atropine, lidocaine, naloxone, flumazenil, dextrose (25% or 50%), racemic epinephrine, diphenhydramine, methylprednisolone, and albuterol. Drugs that allow the deep sedation and general anesthesia states required for emergency tracheal intubation such as midazolam, fentanyl, ketamine, etomidate, propofol, rocuronium or vecuronium, and succinylcholine may be emergently needed.

Pediatric sedation equipment should include supplies for IV catheter placement, monitoring equipment, and emergency equipment and medication. The AAP and AAPD recommend using the acronym SOAPME while preparing a site for pediatric sedation:

S: suction
O: oxygen
A: airway
P: pharmacy
M: monitors
E: equipment (Figure 6.3.2).

S-suction

- Suction catheters (size appropriate)
- Suction apparatus

O-oxygen

- Oxygen supply
- Oxygen delivery devices

A-airway

- laryngoscope blades (checked)
- ETT (2.5–6.0 uncuffed and 6.0–8.0 cuffed)
- Stylets
- Ambu bag
- Nasopharyngeal, oropharyngeal airways (size appropriate)

P-pharmacy

- Emergency life support drugs
- Sedation antagonist

M-monitors

- Pulse ox
- Capnography
- BP cuff (age/size appropriate)
- ECG (3 lead)
- Stethoscope

E-equipment

- Special equipment/drugs for procedure
- Defibrillator

FIGURE 6.3.2.

Checklist of equipment and medication availability during pediatric moderate and deep sedation

This acronym encourages the sedation team to ensure the presence of all equipment and medications needed during a pediatric sedation to enhance team function during an emergent situation.

Checklists as a Tool for Safety in Pediatric Sedation

The SOAPME acronym is an example of a checklist approach focused on equipment availability. Checklists in the medical arena have proven beneficial in reducing errors and harms to patients, particularly in the operating room,[3,4] which of course has many similarities to a procedural sedation event—that is, team-based care with a risk of communication breakdown and medical care associated with high risk of serious complication. In an early study, Haynes et al. found a significant decrease in total complications, mortality, surgical site infections, and unplanned reoperations with use of a surgical safety checklist.[4] Using a checklist increased the number of safety measures addressed with each patient, including:

- Objective airway evaluation
- Pulse oximeter use
- Appropriate IV access
- Appropriate prophylactic antibiotics given
- Oral confirmation of patient identity and operative site
- Sponge count completed at the end of the surgery.

Obviously, many of these types of safety measures apply during procedural sedation. Opponents of safety checklists cite increased time, increased cost, and lack of resources as reasons to avoid their use. The use of a checklist has been shown to cause a slight increase in time required for postoperative handover (59.5 seconds without a checklist to 120.5 seconds).[5] Cost during cardiac surgery has been decreased with the use of a checklist approach.[6] A study that did not show decreased complication or mortality rates in fact highlighted the importance of team-specific implementation and modification of the checklist to meet specific team needs.[7] The vast majority of medical personnel in a follow-up study by Haynes et al. felt that use of the checklist prevented errors, improved communication, and improved operating room safety; the checklist was also easy to use. Even more impressively, 93.4% of personnel polled said they would want the checklist used on themselves if they were having surgery.[8]

Figure 6.3.3 is a modified pediatric sedation checklist created using the World Health Organization Surgical Safety Checklist and the South Carolina Safe Surgery 2015 Checklist templates.[7,9] It is meant to be applied immediately before every procedural sedation event.

Procedural Safety Checklist

Step 1: Prior to Procedure

ALL team members STOP activity and begin checklist

- ☐ Introductions
- ☐ Verify hand hygiene by all
- ☐ Timeout: name, DOB, procedure(s), verify consent(s)
- ☐ Weight (kg)
- ☐ Allergies
- ☐ Airway concerns
- ☐ Pre-meds
- ☐ Confirm equipment available, verify expiration dates
- ☐ Mark/confirm site
- ☐ If procedure based on image: imaging displayed
- ☐ If new/different: procedure description
- ☐ If diabetic: glucose

MD says: "Any concerns? If you see anything that concerns you, please speak up."

Step 2: Debriefing at end of procedure

- ☐ Confirm specimens
- ☐ Equipment issues & areas for improvement
- ☐ Key concerns for recovery (airway, vomiting, pain)

FIGURE 6.3.3.

Adapted procedural checklist using WHO Surgical Safety Checklist and South Carolina Safe Surgery 2015 Checklist

References

1. Coté CJ, Wilson S. Guidelines for monitoring and management of pediatric patients during and after sedation for diagnostic and therapeutic procedures: an update. *Pediatrics.* 2006;118(6):2587–2602.
2. Eichhorn V, Henzler D, Murphy MF. Standardizing care and monitoring for anesthesia or procedural sedation delivered outside the operating room. *Current Opin Anaesthesiol.* 2010; 3:494–499.
3. Lubbeke A, Hovaguimian F, Wickboldt N, et al. Effectiveness of the surgical safety checklist in a high standard care environment. *Medical Care.* 2013;51(5):425–429.
4. Haynes AB, Weiser TG, Berry WR, et al. A surgical safety checklist to reduce morbidity and mortality in a global population. *N Engl J Med.* 2009;360(5):491–499.
5. Salzwedel C, Hans-Jurgen B, Kuhnelt I, et al. The effect of a checklist on the quality of post-anesthesia patient handover: a randomized control trial. *Int J Qual Health Care.* 2012;25(2):176–181.
6. Semel ME, Resch S, Haynes AB, et al. Adopting a surgical safety checklist could save money and improve the quality of care in U.S. hospitals. *Health Aff (Millwood).* 2010;29(9):1593–1599.
7. Molina G, et al. Implementation of the surgical safety checklist in South Carolina hospitals is associated with improvement in perceived perioperative safety. *Am Coll Surg.* 2016;222:725–736.
8. Haynes AB, Weiser TG, Berry WR, et al. Changes in safety attitude and relationship to decreased postoperative morbidity and mortality following implementation of a checklist-based surgical safety intervention. *BMJ Qual Saf.* 2010;20:102–107.
9. World Patient Safety Alliance. Safe Surgery Saves Lives. Geneva: World Health Organisation; June 2009. Available from: http://www.who.int/patientsafety/safesurgery/knowledge_base/SSSL_Brochure_finalJun08.pdf (accessed December 2013).

6.4

Fasting and Aspiration Risk in Procedural Sedation

MAALA BHATT AND MARK G. ROBACK

Definitions

Pulmonary aspiration **involves** inhalation of oropharyngeal or gastric contents into the larynx and lower respiratory tract. *Clinically apparent pulmonary aspiration* involves oropharyngeal or gastric contents in the trachea and the appearance of new cough, crackles/ rales, decreased breath sounds, tachypnea, wheeze, rhonchi, respiratory distress, new or increased oxygen requirement, and new focal infiltrate, consolidation, or atelectasis on chest radiograph. *Aspiration pneumonitis* is an acute lung injury following the inhalation of regurgitated gastric contents.

The American Society of Anesthesiologists (ASA) Physical Status Classification ("ASA class") is as follows:

- Class I—normal healthy patient
- Class II—mild systemic disease
- Class III—severe systemic disease
- Class IV—disease that is a constant threat to life
- Class V—moribund patient not expected to live without operation

TABLE 6.4.1 ASA preprocedure fasting guidelines for elective procedures

Ingested Material	*Minimum Fasting Period*
Clear liquids	2 hours
Breast milk	4 hours
Light meal, infant formula	6 hours
Meal containing fat/meat	8 hours

Preprocedural Fasting Guidelines and Pulmonary Aspiration

The ASA developed the recommendations in Table 6.4.1 designed to reduce the risk of pulmonary aspiration in healthy patients undergoing **elective** procedures. Patients with a "full" stomach are thought to be at risk when deeply sedated as the competence of the lower esophageal sphincter and airway protective reflexes are diminished or absent. Aspiration pneumonitis is thought to be most severe when aspirated contents are acidic and contain particulate (solid) matter.

Risk of Aspiration During Procedural Sedation Versus General Anesthesia

The impact of strict adherence to these guidelines on patient outcomes is not known. The risk of clinically apparent aspiration during general anesthesia is about 3 in 10,000. Principal risk factors for aspiration are planned airway manipulation (intubation/extubation), absence of airway protective reflexes, ASA class III or more, and extremes of age (<12 months, >70 years). The risk of aspiration during sedation is likely less than during general anesthesia due to the absence of principal risk factors.

Findings from a 2017 comprehensive systematic review of pulmonary aspiration during sedation from 1985 to 2016 found the following:

- All ages: 326 cases of aspiration; 292 (90%) during endoscopy
- Pediatrics: 32 cases of aspiration, 7 (22%) during endoscopy
- Death was uncommon (n = 8, no children) and associated with substantial comorbidity; for all others, full recovery occurred.

Non–Emergency Department (ED) Procedural Sedation

- *Best estimate of aspiration risk during elective procedural sedation*:
  - 0.7 cases per 10,000 sedations (approximately one-third to one-half of the risk in general anesthesia), from the Pediatric Sedation Research Consortium
  - 10 cases of clinically apparent pulmonary aspiration in 139,142 pediatric sedations; all 10 children who aspirated had a minimum fasting period of 6 hours for solids prior to sedation.
- *Predictors of major complications (death, pulmonary aspiration, cardiac arrest, unplanned admission)* from highest to lowest risk:
  - Age <1 month
  - Having a bronchoscopy
  - History of obstructive sleep apnea
  - Age 1 month to 1 year
  - Having an endoscopy
  - ASA class III or IV.

Importantly, this study found no association between fasting duration and pulmonary aspiration, and no association between major complications and provider type or medication administered.

ED Procedural Sedation

Adherence to preprocedural fasting guidelines is highly variable. Several prospective ED cohorts have shown **no association** between fasting duration and the occurrence of adverse events or outcomes. The aspiration risk for ED patients may be less than in elective sedation. Most children who receive procedural sedation in the ED are healthy (ASA I or II), and sedations are short in duration for painful procedures. Ketamine (airway protective reflexes intact) is used most frequently for sedation of children in the ED.

Recommendations for Administering Procedural Sedation to Children who Have Not Fulfilled Fasting Guidelines

- Consider using ketamine as a single agent for sedation.
- Recognize that patients with the following: age <12 months, ASA class III or higher, history of sleep apnea, sedation for endoscopy, or bronchoscopy, are at greater risk.

Disadvantages of Waiting to Fulfill Fasting Guidelines Before Sedation

Fasting can promote dehydration and hypoglycemia in children <3 years old. There is some evidence to suggest fasting can lead to irritability and result in more difficulty with or failed sedation.

Recommendations from Specialty Societies

ASA

- Guidelines only apply to elective procedures.
- Follow same preprocedural fasting recommendations as for general anesthesia.

American College of Emergency Physicians

- Guidelines are only intended for emergency procedures.
- Recommend no delay in ED procedural sedation based solely on fasting time. There is no evidence to support a correlation between fasting, emesis, and pulmonary aspiration in healthy children or adults in this setting.
- Must weigh risks and benefits for each patient (see the section "Clinical Practice Advisory").

American Academy of Pediatrics

- Elective procedures: Follow the same fasting guidelines as for general anesthesia.
- Emergency procedures: Weigh the risk of sedation prior to fulfilling fasting guidelines against the benefit. Lightest effective sedation should be used; consider using ketamine (less risk of depressing airway protective reflexes).

Clinical Practice Advisory for Emergency Procedures

This 3-step, practical approach helps determine the prudent depth of sedation based on presedation aspiration risk (Figure 6.4.1):

Step 1: Assess Patient Risk (if "**yes**" to any, patient is at **higher risk**)

- Is there potential for difficult ventilation should an airway complication occur (e.g., small mandible/micrognathia, large tongue, laryngo/tracheomalacia, congenital airway anomalies, prior difficult intubation, sleep apnea)?
- Are there conditions predisposing to esophageal reflux (e.g., increased intracranial pressure, esophageal disease, bowel obstruction, chronic constipation)?
- Is the patient <12 months old?

Standard-risk patient[a]

Oral intake in the prior 3 hours	Procedural Urgency[b]			
	Emergent Procedure	*Urgent Procedure*	*Semi-Urgent*	*Non-Urgent*
Nothing	All levels of sedation	All levels of sedation	All levels of sedation	All levels of sedation
Clear liquids only	All levels of sedation	All levels of sedation	Up to and including brief deep sedation	Up to and including extended moderate sedation
Light snack	All levels of sedation	Up to and including brief deep sedation	Up to and including dissociative sedation; non-extended modearte sedation	Minimal sedation only
Heavier snack or meal	All levels of sedation	Up to and including extended moderate sedation	Minimal sedation only	Minimal sedation only

Higher-risk patient[a]

Oral intake in the prior 3 hours	Procedural Urgency[b]			
	Emergent Procedure	*Urgent Procedure*	*Semi-Urgent*	*Non-Urgent*
Nothing	All levels of sedation	All levels of sedation	All levels of sedation	All levels of sedation
Clear liquids only	All levels of sedation	Up to and including brief deep sedation	Up to and including extended moderate sedation	Minimal sedation only
Light snack	All levels of sedation	Up to and including dissociative sedation; non-extended modearte sedation	Minimal sedation only	Minimal sedation only
Heavier snack or meal	All levels of sedation	Up to and including dissociative sedation; non-extended modearte sedation	Minimal sedation only	Minimal sedation only

	Procedural sedation and analgesia targeted depth and duration[c]
↓ Increasing potential aspiration risk ↓	Minimal sedation only
	Dissociative sedation; brief or intermediate-length moderate sedation
	Extended moderate sedation
	Brief deep sedation
	intermediate or extended-length deep sedation

Brief: <10 minutes
intermediate: 10–20 minutes
Extended: >20minutes

Figure. Prudent limits of targeted depth and length of ED procedural sedation and analgesia according to presedation assessment of aspiration risk

FIGURE 6.4.1.

Prudent limits of targeted depth and length of sedation based on patient risk

- Does the patient have severe systemic disease (ASA class III or higher)?
- Are there other findings that increase patient risk (e.g., altered level of consciousness)?

Step 2: Assess Timing and Nature of Recent Oral Intake (vertical axis of matrix)

- In the 3 hours prior to sedation, what has the patient consumed (nothing, clear liquids, light snack, full meal)?

Step 3: Assess the Urgency of the Procedure (horizontal axis of matrix)

- **Emergency**: cardioversion, reduction of severely angulated fracture or dislocation with soft tissue/vascular compromise, intractable pain or suffering
- **Urgent**: care of dirty wounds, animal/human bites, abscess incision and drainage, fracture reduction, trauma imaging
- **Semi-urgent**: care of clean wounds, foreign body removal, sexual assault examination
- **Nonurgent or elective:** nonorganic foreign body, planned procedure

Summary of Evidence

- Adherence to the ASA preprocedural fasting guidelines does not guarantee protection against clinically apparent pulmonary aspiration in elective or emergent procedures.
- There is no preprocedural fasting duration after which the risk of serious adverse events has been shown to decrease.
- Patient and procedure factors are the most important determinants in predicting major complications from

sedation; the risks for a given patient and procedure should be assessed on a case-by-case basis.

- Special consideration should be given to patients at higher risk (ASA class III or higher, very young age, sedation for endoscopy or bronchoscopy).
- It is prudent to follow preprocedural fasting guidelines when procedures are elective, but use caution in young children, who can experience dehydration, hypoglycemia, and irritability with prolonged fasting.

Suggested Reading

Agrawal D, Manzi SF, Gupta R, et al. Preprocedural fasting state and adverse events in children undergoing procedural sedation and analgesia in a pediatric emergency department. *Ann Emerg Med.* 2003;42:636–646.

American Society of Anesthesiologists. Practice guidelines for sedation and analgesia by non-anesthesiologists. *Anesthesiology.* 2002;96:1004–1017.

Andersson H, Zaren B, Frykholm P. Low incidence of pulmonary aspiration in children allowed intake of clear fluids until called to the operating suite. *Paediatr Anaesth.* 2015;25:770–777.

Beach ML, Cohen DM, Gallagher SM, Cravero J. Major adverse events and relationship to nil per os status in pediatric sedation/anesthesia outside the operating room. *Anesthesiology*. 2016;124(1):80–88.

Bhatt M, Johnson DW, Taljaard M, et al. Association of Preprocedural Fasting With Outcomes of Emergency Department Sedation in Children. *JAMA Pediatr* 2018; Online May 7, 2018.

Bhatt M, Kennedy R, Osmond MH, et al. Consensus-based recommendations for standardizing terminology and reporting adverse events for emergency department procedural sedation and analgesia in children. *Ann Emerg Med.* 2009;53:426–435.

Coté CJ, Wilson S, American Academy of Pediatrics, American Academy of Pediatric Dentistry. Guidelines for monitoring and management of pediatric patients before, during, and after sedation for diagnostic and therapeutic procedures: update 2016. *Pediatrics.* 2016;138(1):e20161212

Godwin SA, Burton JH, Gerardo CJ, et al. Clinical policy: procedural sedation and analgesia in the emergency department. *Ann Emerg Med.* 2014;63(2):247–258.

Green SM. Fasting is a consideration—not a necessity—for emergency department procedural sedation and analgesia. *Ann Emerg Med.* 2003;42:647–650.

Green SM, Krauss B. Pulmonary aspiration risk during emergency department procedural sedation—an examination of the role of fasting and sedation depth. *Acad Emerg Med* 2002;9(1):35–42.

Green SM, Mason KP, Krauss B. Pulmonary aspiration during procedural sedation: a comprehensive systematic review. *Br J Anaesth.* 2017;118(3):344–354.

Green SM, Roback MG, Miner JR, et al. Fasting and emergency department procedural sedation and analgesia: a consensus-based clinical practice advisory. *Ann Emerg Med.* 2007;49:454–461.

Marik PE. Aspiration pneumonitis and aspiration pneumonia. *N Engl J Med.* 2001; 344:665–671.

Roback MG, Bajaj LB, Wathen J, et al. Preprocedural fasting and adverse events in procedural sedation and analgesia in a pediatric emergency department—are they related? *Ann Emerg Med.* 2004;44:454–459.

7

Monitoring

7.1

Noninvasive Blood Pressure Monitoring and Electrocardiography

MELISSA LANGHAN AND SETH WOLF

Understanding the cardiovascular changes that occur at each level of sedation will allow providers to recognize and manage possible complications. The following points outline cardiovascular function impairment at different levels of sedation:

- Minimal sedation (anxiolysis): maintained
- Moderate sedation: usually maintained
- Deep sedation: usually maintained
- General anesthesia: may be impaired

In addition to the changes in cardiovascular function as a result of the level of sedation, many of the medications used for procedural sedation and analgesia (PSA) have cardiovascular side effects. Providers must have a clear understanding of these pharmacokinetic and pharmacodynamic effects, as well as the possible drug interactions. Prompt detection of abnormalities in a patient's blood pressure (BP) or heart rate allows the provider to consider appropriate interventions to avoid further adverse events.

Discussion

There is a lack of data regarding the benefits of hemodynamic monitoring modalities during pediatric PSA. Many of the published guidelines rely on expert opinion and not on robust quantitative information. This lack of evidence-based data has resulted in a difference in practice among providers and in organizational recommendations. Table 7.1.1 is a summary of recommendations from various organizations for pediatric PSA.

It is generally accepted that a baseline determination of heart rate and BP should be documented prior to the administration of the sedative medication. For minimal sedation, or anxiolysis, such as with midazolam only, the patient's cognitive function and coordination may be impaired, but the patient should maintain cardiovascular function. Thus, among patients who receive minimal sedation, cardiovascular monitoring is not required. A higher

TABLE 7.1.1 Summary of monitoring recommendations for procedural sedation by professional organizations

Organization	*Heart Rate*	*BP*
American Academy of Pediatrics and American Academy of Pediatric Dentistry	Continuous	Intermittent
American Society of Anesthesiologists for non-anesthesiologists	Continuous	Intermittent
American College of Emergency Physicians	Consider	Unknown frequency
European Board of Anaesthesiology of the European Union of Medical Specialists	Continuous	Intermittent

level of cardiovascular monitoring is required for deeper sedation, however.

Before administering PSA, it is important to take an appropriate history from the patient, paying particular attention to any underlying heart disease, congenital defects, or cardiac risk factors. Various studies have shown that significant cardiovascular complications and adverse events, such as cardiac arrest, life-threatening arrhythmias, hypotension with poor perfusion, or severe bradycardia, are extremely rare during PSA, even in patients with heart disease. However, in patients with complex medical problems or American Society of Anesthesiologists (ASA) class III or IV, providers should consider a consultation from appropriate subspecialists or anesthesiologists before administering any sedation deeper than minimal sedation.

As mentioned earlier, the data regarding electrocardiogram (ECG) and BP monitoring during sedation is limited and the incidence of severe cardiovascular adverse events, such as ventricular tachycardia or the need for vasopressors, is low. Other significant physiologic changes, such as hypercapnia and hypoxemia, typically occur before any changes in BP or heart rate. Monitoring of the heart rate via pulse oximetry is often acceptable given that the majority of abnormalities are reflected in changes in heart rate, not rhythm. That being said, it is reasonable to use a 3-lead (I, II, and III) ECG to monitor heart rate and rhythm and an appropriate-sized arterial BP cuff as monitoring modalities during the sedation due to their noninvasive nature and high availability. From various sources, the most common time interval for taking BP during sedation is every 5 minutes. For patients with comorbid conditions or heart disease, the use of a 5-lead ECG will allow providers more in-depth cardiac monitoring and improved rhythm analysis.

A caveat to recording the BP intermittently during a sedation is that the cuff insufflation may lead to patient arousal and movement. This is important during certain procedures, such as MRI, where image quality can be compromised by movement. Providers should use discretion when monitoring during these types of procedures.

Providers must also be cognizant about the location of the BP cuff, as it can lead to abnormalities with pulse oximetry during insufflation if they are on the same extremity.

Another benefit of cardiovascular monitoring during sedation is that a provider can use heart rate and BP changes or trends to assess the adequacy of sedation. For example, during a painful procedure, a rising heart rate may indicate that the patient is uncomfortable or that the sedative agent is wearing off. Used in conjunction with other monitoring modalities, such as attentive visual inspection of the patient, the provider may decide to administer additional sedative medication.

The choice of sedative agent can impact hemodynamics, as many of the medications have cardiovascular side effects. Severe cardiovascular adverse effects are rare, but changes in heart rate and BP are common with many sedative medications. Medications generally alter BP by affecting autonomic responses. Many medications affect heart rate through changes in vagal tone and inotropic and chronotropic properties. Table 7.1.2 lists common sedative medications and the possible associated cardiovascular side effects.

Another consideration for providers supervising sedation and analgesia is the use of local anesthetic agents, many of which can depress cardiac function and conduction. Examples include the amide anesthetics, such as lidocaine or bupivacaine, and the ester anesthetics, such as tetracaine or procaine. Providers should pay attention so that the appropriate dose is given in the proper location.

Cardiovascular monitoring should continue until an appropriate level of awareness is obtained during the recovery period. Recovery can be assessed by using various parameters, including stable cardiovascular function, a patent airway, intact protective reflexes, an appropriate level of responsiveness and interaction for age, and an adequate state of hydration.

TABLE 7.1.2 Cardiovascular side effects of common sedative medications

	Heart Rate	*BP*
Elevated (tachycardia, Hypertension)	More common drugs: ketamine Less common drugs: dexmedetomidine	More common drugs: ketamine Less common drugs: propofol, dexmedetomidine
Lowered (bradycardia, hypotension)	More common drugs: propofol, opioids/opiates, barbiturates, dexmedetomidine Less common drugs: ketamine, etomidate	More common drugs: propofol, benzodiazepines, opioids/opiates, barbiturates, dexmedetomidine, nitrous oxide Less common drugs: ketamine

Summary

Noninvasive intermittent BP and ECG monitoring should be used to monitor patients during higher levels of PSA. BP and ECG monitoring are very low risk to the patient and can help identify medication side effects, adequacy of sedation, and rare life-threatening conditions. Obtaining baseline measurements prior to the sedation and obtaining continuous 3-lead ECG and intermittent BP readings throughout the sedation and during recovery are important to monitor the safety of the patient.

Suggested Reading

Coté CJ, Wilson S, American Academy of Pediatrics, American Academy of Pediatric Dentistry. Guidelines for monitoring and management of pediatric patients before, during, and after sedation for diagnostic and therapeutic procedures: update 2016. *Pediatrics*. 2016;138(1):e20161212.

Hartling L, Milne A, Foisy M, et al. What works and what's safe in pediatric emergency procedural sedation: an overview of reviews. *Acad Emerg Med*. 2016;23(5):519–530.

Tobias JD, Cravero JP. *Procedural Sedation for Infants, Children, and Adolescents*. Elk Grove Village, IL: American Academy of Pediatrics, 2015.

7.2

Pulse Oximetry

STORM LIEBLING AND MELISSA LANGHAN

Pulse oximetry is a reliable, noninvasive method for monitoring a patient's peripheral oxygen saturation (SpO_2) of hemoglobin during procedural sedation and analgesia (PSA). Its use is recommended in the monitoring of children undergoing various levels of sedation. Its measurement is an estimation of the patient's arterial oxygen saturation (SaO_2) and usually falls within 4% of the patient's true oxygen saturation. As is the case with other methods of surrogate monitoring, understanding the indications and limitations of pulse oximetry will allow the user to safely monitor a patient's oxygen saturation during PSA.

Discussion

Pulse oximetry is the most common monitoring method used during PSA. Continuous pulse oximetry should be routinely used during minimal, moderate, and deep sedation as a means to detect hypoxemia and decrease the likelihood of adverse outcomes, including cardiopulmonary arrest and death. Given the robust evidence for its use, this recommendation is supported in several major consensus guidelines on monitoring during PSA. Oxygen desaturation events are the most common adverse events during PSA, occurring in >5% of procedural sedations, and are primarily identified by pulse oximetry. While all sedative agents may cause oxygen desaturation and hypoxemia, ketamine is generally associated with the lowest likelihood of oxygen desaturation events. Oxygen desaturation events are more likely to occur when multiple agents are used synchronously.

Proper placement of the pulse oximeter probe through a thin section of a child's body allows the device to sense various wavelength absorbances (infrared and red light) through a pulsatile vascular bed. Several different types of pulse oximetry probes are available; the provider should choose an appropriate probe for the age and location on the patient. The fingertip is generally considered the preferred location for probe placement, although other acceptable locations include the toe, earlobe, or across a foot in an infant. There are also newer forehead probes that are less sensitive to motion artifact. Appropriate placement of the probe is essential to accurate SpO_2 readings; a probe that is too tight may constrict the circulation, while a probe that is too loose may allow for motion artifact or may even fall off during the procedure. Table 7.2.1 lists other limitations of pulse oximetry.

Although normal values typically range between 95% and 100%, the child's premorbid condition (including baseline cardiopulmonary status) will affect the measurement. In addition to absolute measurements, users must be aware that sudden changes in SpO_2 may indicate an acute desaturation event even if the reading falls within the "normal" range.

Several conditions exist in which the SpO_2 will be erroneously displayed by the pulse oximeter. As such, one must interpret the SpO_2 within the context of the clinical setting. Table 7.2.1 also lists various conditions that may affect SpO_2 readings.

In addition to monitoring the SpO_2 value at a given point in time, proper interpretation of this value hinges upon recognition of the associated waveform on plethysmography. Figure 7.2.1 displays the various waveforms one may encounter with pulse oximetry. The provider should note that one may interpret the individual value only if the waveform shows a normal signal with a clear dicrotic notch. Pulse oximetry equipment that does not display a plethysmograph, but shows only a numeric value, may make the SpO_2 reading more difficult to interpret and ensure accuracy.

TABLE 7.2.1 Conditions that may limit the accuracy of the pulse oximeter reading

Falsely Overestimated
Anemia (severe)
Carboxyhemoglobinemia
Falsely Underestimated
Vasoconstriction/poor peripheral circulation (shock, hypothermia)
Methemoglobinemia
Nail polish (black, dark blue, purple)/synthetic fingernails
Blood pressure cuff on monitored arm
Movement/shivering (poor signal/waveform)
No Effect
Skin pigmentation
Ambient room lighting

For patients breathing in room air, changes in SpO_2 measurements will be detected within 30 to 60 seconds of SaO_2 change; therefore, this is not a substitute for additional cardiorespiratory monitoring during PSA. In particular, since oxygenation and ventilation are separate physiologic processes, pulse oximetry is not adequate as the sole device to assess a patient's ventilatory status. The administration of supplemental oxygen will exaggerate this discrepancy. For instance, when a patient experiences hypoventilation or apnea, changes in SpO_2 may not become apparent for several minutes when supplemental oxygen is being provided.

Declines in pulse oximetry are often the first warning sign of a serious adverse event. Despite proper monitoring by pulse oximetry, failure to rescue the patient with adequate intervention or delay in arrival of other skilled professionals is associated with negative

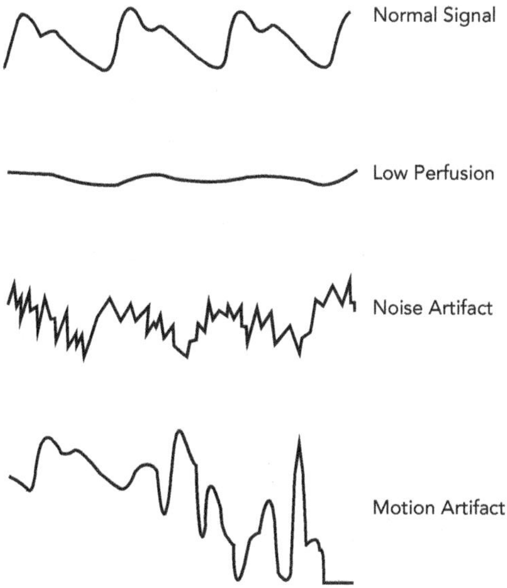

FIGURE 7.2.1.

Various waveforms identified by plethysmography.

outcomes during PSA. The practitioner must intervene immediately when a decline in SpO_2 is noted. Once pulse oximetry readings fall below 90%, SpO_2 may decline more precipitously, as there is a much steeper slope on the oxygen–hemoglobin dissociation curve at this level. For any event in which the SpO_2 falls below 95%, consider the following approaches:

- Examine the patient: check airway, breathing, and circulation and take action immediately.
- Examine the waveform and equipment: reposition or replace device if necessary.

Given the inherent delay in SpO_2 reading, it may take 30 to 60 seconds for the reading to reflect the patient's current status.

Summary

Pulse oximetry is a reliable method for monitoring a patient's SpO_2 during PSA and should be continuously employed during minimal, moderate, and deep sedation. Oxygen desaturation events are the most common adverse events during PSA and are primarily identified by pulse oximetry. Several conditions will limit the accuracy of the SpO_2 measurement and should be recognized and addressed prior to the procedure. When a desaturation event is identified, the provider should examine the patient by checking airway, breathing, and circulation and take immediate action if necessary.

Suggested Reading

Bhatt M, Johnson DW, Chan J, et al. Risk factors for adverse events in emergency department procedural sedation for children. *JAMA Pediatr.* 2017;171(10):957–964.

Coté CJ, Wilson S, American Academy of Pediatrics, American Academy of Pediatric Dentistry. Guidelines for monitoring and management of pediatric patients before, during, and after sedation for diagnostic and therapeutic procedures: update 2016. *Pediatrics.* 2016;138(1):e20161212.

Cravero JP, Beach ML, Blike GT, et al. Pediatric Sedation Research Consortium. The incidence and nature of adverse events during pediatric sedation/anesthesia with propofol for procedures outside the operating room. *Anesth Analg.* 2009;108(3);795–804.

7.3

Ventilation—Observation, Capnography, and Precordial Stethoscope

KEVIN G. COULOURES

Ensuring adequate oxygenation and ventilation is a paramount safety concern during procedural sedation. Close monitoring of these two parameters has increased the safety of sedation/anesthesia over 10-fold during the past 2 decades. This section will cover the following methods of assessing adequate ventilation: visual observation, precordial/pretracheal stethoscope, and end-tidal CO_2 monitoring (capnography).

Discussion

The oldest and least expensive of these methods is direct observation. Direct observation has been used since the time of Hippocrates, who used both his eyes and ears to assess the respiratory cycle. The American Society of Anesthesiologists (ASA) has outlined the use of direct observation for anesthesia practitioners in its standards for basic anesthesia monitoring, stating that the adequacy of ventilation will be continually evaluated. Qualitative clinical signs such as chest excursion and auscultation of breath sounds are useful and can help guide correct positioning of the patient's head and neck along with recognition of changes in the quality of respiration as the depth of sedation is varied. However, direct observation may be difficult to perform in darkened rooms, when the patient has a body drape in place, or when the physician is outside of the procedural/imaging area, such as during a CT or MRI study. Continuous direct observation may also be difficult when the patient is being repositioned for a procedure, medications are being drawn up or during their administration. Subtle variations in the depth of respiratory excursion, particularly in younger children, may not be apparent to the novice practitioner.

Limitations in the ability to detect inadequate ventilation via direct observation led to the development of the precordial or pretracheal stethoscope. The original method utilizes an earpiece molded to the practitioner's ear and then connected to a bell taped over the chest with ~4 feet of tubing connecting the earpiece and bell. This allows the practitioner to constantly monitor the quality of respiration but effectively tethers the practitioner to the patient (Figure 7.3.1). More modern versions of the device utilize a Bluetooth-enabled precordial amplifier

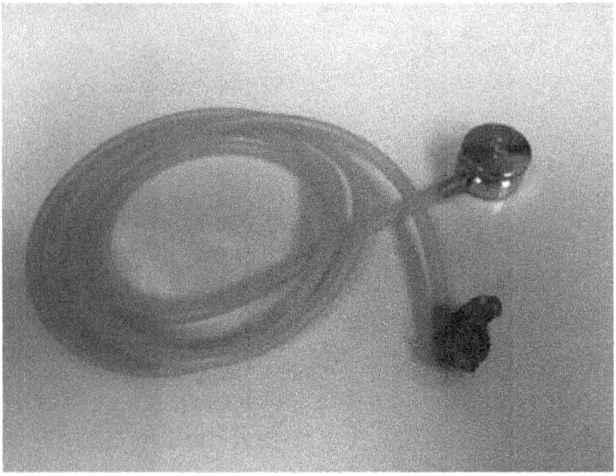

FIGURE 7.3.1.

Precordial/pretracheal stethoscope.

connected to the stethoscope bell. The amplifier then sends a wireless signal to an earpiece. The use of the Bluetooth earpiece increases the sedationist's mobility without interrupting breath sound monitoring.

Both models allow the practitioner to auscultate breath sounds and note the depth of respiration, the presence of snoring or gurgling (which may suggest partial airway obstruction), or faint vocalizations, which may indicate that sedation needs to be deepened. The American Academy of Pediatric Dentistry and the American Academy of Pediatrics recognize that the use of a precordial/pretracheal stethoscope may be preferred in children who will not allow a mask or nasal cannula to be placed over their nose/mouth area or when the procedure involves the oral airway and measurement of end-tidal CO_2 may be difficult or inaccurate.

End-tidal CO_2 monitoring (capnography) is the preferred method of ventilatory monitoring for patients who can tolerate a nasal cannula or face mask. The growth of end-tidal CO_2 monitoring in procedural sedation has mirrored the mandated use in assessing patients with an endotracheal tube or laryngeal mask airway in place. The need for both real-time ventilatory assessment and detection of displaced endotracheal tubes prompted the development of monitors that can graph the relationship of the end-tidal CO_2 concentration over time. For the non-intubated patient undergoing sedation, end-tidal CO_2 monitoring involves a specialized nasal cannula with sidestream gas sampling technology. As the patient exhales, a small amount of the gas is sent via a small cannula to an infrared detector within the monitor that analyzes the sampled gas. Molecules of CO_2 absorb infrared light at specific wavelengths, with the amount of light absorbed proportional to the amount of CO_2 present. The photodetector then converts the amount of light absorbed into a signal that is displayed as the end-tidal CO_2 value. The graphing of these values over time creates the capnogram displayed on the patient's vital sign monitor with both absolute CO_2 values and dynamic airway/ventilatory information in the shape of a waveform. An example of a normal capnogram is shown in Figure 7.3.2, followed by an example

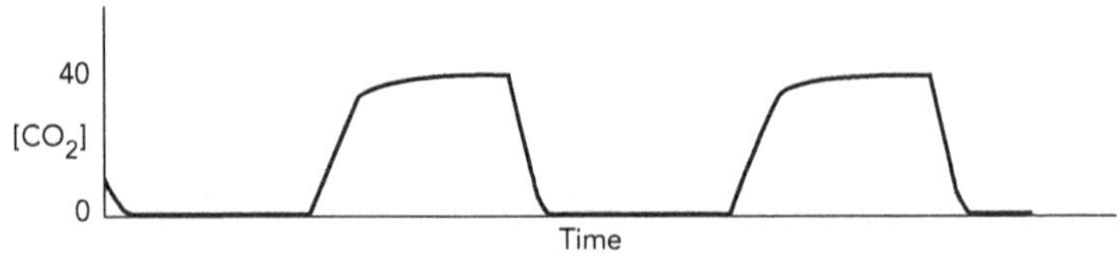

FIGURE 7.3.2.

Capnogram showing normal ventilation.

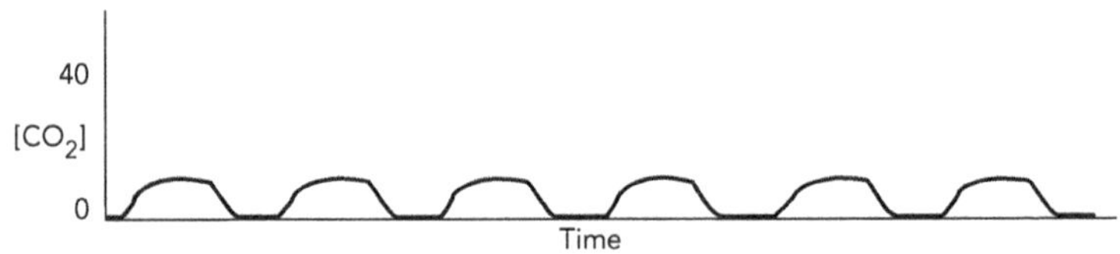

FIGURE 7.3.3.

Capnogram showing hyperventilation.

of hyperventilation (Figure 7.3.3), and normal ventilation followed by hypoventilation (Figure 7.3.4).

Capnography offers the advantage of allowing noninvasive ventilatory assessment with breath-to-breath information in procedural setting patient monitors, including those that are MRI-compatible. Technical challenges yielding inaccurate capnography include thin

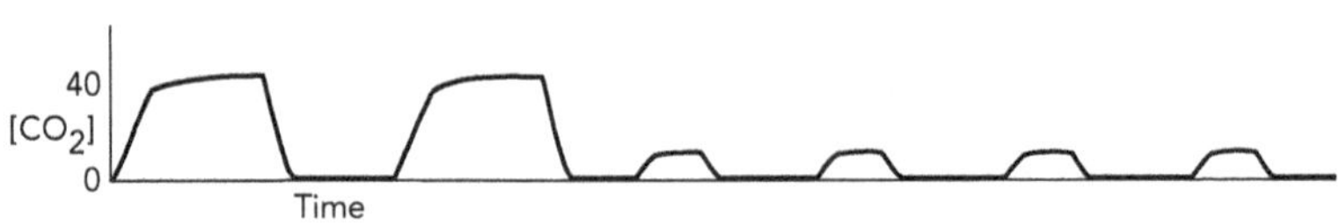

FIGURE 7.3.4.

Capnogram showing normal ventilation followed by hypoventilation.

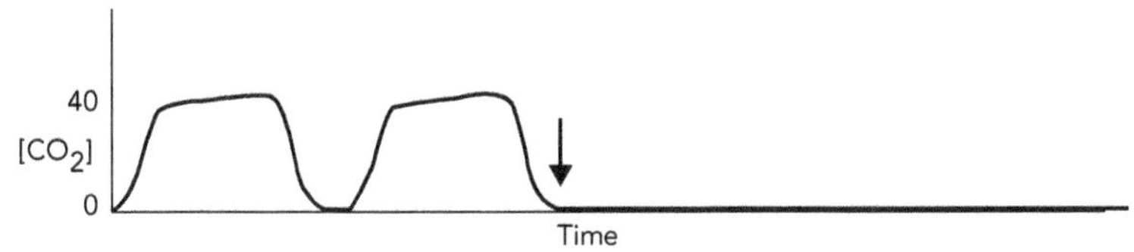

FIGURE 7.3.5.

Capnogram showing normal ventilation followed by complete obstruction or apnea.

cannula tubing easily obstructed by mucus and mouth breathing, which diminishes nasal exhalation gas sampling.

Despite these potential limitations, capnography can detect when the airway is obstructed or decreased ventilation when there is still chest wall movement. The transition from normal ventilation to apnea or complete airway obstruction is demonstrated in Figure 7.3.5. The arrow in the figure marks when the obstruction or apnea begins. Capnography can also help detect low tidal volumes due to respiratory depression that may be subtle and do not initially affect oxygenation. Figure 7.3.6 demonstrates hypoventilation with periodic breathing in an infant.

Use of end-tidal CO_2 monitoring and resultant waveform capnography has been shown to detect abnormalities in ventilation earlier in both emergency department and endoscopic settings. The visual representation of end-tidal CO_2 values as a graph may be superior to monitors that display only the numeric value.

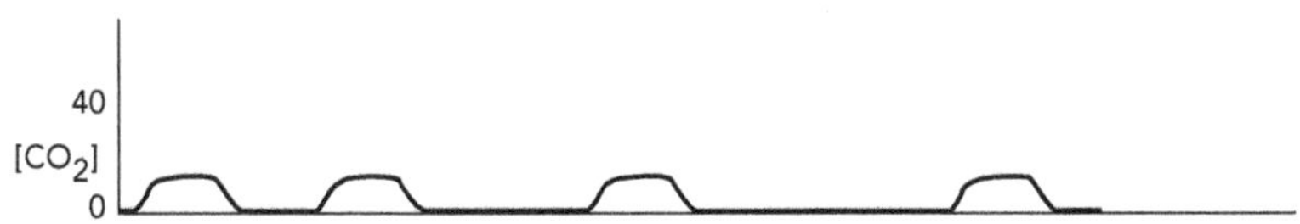

FIGURE 7.3.6.

Capnogram showing hypoventilation with periodic breathing.

A low-flow (50 mL/min) monitor is available and should be used for patients whose low tidal volumes are insufficient for a high-flow (150 mL/min) device.

Summary

The most important aspect of any of these modalities is to use them and alter care as needed. Universal incorporation of capnography into procedural sedation monitoring has yet to occur, with variation perhaps accounted for by differences in guidance from the societies involved in sedation. But in those cases where the equipment is available and the patient can tolerate the nasal cannula, end-tidal CO_2 monitoring will give the practitioner the most information about the ventilatory status of the sedated patient. The expenses associated with purchase of a new monitor (or monitor upgrade) and a specialized sidestream end-tidal CO_2 nasal cannula (Figure 7.3.7) are not insignificant, but the critical ventilation information that

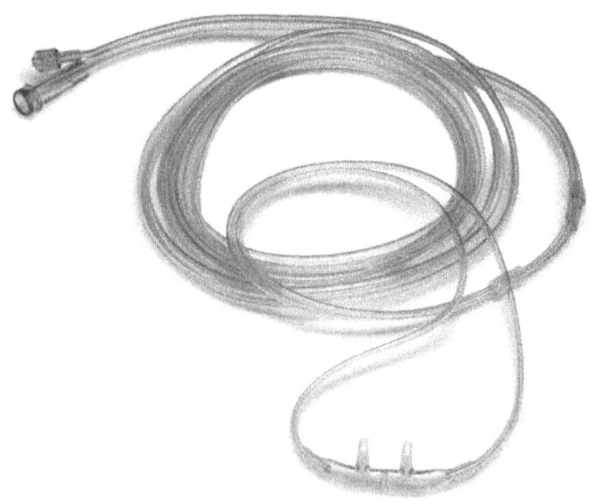

FIGURE 7.3.7.

Nasal cannula with separate line for end-tidal CO_2 monitoring.

end-tidal CO_2 monitoring provides is worth the investment to prevent sedation-associated adverse events (see Chapter 9).

Suggested Reading

Coté CJ, Wilson S, American Academy of Pediatrics, American Academy of Pediatric Dentistry. Guidelines for monitoring and management of pediatric patients before, during, and after sedation for diagnostic and therapeutic procedures: update 2016. *Pediatrics*. 2016;138(1):e2016121.2

Krauss B, Hess DR. Capnography for procedural sedation and analgesia in the emergency department. *Ann Emerg Med*. 2007;50:172–181.

Langhan ML, Shabanova V, Li F, et al. A randomized controlled trial of capnography during sedation in the pediatric emergency setting. *Am J Emerg Med*. 2015;33(1):25–30.

7.4

Observation

DEBRA J. FAULK

Sedation is a service best delivered by a multispecialty team, and several organizations have put forth guidelines and definitions regarding the provision of sedation for diagnostic and therapeutic procedures in children. The American Academy of Pediatrics (AAP), the American Society of Anesthesiologists (ASA), the Joint Commission (JCAHO), the American Academy of Pediatric Dentistry (AAPD), and the Centers for Medicare and Medicaid Services (CMS) have consensus definitions for levels of sedation (see Chapter 3).

Clinically, children transition between levels of sedation while receiving sedative medications for procedures. Deeper levels of sedation place patients at greater risk of altered cardiorespiratory function. Children—especially those younger than 6 years of age—often require deeper levels of sedation than adults. Adverse events are most commonly respiratory in nature and can progress to cardiac arrest if not addressed (see Chapter 9). Proper monitoring and prompt recognition of physiologic compromise are crucial for early support and intervention to prevent potentially catastrophic clinical deterioration.

Safe conduct of sedation includes observational assessment of the patient's condition and utilizes a variety of scales that assess the responsiveness of the sedated patient. Many of these were developed to assess patients requiring sedation in intensive care unit settings. However, the provision of procedural sedation presents distinctive goals and challenges that differ from the needs for sedation care of the critically ill patient. This section will review some of the more commonly used or well-known scales for assessing sedation or responsiveness during procedural sedation.

When considering tools to assess the sedated child undergoing diagnostic or therapeutic procedures, the ideal scale would be:

- Applicable to all ages and procedures
- Simple and intuitive to use
- Applicable for healthcare providers of differing training and specialties
- Able to be rapidly and repeatedly administered
- Objective in nature
- Validated with good interrater reliability.

It would also speak to the efficacy, efficiency and safety of sedation being provided. Available scales lack many of these criteria and measure only one dimension of sedation: level of consciousness (LOC). LOC is used as a surrogate measure for safety as it is well recognized that deeper levels of sedation place patients at greater risk of cardiorespiratory compromise. However, LOC is not indicative of the quality of sedation or other factors that can impact safety such as movement, pain, or stress. Responsiveness scales are designed to assess a single point in time but are limited in their capacity to account for change in sedation level over time. Users of such scales may effectively distinguish minimal from deep sedation or general anesthesia but struggle to discriminate between intermediate levels of sedation (e.g., moderate to deep, deep to general anesthesia), where increased risk may be imposed. Scales such as the COMFORT scale[1] and the Dartmouth Operative Conditions Scale (DOCS)[2] may enhance discernment between intermediate levels of sedation, but their complexity hinders repeated administrations in the clinical setting of procedural sedation.

The recently developed Pediatric Sedation State Scale (PSSS) is a validated pediatric scale developed specifically to assess patient state and appropriateness of conditions during pediatric procedural sedation regardless of the sedation/analgesia technique or procedure being performed. Future use of this scale may help fill the gap that exists among the currently available scales linking observational assessment to sedation quality and patient outcomes.

Available scales include the following:

- *Ramsay Sedation Scale (RSS)*[4]: This is the most widely used scale in clinical sedation and research. It describes 6 categories but does not clearly delineate between purposeful and nonpurposeful movement, thereby creating ambiguity in determining moderate versus deep levels of sedation.
- *Modified Ramsay Sedation Scale*[4,5]: The original 6 categories of the RSS were modified to 8 categories, more clearly coinciding with the currently accepted definitions of sedation as adopted by the AAP, ASA, JCAHO, AAPD, and CMS.
- *Observer's Assessment of Alertness/Sedation Scale (OAA/S)*[6]: Developed to measure the level of alertness in adults sedated with midazolam.
- *Modified OAA/S (MOAA/S)*[6]: Uses only the responsiveness category of the OAA/S, which was seen to contribute most heavily to the composite score. This category has not been validated in children.
- *Extended OAA/S (EOAA/S)*[7]: Adapted from MOAA/S to extend evaluation into the realm of light to deep general anesthesia.
- *University of Michigan Sedation Scale (UMSS)*[8]: Developed to provide a simple, reliable, valid tool for rapid assessment and documentation of sedation depth in children receiving sedative medication for diagnostic and therapeutic procedures.
- *Richmond Agitation Sedation Scale (RASS)*[9,10]: Developed by a multidisciplinary team of physicians, nurses, and pharmacists to assess sedation in adult intensive care unit (ICU) patients. Validated to assess sedation in pediatric ICU patients.
- *COMFORT Scale*[1]: A physiologic scale developed in the pediatric ICU setting that considers pain/discomfort. Complex

and time-consuming to use. More appropriate for ICU setting where assessments are needed less often.

- *Dartmouth Operative Conditions Scale (DOCS)*[2]: Designed as a research tool to evaluate and improve sedation practices between individual providers, service lines, and institutions. Codifies observations of patient movement, stress, pain, and respiratory changes through video review with the goal of optimizing provider, pharmacologic, and nonpharmacologic interventions to create ideal procedural sedation conditions.
- *Pediatric Sedation State Scale*[3]: Validated to assess patient state during procedural sedation rather than simply level of consciousness. Considers factors such as movement, stress, and pain to evaluate the efficiency, efficacy, and safety of the sedation being provided.

While assessment of a child's level of sedation or consciousness is vital for the safe conduct of procedural sedation, stimulation of the patient for this assessment may be in direct opposition to the goal of sedation itself—to have a calm, motionless patient. As such, there is interest in the utility of noninvasive, objective measures of sedation and investigations into processed electroencephalographic (EEG) systems such as the Bispectral Index™ monitor (BIS), state entropy index, and the Narcotrend® index. The most studied of these systems is the BIS.

The BIS is a brain function monitor developed from EEG recordings of healthy adult volunteers that gained approval from the U.S. Food and Drug Administration in 1996 for hypnotic monitoring. The processed EEG data from a single lead is digitized, analyzed, and transformed into a single, dimensionless number on a scale from 100 (awake) to 0 (isoelectric EEG). BIS output has been shown to correlate with observational scales to varying degrees.[11–13] The freedom the BIS offers from avoiding stimulation of the comfortably sedated patient must be weighed against the potential for inaccuracy, as the dominant amplitude and frequency of EEG waves change with ongoing neurodevelopment in children.[14,15] This is especially true in patients from newborns to 1-year-olds. This monitor has been seen to face the same challenge of poor discrimination between intermediate levels of sedation.[11,16,17] BIS may overestimate or underestimate sedation due to age variation in the EEG and with certain medications or comorbid conditions.[18] The reliability and utility of the BIS in pediatric sedation are therefore questionable, and it does not have clear advantages over currently accepted observational methods.[19]

Regardless of the intended level of sedation, providers should increase the vigilance and intensity of their monitoring appropriate to the actual level of sedation achieved. In lieu of noninvasive means of monitoring, and considering the undesirable results from stimulating children to assess their clinical level of consciousness during procedural sedation, this author recommends appropriate physiologic monitoring to confirm clinical stability at intervals that assume the patient has fallen to a deeper level of sedation.

Observation and monitoring are made especially challenging when hazardous exposures require separation from the sedated patient for an extended period. Prime examples are the limited visualization of a child in the bore of an MRI magnet, or the shielding needed for high-energy external beam radiation therapy. Extra vigilance in monitoring and observation is critical, the main concern being maintenance of airway patency and respiratory function. Considerations when physical separation is necessary include the following:

- Meticulous attention to airway positioning and patency is essential prior to separation from the patient for the beginning of the procedure.
- Vital signs should be monitored at intervals that assume deeper levels of sedation.
- Closed-circuit video monitoring should be used to visually assess breathing and to alert providers to unwanted or dangerous movement. Cameras that can zoom to a particular view of the patient or equipment should be used. (Note: camera views may not provide sufficient visualization of adequate chest excursion and respiratory effort.)

- Microphones can be used to transmit pulse oximetry tones.
- Monitors with VGA output can be wired to control room monitors via cables passed through ports in the wall for remote viewing.
- When adequate visualization of respirations is not possible, quantitative measurement of expired carbon dioxide is essential. In the unintubated patient, a nasal cannula with a side-stream capnograph can confirm the presence of end-tidal carbon dioxide ($ETCO_2$) and the adequacy of ventilation, and can immediately alert the provider to inadequate ventilation or apnea, which could be missed due to poor visualization or might otherwise be masked by supplemental oxygen administration.
- Appropriate emergency equipment should be readily available either in the room with the patient, or directly adjacent.

It will likely take extra time to access the patient in distress when the sedationist is monitoring the patient from the adjacent control center. Removal from a dangerous environment for resuscitation, such as the MRI magnet room, or waiting for a slow-moving lead-lined door to open to enter the radiation therapy vault should be considered in your response times. Proactivity in planning responses is essential.

Suggested Reading

Coté CJ, Wilson S, American Academy of Pediatrics, American Academy of Pediatric Dentisty. Guidelines for monitoring and management of pediatric patients before, during, and after sedation for diagnostic and therapeutic procedures: update 2016. *Pediatrics.* 2016;138(1):20161212.

Cravero JP, Beach ML, Blike GT. Incidence and nature of adverse events during pediatric sedation/anesthesia for procedures outside the operating room: report from the Pediatric Sedation Research Consortium. *Pediatrics.* 2006;118(3):1087–1096.

References

1. Ambuel B, Hamlett KW, Marx CM, Blumer JL. Assessing distress in pediatric intensive care environments: the COMFORT scale. *J Pediatr Psychol.* 1992;17(1):95–109.
2. Cravero JP, Blike GT, Surgenor SD, Jensen J. Development and validation of the Dartmouth Operative Conditions Scale. *Anesth Analg.* 2005;100(6):1614–1621.
3. Cravero JP, Askins N, Sriswadi P, et al. Validation of the Pediatric Sedation State Scale. *Pediatrics.* 2017;139(5):e20162897.
4. Ramsay MA, Savege TM, Simpson BR, Goodwin R. Controlled sedation with alphaxalone-alphadolone. *Br Med J.* 1974;2(5920):656–659.
5. Agrawal D, Feldman HA, Krauss B, Waltzman ML. Bispectral index monitoring quantifies depth of sedation during emergency department procedural sedation and analgesia in children. *Ann Emerg Med.* 2004;43(2):247–255.
6. Chernik DA, Gillings D, Laine H, et al. Validity and reliability of the Observer's Assessment of Alertness/Sedation Scale: study with intravenous midazolam. *J Clin Psychopharmacol/* 1990;10(4):244–251.
7. Kim TK, Niklewski PJ, Martin JF, et al. Enhancing a sedation score to include truly noxious stimulation: the Extended Observer's Assessment of Alertness and Sedation (EOAA/S). *Br J Anaesth.* 2015;115(4):569–577.
8. Malviya S, Voepel-Lewis T, Tait AR, et al. Depth of sedation in children undergoing computed tomography: validity and reliability of the University of Michigan Sedation Scale (UMSS). *Br J Anaesth.* 2002;88(2):241–245.
9. Sessler CN, Gosnell MS, Grap MJ, et al. The Richmond Agitation-Sedation Scale: validity and reliability in adult intensive care unit patients. *Am J Respir Crit Care Med.* 2002;166(10):1338–1344.
10. Kerson AG, De Maria R, Mauer E, et al. Validity of the Richmond Agitation-Sedation Scale (RASS) in critically ill children. *J Intensive Care.* 2016;4:65.
11. Malviya S, Voepel-Lewis T, Tait AR. A comparison of observational and objective measures to differentiate depth of sedation in children from birth to 18 years of age. *Anesth Analg.* 2006;102(2):389–394.
12. Gill M, Green SM, Krauss B. A study of the Bispectral Index Monitor during procedural sedation and analgesia in the emergency department. *Ann Emerg Med.* 2003;41(2):234–241.

13. Overly FL, Wright RO, Connor FA Jr., et al. Bispectral analysis during pediatric procedural sedation. *Pediatr Emerg Care.* 2005;21(1):6–11.
14. Davidson AJ, McCann ME, Devavaram P, et al. The differences in the bispectral index between infants and children during emergence from anesthesia after circumcision surgery. *Anesth Analg.* 2001;93(2):326–330.
15. Bannister CF, Brosius KK, Sigl JC, et al. The effect of bispectral index monitoring on anesthetic use and recovery in children anesthetized with sevoflurane in nitrous oxide. *Anesth Analg.* 2001;92(4):877–881.
16. Malviya S, Voepel-Lewis T, Tait AR, et al. Effect of age and sedative agent on the accuracy of bispectral index in detecting depth of sedation in children. *Pediatrics.* 2007;120(3):e461–e470.
17. Mason KP, Michna E, Zurakowski D, et al. Value of bispectral index monitor in differentiating between moderate and deep Ramsay Sedation Scores in children. *Paediatr Anaesth.* 2006;16(12):1226–1231.
18. Dahaba AA. Different conditions that could result in the bispectral index indicating an incorrect hypnotic state. *Anesth Analg.* 2005;101(3):765–773.
19. Dag C, Bezgin T, Ozalp N, Golcuklu Aydin G. Utility of bispectral index monitoring during deep sedation in pediatric dental patients. *J Clin Pediatr Dent.* 2014;39(1):68–73.

8

The Recovery Phase of Sedation

8.1

Monitoring

LORIE REILLY

The recovery phase of sedation can be divided into a timeline that consists of the immediate, early, and late phases. In the immediate phase, the patient begins to awaken and recover protective airway reflexes and begins to move purposefully. This typically starts once the procedure is completed. When the early phase begins, the patient moves closer to baseline and vital signs stabilize. Physiologic and psychological effects of the sedation medications resolve during the late phase. There is no definitive time period that marks completion of the late phase.

Patients are closely monitored during these phases, and providers need to be aware of adverse events that may occur during each phase. For example, in the immediate phase, the patient may not have fully regained airway protective reflexes and may continue to need airway support and monitoring for respiratory depression, hypoxia, airway obstruction, and apnea. In the early phase, as the child begins to awaken and emerge from the effects of the sedatives, agitation and excitation may occur. Patient safety through close observation and monitoring needs to be maintained, as the child may be at risk of thrashing and self-harm. Patients in the late phase of recovery may experience a more prolonged recovery period with delayed wakefulness if they had received longer-acting sedation medications or were sedated closer to their naptime, or later in the day closer to their nightly bedtime. Patients with comorbidities such as obstructive sleep apnea and hypotonia may also experience a prolonged recovery from sedation. The recovery area may provide them with a quiet, nonstimulating environment and therefore promote sleep.

Induction and recovery from sedation are associated with risks. The procedure may be brief, and the half-life of the sedation medications may extend far beyond the length of the procedure. Monitoring and resuscitation equipment of the same high standard should be available in all sedated patient care areas: the induction location (if distinct), the procedural suite, and the recovery area.

Direct observation is critical in monitoring the sedated patient during the recovery phase. In general, the parameters that are monitored in the recovery phase include the following:

- Level of consciousness
- Oxygen saturation
- Heart rate
- Respiratory rate
- Temperature
- Pain score

The monitoring of the pediatric patient during the recovery phase is continuous. Patients should be monitored until they return to their presedation state. The Aldrete score (Table 8.1.1) and the Vancouver Sedative Recovery Scale (Table 8.1.2) are two examples of sedation recovery scales, providing objective measurements of the patient's recovery status and readiness to be transferred or discharged from the sedation recovery area.

TABLE 8.1.1 The aldrete score

Activity	Able to move all extremities voluntarily or on command	2
	Able to move 2 extremities voluntarily or on command	1
	Unable to move extremities voluntarily or on command	0
Respiration	Able to breathe deeply and cough freely	2
	Dyspnea or limited breathing	1
	Apneic	0
Circulation	BP ± 20% of preanesthetic level	2
	BP ± 20–49% of preanesthetic level	1
	BP ± 50% of preanesthetic level	0
Consciousness	Fully awake	2
	Arousable on calling	1
	Not responding	0
Oxygen Saturation	Able to maintain O_2 saturation >92% on room air	2
	Needs O_2 inhalation to maintain O_2 saturation >90%	1
	O_2 saturation <90% even with O_2 supplement	0
Total		

Maximum score 22 (fully awake); minimum score 0 (unable to arouse)

Reprinted with permission from JA Aldrete. The post-anesthesia recovery score revisited. Table 1. *Journal of Clinical Anesthesia*, 1995,7, 89–91. Published by Elsevier.

TABLE 8.1.2 The vancouver sedative recovery scale

Response	A	(i)	Awake/alert	4
		(ii)	Awake/drowsy	3
		(iii)	Asleep/easily aroused	2
		(iv)	Asleep/difficult to arouse	1
If child scores 0 on above, do not proceed		(v)	Asleep/unable to arouse	0
	B	(i)	Responds fully to stimuli in an age-appropriate manner	2
		(ii)	Delayed response to stimuli	1
		(iii)	Absent response to stimuli	0
	C	(i)	Alert facial expression	1
		(ii)	Flat facial expression	0
Eyes	D	(i)	Bright eyes	1
		(ii)	Dull eyes; glazed	0
	E	(i)	Looks "at you"	1
		(ii)	Looks "through" you	0
	F	(i)	Accommodates	1
		(ii)	Does not accommodate	0
	G	(i)	Recognition of stimulus	1
		(ii)	Limited or no recognition of stimulus	0
	H	(i)	Purposeful and spontaneous eye movement	1
		(ii)	Little or no spontaneous or purposeful eye movement	0

(Continued)

TABLE 8.1.2 Continued

Movement	I	(i)	Spontaneous and varied central activity	4
		(ii)	Spontaneous and varied peripheral activity	3
		(iii)	Central activity in response to activity	2
		(iv)	Peripheral activity in response to stimuli	1
		(v)	No movement	0
	J	(i)	Absence of tremor or ataxia	2
		(ii)	Minor ataxia or tremor	1
		(iii)	Major ataxia or tremor	0
	K	(i)	Coordinated spontaneous movement	2
		(ii)	Weak/coarse spontaneous movement	1
		(iii)	No purposeful spontaneous movement	0
	L	(i)	Shows age-appropriate manual dexterity	2
		(ii)	Awkward or clumsy hand movement	1
		(iii)	No fine hand movement	0

Reprinted with permission from J Macnab et al. The Vancouver Sedative Recovery Scale for children: validation and reliability of scoring based on videotaped instruction. *Canadian Journal of Anaesthesia*, 1994, 41:10. 913–918. Published by Springer.

Suggested Reading

Aldrete JA. The post-anesthesia recovery score revisited. *J Clin Anesth.* 1995;7:89–91.

Coté CJ, Wilson S, American Academy of Pediatrics, American Academy of Pediatric Dentistry. Guidelines for monitoring and management of pediatric patients before, during and after sedation for diagnostic and therapeutic procedures: update 2016. *Pediatrics.* 2016;138(1):e20161212.

Horeczko T, Mahmoud MA. The sedation mindset: philosophy, science and practice. *Curr Opin Anaesth.* 2016;29:s48–s55.

Macnab AJ, Levine M, Glick N, et al. The Vancouver Sedative Recovery Scale for children: validation and reliability of scoring based on videotaped instruction. *Can J Anaesth.* 1994;41(10):913–918.

8.2

Discharge Considerations

MICHELLE M. RHOADS AND TRACY CAMPBELL

The increase in therapeutic and diagnostic procedures being done outside of the operating room has been a driving force in the need for development of formalized sedation services including the need for more defined criteria for discharge. Having defined criteria for discharge minimizes the incidence of adverse events, poor patient outcomes, and decreased patient and family satisfaction. A successful discharge with positive patient outcomes is also affected by the use of a validated scoring system, team collaboration, effective communication, and use of evidence-based policies and procedures. A prolonged recovery resulting from pain, postoperative nausea and vomiting (PONV), drowsiness, or intolerance of the procedure can lead to poor patient outcomes. Using criteria to anticipate the needs of the patient and providing an individualized plan of care will reduce the risk of adverse events and poor patient outcomes. The resulting safe, high-quality, timely patient care ultimately increases the patient/family experience and satisfaction rate.

Based on the most current validated discharge scoring systems, a patient who regains baseline motor control, baseline vital signs, and adequate pain management meets criteria for discharge.[1] A scoring system is an objective measure of the patient's progress toward discharge. Three commonly used, validated discharge scoring systems are the Modified Aldrete Score, the Post-Anesthesia Recovery Score (PARS), and the Post-Anesthesia Discharge Scoring System (PADSS).

Broad acceptance of a postanesthesia discharge scoring system among nurses and physicians promotes consistent communication as to the patient's condition and readiness for discharge. In addition to fulfilling the criteria of the validated scoring system, the dischargeable patient must also display the following[2]:

1. Return to presedation baseline level of consciousness
2. Regained verbal capacity (if appropriate)
3. The capacity to sit up (if appropriate)
4. Wakefulness for 20 minutes when unstimulated
5. Stable and adequate vital signs
6. Adequate hydration status
7. Adequate pain relief.

Adequate hydration status of a patient does not necessarily require oral intake (depending on the organization's policy) in order for the patient to be discharged. The family should be educated on whom to contact or where to go should the child exhibit signs and symptoms of dehydration.

The child's inability to remain awake and maintain head control for the trip home may result in positional airway obstruction.[2] The family must be made aware of this risk.

Once the child meets all of the discharge criteria, the sedation provider needs to evaluate and clear the patient for discharge. Any variance or delay in discharge should be communicated with the sedation provider to address any further interventions.

In addition to the clinical presentation of the patient's readiness for discharge, postprocedural considerations should include PONV, pain management, and education/discharge instructions.

Postoperative Nausea and Vomiting

A common postsedation side effect that may delay discharge is PONV. The current literature suggests that the earlier practice of forcing oral fluid intake before discharge has widely changed. Sedation personnel should be familiar with risk factors, etiology, assessment, and treatment modalities to prevent and treat PONV. Common risk factors associated with PONV include the following[4,5]:

- History of PONV
- Motion sickness
- Use of periprocedural opioids
- Type and duration of procedure
- Type and duration of sedation medications
- Age (in children >3 years old)
- Female gender

Prehydration for at-risk patients can decrease the incidence of PONV, especially for cases scheduled later in the day. A multimodal approach using hydration and pharmacologic and nonpharmacologic modalities should be considered for those at high risk for PONV. Other factors that can precipitate PONV include pain, motion, visual and auditory stimulation, and hypotension. Nurses should evaluate and treat any contributing factors by using antiemetic medications and nonpharmacologic modalities such as deep breathing, distraction, and a cool washcloth to the forehead. Clear and concise clinical practice guidelines regarding presedation treatment of patients at risk for PONV should be defined and readily available to staff.

Pain Management

Adequate pain management is crucial to a timely discharge. Factors contributing to postprocedural pain may include both procedural pain and anticipated pain. Early detection and treatment are key components to efficient and effective management of the needs of the patient and family. A proactive multimodal approach that includes pharmacologic and nonpharmacologic methods should be used in evaluating and managing procedural pain. An age-appropriate assessment and treatment of pain should begin during the procedure and continue through the recovery phase. Engagement with the family fosters individualization of the patient's pain care strategy. The home-care pain management needs of the patient should be identified and communicated with the family prior to the procedure and reinforced prior to discharge. Inability to identify and address postprocedural pain may result in prolonged recovery, an increased rate of readmission, decreased patient/family satisfaction, and an overall poor procedural outcome that potentially leads to long-term negative effects.[3]

Education/Discharge Instructions

Patient and family education is a continuum that should begin at the first contact with the family and conclude in the recovery phase.[4,5] While all discharge instructions are reviewed verbally during the recovery phase, written discharge instructions should be provided for the patient and family to refer to at home. Patients and families who are educated throughout the process are better prepared for discharge to home and can form more realistic expectations to alleviate unnecessary stress and anxiety.[4] Parental understanding should be verbalized and validated with a signature, including the date and time. Patients and families should be educated on when/how to call the sedation provider. Instructions should also include postprocedure education and expectations, management of PONV, signs and symptoms of dehydration, and signs and symptoms of excess drowsiness. For emergencies, including the inability to arouse the child, difficulty breathing, or any other life-threatening concerns, the family should be instructed to call 911.

Conclusion

Discharge planning begins during the initial contact with the patient and family and continues throughout the sedation process.[5] It is most effective when a collaborative, family-centered approach is used that includes communication between all disciplines and the family. Development of structured guidelines, use of evidence-based practice, and discharge scoring systems will ensure a standardized approach to patient discharge, minimize unnecessary variability, improve outcomes, and prepare the patient/family for a smooth, uneventful discharge to home.

Suggested Reading

Ead H. From Aldrete to PADSS: reviewing discharge criteria after ambulatory surgery. *J Perianesth Nurs.* 2006;21(4):259–267.

Perianesthesia Nursing Standards Practice Recommendations and Interpretive Statements. Cherry Hill, NJ: American Society of Perianesthesia Nurses, 2017.

Sessler C, Grap M, Brophy G. Multidisciplinary management of sedation and analgesia in critical care. *Semin Respir Crit Care Med.* 2001;22(2):211–226.

References

1. Practice Recommendation 2. In: *Perianesthesia Nursing Standards Practice Recommendations and Interpretive Statements.* Cherry Hill, NJ: American Society of Perianesthesia Nurses, 2017:38–45.
2. Guideline for managing the patient receiving moderate sedation/analgesia. In: *Guidelines for Perioperative Practices.* Denver, CO: Association of Perioperative Registered Nurses, 2015:553–561.
3. Maurice E. Timely patient discharge from the ambulatory setting. *AORN.* 2015;102(2):185–191.

4. Clinical Practice Guideline 3. In: *Perianesthesia Nursing Standards and Practice Recommendations.* Cherry Hill, NJ: American Society of Perianesthesia Nurses, 2010:47–66.
5. Position Statement 7. In: *Perianesthesia Nursing Standards Practice Recommendations and Interpretive Statements.* Cherry Hill, NJ: American Society of Perianesthesia Nurses, 2017:109–110.

8.3

Follow-up

LORIE REILLY

Follow-up is an important part of the pediatric sedation process. Follow-up may be performed in several different ways, such as a telephone call, direct contact with the patient and family, a mailed questionnaire, or an in-person visit (e.g., inpatient). Adverse events that occur after the postsedation discharge and are reported during the follow-up process should be documented in the medical record, because this is important and useful information for future sedation encounters. During follow-up some of the topics for discussion with the parent may include any change in the child's activity level, appetite, sleep pattern, or behavior.

Periodic review of issues identified in the presedation/triage process, sedation, and recovery phases should be included as part of the follow-up process and may be considered for discussion during multidisciplinary conference. The follow-up should also have a mechanism in place to evaluate patient/family satisfaction. Recommendations for future sedation encounters based on information obtained in the follow-up should be noted in the medical record.

Suggested Reading

Coté CJ, Wilson S, American Academy of Pediatrics, American Academy of Pediatric Dentistry. Guidelines for monitoring and management of

pediatric patients before, during and after sedation for diagnostic and therapeutic procedures: update 2016. *Pediatrics.* 2016;138(1):e20161212.
Horeczko T, Mahmoud MA. The sedation mindset: philosophy, science and practice. *Curr Opin Anaesthesiol.* 2016;1:S48–S55.
Newman DH, Azer M, Pitetti RD, Singh S. When is a patient safe for discharge after procedural sedation? The timing of adverse effect events in 1367 pediatric procedural sedations. *Ann Emerg Med.* 2003;42:627–635.

9

Adverse Events of Sedation

9.1

Definition and Incidence of Adverse Events

DAVID FAGIN

To perform effective and safe procedural sedation, one must be knowledgeable about the adverse events that can occur with the administration of various sedatives and analgesics. Actually, labeling many of these sedation-related events as "adverse" may be misleading by implying that they are unexpected and are likely to result in harm. On the contrary, although adverse events are statistically infrequent, sedationists, if aware of the risk and trained and prepared to intervene with appropriate support, can prevent an event from having a lasting impact on the patient outcome.

There has been a great deal of discussion and a lack of consistency in the medical and nursing literature about the definition of adverse sedation events. Hypoxemia (itself ill defined—duration? depth?), noted with monitoring, may have been caused by an obstructed airway. It is often easily relieved with the administration of oxygen and repositioning of the patient to open the airway. Is the adverse event the hypoxemia or the airway obstruction? It is more important to understand the risk factors associated with the medications used, the procedure being performed, and the particular patient factors involved so the sedationist may prevent the airway obstruction or at the very least be prepared to rescue the patient from the hypoxemia. In a collaborative effort between emergency physicians and anesthesiologists, Bhatt et al.[1] chose to include in the definition of adverse sedation events any interventions taken during an event so as to better define it.

Indeed, serious adverse events causing long-term patient harm do occur. In 2000, Coté et al.[2] reviewed 95 adverse events from several national databases. Sixty of these occurrences resulted in death or permanent neurologic injury. The events were associated with various routes of drug administration and included various classes of drugs. In addition, these events were associated with inadequate patient monitoring and resuscitation. Although the events occurred more frequently in non–hospital-based facilities, some of them did occur in the hospital. This and other reports have led the American Academy of Pediatrics and other national organizations to develop guidelines for caring for patients requiring procedural sedation[3] with the intent of informing sedationists of the risks involved in sedation care and the skills and equipment needed to ameliorate or prevent patient harm.

In an effort to collect more comprehensive data regarding sedation adverse events, the Pediatric Sedation Research Consortium (PSRC) was established in 2003. The consortium initially consisted of 35 fairly uniformly high-performing, organized institutions sharing data on sedation encounters. Initial results from over 30,000 sedation encounters were published in 2006.[4] This represented a large enough population of sedated patients to begin to statistically support statements about the safety of certain systems of sedation care (Table 9.1.1). Initial data revealed that major adverse events are rare in procedural sedation. The data also showed that moderate respiratory events such as stridor, laryngospasm, wheezing, or apnea were not as infrequent: 1 in 400 sedation encounters was associated with stridor, laryngospasm, wheezing, or apnea. Further PSRC data have been published with well over 100,000 encounters.[5,6] The results of these studies showed a somewhat increased need for airway interventions when looking at over 50,000 propofol sedations but have also revealed similar safety results among different specialty-trained providers (e.g., emergency medicine, intensive care, anesthesiology). These and other studies have helped support the creation of sedation services in many pediatric institutions with dedicated staff whose goal is to provide safe and effective pediatric procedural sedation.

TABLE 9.1.1 Complications

	Incidence per 10,000	*n*	*95%CI*
Adverse events			
Death	0.0	0	0.0–0.0
Cardiac Arrest	0.3	1	0.0–1.9
Aspiration	0.3	1	0.0–1.9
Hypothermia	1.3	4	0.4–3.4
Seizure (unanticipated) during sedation	2.7	8	1.1–5.2
Stridor	4.3	11	1.8–6.6
Laryngospasm	4.3	13	2.3–7.4
Wheeze (new onset during sedation)	4.7	14	2.5–7.8
Allergic reaction (rash)	5.7	17	3.3–9.1
Intravenous-related problems/complication	11.0	33	7.6–15.4
Prolonged sedation	13.6	41	9.8–18.5
Prolonged recovery	22.3	67	17.3–28.3
Apnea (unexpected)	24.3	73	19.1–30.5
Secretions (requiring suction)	41.6	125	34.7–49.6
Vomiting during procedure (nongastrointestinal)	47.2	142	39.8–557
Desaturation below 90%	156.5	470	142.7–171.2
Total adverse events	339.6 (1 per 29)	1020	308.1–371.5
Unplanned treatments			
Reversal agent required (unanticipated)	1.7	5	0.6–3.9

TABLE 9.1.1 Continued

	Incidence per 10,000	*n*	*95%CI*
Emergency anesthesia consult for airway	2.0	6	0.7–4.3
Admission to hospital (unanticipated; sedation related)	7.0	21	4.3–10.7
Intubation required (unanticipated)	9.7	29	6.5–13.9
Airway (oral; unexpected requirement)	27.6	83	22.0–34.2
Bag-mask ventilation (unanticipated)	63.9	192	55.2–73.6
Total unplanned treatments	111.9 (1 per 89)	336	85.3–130.2
Conditions present during procedure			
Inadequate sedation, could not complete	88.9 (1 per 338)	267	78.6–100.2

Reprinted from: Cravero J, Blike G, Beach M, et al. Incidence and nature of adverse events during pediatric sedation/anesthesia for procedures outside the operating room: report from the Pediatric Sedation Research Consortium. Pediatrics. 2006;118(3):1094.

The following sections of this chapter will further classify adverse events as follows:

Minor events, such as postsedation vomiting and prolonged recovery times, are preventable with preparation and are unlikely to cause more than patient inconvenience or discomfort.

Moderate events, such as airway obstruction and laryngospasm, may lead to more significant risk to the patient (prolonged hypoxemia), particularly if the sedationist is not prepared to respond and limit their impact.

Major events are those that have a significant impact on the patient due to lack of recognition of minor or moderate events, failure to rescue, or failure to recognize a particular patient factor that places him or her particularly at risk (e.g., pulmonary hypertension). Major events include cardiovascular collapse, true respiratory failure, and significant aspiration.

References

1. Bhatt M, Kennedy RM, Osmond MH, et al. Consensus-based recommendations for standardizing terminology and reporting adverse events for emergency department procedural sedation and analgesia in children. *Ann Emerg Med.* 2009;53:426–435.
2. Coté CJ, Notterman DA, Karl HW, et al. Adverse sedation events in pediatrics: a critical incident analysis of contributing factors. *Pediatrics.* 2000;105:805–814.
3. Coté CJ, Wilson S, American Academy of Pediatrics, American Academy of Pediatric Dentistry. Guidelines for monitoring and management of pediatric patients before, during and after sedation for diagnostic and therapeutic procedures: update 2016. *Pediatrics.* 2016;138(1):e20161212.
4. Cravero JP, Blike GT, Beach M, et al. Incidence and nature of adverse events during pediatric sedation/anesthesia for procedures outside the operating room: report from the Pediatric Sedation Research Consortium. *Pediatrics.* 2006;118:1087–1096.
5. Cravero JP, Beach MI, Blike GT, et al. The incidence and nature of adverse events during pediatric sedations/anesthesia with propofol for procedures outside the operating room: a report from the Pediatric Sedation Research Consortium. *Anesth Analg,* 2009;108:795–804.
6. Coulores KG, Beach M, Cravero JP, et al. Impact of provider specialty on pediatric procedural sedation complication rates. *Pediatrics.* 2011;127(5):e1154–e1160.

9.2

Minor Adverse Events

CORRIE E. CHUMPITAZI

The incidence of sedation-related adverse events depends on (1) the types of medications used; (2) the type, duration, invasiveness, and location of the procedure; and (3) patient factors (e.g., age, medical condition, psychological factors). For the purposes of this chapter, we will define "minor adverse sedation-related events" as those that may present inconvenience or transient discomfort to the patient and that, if recognized and supported in a timely manner by the sedationist, will not usually result in physiologic or psychological harm to the patient. Large safety studies of pediatric sedation events from the Pediatric Sedation Research Consortium suggest that events of this type occur in 1 of every 200 sedation episodes; these data offer significant impetus for effective preparation and training for sedationists to effectively respond to or preempt minor adverse events,[1] because some of these "minor" events can progress to more significant harm.

Nausea

Nausea is a relatively common side effect in sedation and anesthesia. Postsedation nausea is particularly associated with the use of opioids for analgesia, and the incidence is increased in patients receiving ketamine. Patients undergoing procedures involving manipulation of the gastrointestinal tract are also prone to nausea.

Vomiting

Postprocedural vomiting, like nausea, is associated with the use of opioids, with the use of ketamine (perhaps dose-dependent and more likely to occur in children >12 years old), and in procedures involving gastrointestinal tract manipulation. Vomiting may be mitigated by preprocedure administration of ondansetron. Nitrous oxide is also associated with a dose- and duration-related incidence of postprocedure vomiting. Postprocedure vomiting when the patient is able to protect his or her airway is a minor adverse event, but emesis while moderately or deeply sedated places the patient at risk for aspiration leading to respiratory distress or failure. Aspiration is a major adverse event mostly associated with endoscopy but also occurs in patients with gastrointestinal pathology and gastric emptying abnormalities. Avoiding the use of medications associated with an increased incidence of postprocedure vomiting in patients with gastrointestinal tract involvement may reduce the chance of intraprocedure vomiting.

Oxygen Desaturation and Hypoxemia

Hypoxemia or oxygen desaturation in the normal individual is generally defined as a $pO_2 < 60$ mm Hg or an $O_2Hb < 90\%$ when breathing room air. When hypoxemia begins to manifest adverse effects depends on the patient's intrinsic ability to increase oxygen delivery and the length of time the patient is hypoxemic. Many studies of sedation and anesthesia safety report hypoxemia (usually monitored by pulse oximetry) lasting >30 seconds as an "adverse event." As most providers would not allow saturations to decline without intervening, a more prudent way to evaluate this adverse event would be to examine the intervention needed to reverse the issue. Hypoxemia in procedural sedation is usually the result of partial airway obstruction or medication-induced central hypoventilation or apnea. Thus, hypoxemia generally responds to interventions such as the following:

- Stimulation: auditory and/or tactile
- Airway repositioning (e.g., chin lift, jaw thrust, neck extension, midline repositioning)
- Suctioning
- Supplemental or increased oxygen delivery
- Oral or nasal airway placement
- Application of positive pressure with bag-mask ventilation

Bradycardia and Hypotension

Sedative and analgesic agents can depress the central and peripheral autonomic nervous system, blunt the compensatory baroreceptor reflexes, depress the myocardium, and decrease both preload and afterload. Hypotension is generally considered significant when the systolic pressure is 30% less than baseline. Infant cardiac output is quite rate-dependent, but older children with healthy cardiovascular systems are relatively resilient and rarely require more than adjustment of drug dosing or isotonic fluid bolus in response to hypotension. Dexmedetomidine, an α_2-adrenoceptor agonist, is particularly associated with bradycardia, but slow intravenous administration of the bolus is usually effective in reducing the magnitude of bradycardia.

Hypersensitivity (Allergic) Reaction

Development of a rash may occur idiosyncratically with medications such as ketamine and opioids, but severe anaphylactic reactions are rare. In the case of an anaphylactic reaction, stop the medication and provide standard management with rapid attention to airway, breathing, and circulation.

Agitation/Delirium/Abnormal Movements

Children often emerge the way they are induced, so every effort to provide a calm induction can help produce a smooth recovery. Recovery agitation has been reported with many medications, including nitrous oxide, benzodiazepines, ketamine, propofol, and pentobarbital. "Propofol frenzy" has been described as transient but repetitive violent motor activity and impaired consciousness with clinical manifestations that looks similar to seizure activity. The incidence of recovery agitation is higher in patients with neuropsychiatric disorders. If patients are not responsive to calming measures such as turning down the lights and decreasing stimulation, benzodiazepines may be helpful. Flumazenil will reverse agitation associated with benzodiazepines. Myoclonus, muscle rigidity, and generalized motor seizure have been reported with procedural sedation. These side effects should be considered adverse events if they interrupt, prolong, or require additional medication administration to complete the procedure. Expected side effects, such as lateral nystagmus with ketamine, should be fully explained to the family, especially if they will be present during the procedure.

Prolonged Recovery

Prolonged recovery time not only affects patient and parent satisfaction but can also contribute to overall decreased efficiency and quality of sedation care. Every effort should be made to match the sedative medication duration to the anticipated procedure time. Large doses given enterally may prolong sedation and recovery time. Dexmedetomidine is associated particularly with prolonged recovery.

Suggested Reading

Langston WT, Wathen JE, Roback MG, Bajaj L. Effect of ondansetron on the incidence of vomiting associated with ketamine sedation in children: a double-blind, randomized, placebo-controlled trial. *Ann Emerg Med.* 2008;52(1):30–34.

Roback MG, Wathen JE, Bajaj L, et al. Adverse events associated with procedural sedation and analgesia in a pediatric emergency department: a comparison of common parenteral drugs. *Acad Emerg Med.* 2005;12:508–513.

Roback MG, Wathen JE, MacKenzie T, Bajaj L. A randomized, controlled trial of IV versus IM ketamine for sedation of pediatric patients receiving emergency department orthopedic procedures. *Ann Emerg Med.* 2006;48(5):605–612.

Sacchetti A, Stander E, Ferguson N, et al. Pediatric procedural sedation in the community emergency department: results from the ProSCED registry. *Pediatr Emerg Care.* 2007;23:218–222.

Reference

1. Cravero JP, Blike GT, Beach M, et al. Incidence and nature of adverse events during pediatric sedation/anesthesia for procedures outside the operating room: report from the Pediatric Sedation Research Consortium. *Pediatrics.* 2006;118:1087–1096.

9.3

Moderate Adverse Events

CORRIE E. CHUMPITAZI

The incidence of sedation-related adverse events depends on (1) the medications used; (2) the type, duration, invasiveness, and location of the procedure; and (3) patient factors (e.g., age, medical condition, psychological factors). For the purposes of this chapter, moderate adverse sedation-related events represent physiologic change that is extremely likely to lead to significant patient harm if unnoticed or responded to ineffectively by the sedationist. Large safety studies of pediatric sedation events from the Pediatric Sedation Research Consortium suggest that events of this type occur in approximately 1 of every 400 sedation episodes, providing significant impetus for effective preparation and training for sedationists to effectively respond to or preempt these events.[1] Even though they are categorized as "moderate" and may not be associated with harm in and of themselves, these events may certainly progress to produce significant harm.

Respiratory Events

Moderate adverse sedation events are overwhelmingly associated with control of breathing and maintenance of an open airway. Central apnea, bradypnea, inability to clear secretions, partial airway obstruction by loss of airway tone, and more complete obstruction represented by laryngospasm may occur during induction, moderate or deep sedation states, and emergence.

Apnea

Apnea is a cessation or pause in effective respiratory effort. Central apnea occurs when the sedation causes abnormal neural and chemical receptor responses in the respiratory center of the brain to rising carbon dioxide levels or dropping oxygen levels. Obstructive apnea occurs when inspiratory efforts persist yet are ineffective due to the presence of complete or partial upper airway obstruction. Infants, especially premature ones, are particularly susceptible to frank central apnea during and after sedative or opioid administration.

Airway Obstruction

Airway obstruction is a frequent cause of hypoxemia and hypercarbia in children undergoing sedation due to a variety of factors intrinsic to a child's airway. Symptoms of early obstruction are snoring, coughing to clear secretions, tracheal tugging, increased effort without breath sounds, stridor, and rising or falling end-tidal carbon dioxide levels or abrupt change in the waveform. Anatomic factors in children promoting airway obstruction during sedation include the following:

- Large posterior occiput that results in flexion of the neck
- Large tongue
- Decreased muscle tone of the pharynx and larynx, which promotes partial obstruction
- Relatively small airway diameter: partial obstruction creates a significant decrement in air flow.

Please see Chapter 4 for a more complete discussion of the child's airway anatomy and the effect of sedatives on its function.

Laryngospasm

Laryngospasm is defined as partial or complete upper airway obstruction caused by involuntary and sustained closure of the glottis. Positive-pressure ventilation is sometimes ineffective in bypassing the obstruction, so this is one of the most serious of the reversible adverse effects associated with sedation. Laryngospasm is most frequently seen during induction and emergence, so airway manipulation when the patient is lightly sedated must be carefully monitored. A characteristic stridulous noise can be heard with partial laryngospasm but is absent with complete laryngospasm. Laryngospasm has not been shown in meta-analysis to be associated with any specific clinical factors, except a slightly greater risk with unusually high intravenous doses of ketamine. While laryngospasm may be triggered by excessive secretions stimulating an irritable glottis in which normal reflexes may be blunted with sedation, studies have not supported the use of anticholinergic medications as an effective prevention modality, as seen with upper respiratory infections or gastroesophageal reflux.

Unanticipated Consults or Change in Level of Care

When a moderate or severe adverse event related to procedural sedation occurs, even when the rescue response is effective, it may be necessary to change the planned processes of care to include the following:

- Cancellation of the procedure
- Emergent consult with an anesthesiologist
- Hospital admission
- Transfer to a pediatric intensive care unit.

Suggested Reading

Beach ML, Cohen DM, Gallagher SM, Cravero JP. Major adverse events and relationship to nil per os status in pediatric sedation/anesthesia outside the operating room: a report of the Pediatric Sedation Research Consortium. *Anesthesiology*. 2016;124(1):80–88.

Bellolio MF, Puls HA, Anderson JL, et al. Incidence of adverse events in paediatric procedural sedation in the emergency department: a systematic review and meta-analysis. *BMJ Open*. 2016;6(6):e011384.

Grunwell JR, Travers C, McCracken CE, et al. Procedural sedation outside of the operating room using ketamine in 22,645 children: a report from the Pediatric Sedation Research Consortium. *Pediatr Crit Care Med*. 2016;17:1109–1116.

Mallory MD, Travers C, McCracken CE, et al. Upper respiratory infections and airway adverse events in pediatric procedural sedation. *Pediatrics*. 2017;140(1):e20170009.

Srinivasan M, Turmelle M, Depalma LM, et al. Procedural sedation for diagnostic imaging in children by pediatric hospitalists using propofol: analysis of the nature, frequency, and predictors of adverse events and interventions. *J Pediatr*. 2012;160(5):801–806.

Reference

1. Cravero JP, Blike GT, Beach M, et al. Incidence and nature of adverse events during pediatric sedation/anesthesia for procedures outside the operating room: report from the Pediatric Sedation Research Consortium. *Pediatrics*. 2006;118:1087–1096.

9.4

Major Adverse Events

CORRIE E. CHUMPITAZI

The incidence of sedation-related adverse events depends on (1) the medications used; (2) the type, duration, invasiveness, and location of procedure; and (3) patient factors (e.g., age, medical condition, psychological factors). For the purposes of this chapter, major adverse sedation-related events represent extreme physiologic change causing significant patient harm that may be long-lasting or permanent, particularly if responded to ineffectively by the sedationist. Large safety studies of pediatric sedation events from the Pediatric Sedation Research Consortium (PSRC) suggest that events of this type occur very rarely when well-organized, equipped, and trained sedation teams are present.[1] However, sporadic reports of death during pediatric sedation continue to surface, providing significant impetus for effective preparation and training for sedationists so that they can recognize, before sedation, patients whose particular medical conditions place them at risk and can develop effective rescue systems.

Major adverse sedation-related events include aspiration, cardiovascular collapse, respiratory failure, and death.

Aspiration

Aspiration, in the context of sedation care, is defined as an episode where gastric contents or oral secretions are found in the subglottic airway. Signs and symptoms of aspiration include cough, wheeze, increase in respiratory effort, hypoxemia/hypercarbia, reflux or vomiting, and laryngospasm. The aspiration rate associated with procedural sedation has been reported by the PSRC as 0.3 per 10,000 sedations.[1] The PSRC is a group of well-organized, high-functioning pediatric sedation centers, so the risk for aspiration may be higher in less well-regulated sedation situations. Principal risk factors include (1) planned airway manipulation (e.g., intubation or extubation); (2) absence of airway protective reflexes; (3) American Society of Anesthesiologists (ASA) class III or higher; and (4) procedures in or near the airway (e.g., bronchoscopy, endoscopy).

Respiratory Arrest

As noted previously, airway adverse events are common during procedural sedation. When adequate airway protection is not possible such that the patient experiences a respiratory arrest, effective bag-valve-mask ventilation should be performed until a secure airway can safely be obtained. This is most often achieved with an endotracheal tube.

Cardiac Arrest

It is not uncommon to observe hemodynamic perturbations during procedural sedation. Generally, the clinical manifestations are hypotension or bradycardia (see Chapter 9.2). Particularly at risk for hemodynamic disturbance are children with (1) acute illness with fever and dehydration or compensated shock states; (2) congenital heart disease; or (3) preexisting arrhythmia. Nonetheless, it is highly unusual that such changes will result in cardiac arrest, particularly if the sedationist has been careful to use appropriate medications and intravascular fluid support. The more likely scenario in which cardiac arrest occurs is with unrecognized respiratory distress or with ineffectively supported airway obstruction that has progressed to cardiopulmonary arrest. A major adverse event should be documented whenever chest compressions are used or vasoactive medications are administered.

Death

Death related to anesthesia is well studied and documented. Safety practices and the advent of pulse oximetry and end-tidal carbon monoxide monitoring in the operating room have resulted in a dramatic decrease in the number of deaths attributed to general anesthesia in the general population.[1] Since the papers in 2000 by Dr. Coté describing events associated with pediatric sedation deaths, procedural sedation care, particularly in the hospital setting, has become more organized and scrutinized for safety.[2,3] Continued sporadic reports of deaths associated with pediatric sedation, particularly in the outpatient setting, highlight the need for further work to achieve similar confidence in sedation-related care as in the operating room.

Suggested Reading

Green SM, Mason KP, Krauss BS. Pulmonary aspiration during procedural sedation: a comprehensive systematic review. *Br J Anaesth.* 2017;118(3):344–354.

Green SM, Roback MG, Krauss B, et al. Predictors of emesis and recovery agitation with emergency department ketamine sedation: an individual-patient data meta-analysis of 8,282 children. *Ann Emerg Med.* 2009;54:171–180.

Lee H, Milgrom P, Huebner CE, et al. Ethics rounds: death after pediatric dental anesthesia: an avoidable tragedy? *Pediatrics.* 2017;140(6):e20172370.

Woodward ZG, Urman RD, Domino KB. Safety of non-operating room anesthesia: a closed claims update. *Anesthesiol Clin.* 2017;35(4):569–581.

References

1. Cravero JP, Blike GT, Beach M, et al. Incidence and nature of adverse events during pediatric sedation/anesthesia for procedures outside the operating room: report from the Pediatric Sedation Research Consortium. *Pediatrics.* 2006:118:1087–1096.
2. Li G, Warner M, Lang BH, et al. Epidemiology of anesthesia-related mortality in the United States, 1999–2005. *Anesthesiology.* 2009;110(4):759–765.
3. Coté CJ, Notterman DA, Karl HW, et al. Adverse sedation events in pediatrics: a critical incident analysis of contributing factors. *Pediatrics.* 2000;106(4):633–644.

9.5

Risks of Sedation

PETER A. CHIN AND SARA WALLS

A discussion of risks, benefits, and alternatives is an integral part of informed consent for any procedure, including sedation. Many of the risks have been discussed earlier in this chapter and include nausea, vomiting, inadequate sedation, airway obstruction, apnea, and cardiovascular events leading to escalation of care. This section will discuss risks, the sedation consent process, and which risks should be disclosed and will provide a brief review of what is currently known about the neurotoxicity of anesthetic and sedative agents. The latter will include guidance on what to discuss with parents.

Discussion

The aim of sedation is to provide patient comfort, analgesia, and amnesia during stressful procedures while maintaining patient safety. Analgesia may not be required for nonpainful procedures such as magnetic resonance imaging, and complete amnesia may not be needed depending on the procedure and the developmental level of the child. Distraction techniques and age-appropriate preparation can be useful adjuncts to minimize medications required. Assessment of the child's developmental level and emotional maturity and knowledge of the level of immobility required and degree of pain caused by the intended procedure are integral to developing a comprehensive sedation plan.

The sedation plan should be discussed with parents during the consent process. It is not possible to list every single possible complication, but "material" risks should be disclosed.[1] Material risks include both minor but frequent events such as nausea, and rare but severe complications such as cardiac arrest. It has been strongly recommended that written consent should be documented in an anesthesia (or sedation)-specific consent form.[2]

Limits of sedation should also be discussed. Sedation is not a general anesthetic and recall is more possible. Inability to complete the planned procedure due to inadequate sedation is also a possibility and should be disclosed. This can be minimized by careful patient screening.

Some minor but common complications include nausea, vomiting, and prolonged sedation. There is no universally accepted definition of prolonged sedation, but the Pediatric Sedation Research Consortium has used greater than 3 times the "expected" duration.[3]

More severe but rare complications can include aspiration, respiratory obstruction, or arrest with the need for advanced airway placement and escalation of care. Cardiovascular risks include hypotension, bradycardia, arrhythmias and cardiac arrest.

There has been increasing public awareness of anesthetic- and sedative-related neurodegeneration, and this is becoming a question that is frequently asked by parents. The first animal studies were published in 1999 and the 2000s and showed histologic changes of neurodegeneration when immature animals were exposed to various anesthetic agents during the brain growth spurt but not later in life.[4–6]

The initial studies were done in rodents but have been replicated in neonatal monkeys.[7,8] The period of maximal brain growth or rapid synaptogenesis varies in each animal species but is thought to range from the second trimester up to ~2–4 years of age in humans.[9,10] Evidence thus far suggests that both the age at exposure and the dose-duration of exposure are important.

Animal studies have suggested the following:

Ketamine—associated with neuroapoptosis due to *N*-methyl-D-aspartate (NMDA) receptor antagonism, possibly in a dose-dependent fashion[10,11]

Propofol—less studied than volatile agents or ketamine but still shown to have negative effects[12]

Volatile agents—Isoflurane, sevoflurane, and desflurane have been shown to cause apoptosis.[12,13]

Nitrous oxide—similar to ketamine due to shared mechanism of action (NMDA antagonism)[14]

Dexmedetomidine—shown in multiple studies to have a neuroprotective effect in clinical doses,[15,16] but may cause neurodegeneration of its own in very high doses[17]

Opioids—notable absence of animal studies looking at the effects of just opioids. One study suggested that there was no effect of fentanyl compared with a combination of isoflurane, nitrous oxide, and midazolam.[18]

Benzodiazepines—shown to cause apoptosis independently; effect is likely dose-dependent.[19]

Noxious stimulation—conflicting results; may protect against or worsen neuroapoptosis.[20,21]

Questions have been raised about the applicability of these animal studies to humans as well as the high doses and prolonged duration of drugs used and the lack of physiologic monitoring in the initial studies. This led to several retrospective studies looking at a possible correlation between early anesthesia exposure and subsequent neurodevelopmental outcome against matched controls in existing human health datasets (Table 9.5.1).[22-26] These suggest that there may be an association between developmental and/or learning disorders with multiple anesthetic exposures, but probably not with single exposures.

Several human studies either have been recently completed or are underway attempting to answer these questions.[27]

The General Anesthesia Compared to Spinal Anesthesia (GAS Study) is an international, randomized controlled trial. Infants <60 weeks postmenstrual age but born >26 weeks who required inguinal hernia surgery were randomized into two groups. One received regional or local anesthesia only and the other group received general

TABLE 9.5.1 Summary of selected published human retrospective studies

Authors	*Dataset*	*Methods*	*Conclusion*
Flick RP et al. (2011)[22]	Olmstead Co., MN, health and school records	Comparison of children who received surgery/anesthesia age <2 years and a subsequent learning disability or need for an individualized education program (IEP) as determined from school records, with matched controls	Exposure to multiple but not single anesthetics increased the risk of learning disabilities.
DiMaggio C et al. (2011)[23]	New York State Medicaid program	Only twin-sibling pairs were used age <3 years. Comparisons were made between anesthesia-exposure discordant and concordant pairs for subsequent diagnoses of autism, emotional or social conduct disorders, developmental delay, or attention-deficit/hyperactivity disorder.	Exposure to multiple but not single anesthetics increased the risk of developmental or behavioral disorders.

(Continued)

TABLE 9.5.1 Continued

Authors	*Dataset*	*Methods*	*Conclusion*
Hansen TG et al. (2011),[24] (2013)[25]	Danish Civil Registration System	Compared 9th-grade test scores (age 15–16 years) of all children who underwent inguinal hernia repair at age <1 year (2011) and age <3 months for pyloric stenosis (2013) in Denmark with randomly matched controls	No difference in test scores was found when confounding factors were taken into account. Multiple anesthesia exposures were not examined.
Ing C et al. (2012)[26]	Western Australia Pregnancy Cohort Study (originally done to look for long-term effects of prenatal ultrasound)	Children born during that study were divided into 2 groups, those exposed to anesthesia at <3 years of age and those not exposed. Groups were compared on 6 neuropsychological tests.	Diminished language and abstract reasoning skills were found in anesthesia-exposed children with both single and multiple anesthetics.

supplemented by regional or local anesthesia. The primary outcome was neurodevelopmental at age 5 years, but the results at age 2 years was published in 2016.[28] This portion of the study showed no difference between regional and general anesthesia exposure. However, the study was not designed to examine any relationship with repeated or prolonged anesthesia exposure.

The Pediatric Anesthesia and Neurodevelopment Assessment (PANDA Study) used a sibling-matched cohort design that looked for differences in 105 sibling pairs. In each pair, one sibling was exposed to anesthesia prior to age 36 months during the period 2000–2010 and the other was not. Neurodevelopmental testing was performed between ages 8 and 15 years of age. Results published in 2016 showed no difference in global cognition (IQ) or behavior.[29]

In the Mayo Anesthesia Safety in Kids (MASK) study, patients exposed to general anesthesia during 1994 to 2007 were compared with propensity-matched controls. Both groups underwent neuropsychological testing between ages 8 and 12 years or 15 and 19 years between 2012 and 2016.[30] Testing included the National Center for Toxicological Research-Operant Test Battery, which was used to test for neurotoxicity in nonhuman primates.

In December 2016, the U.S. Food and Drug Administration (FDA) issued a Drug Safety Announcement warning that "repeated or lengthy use of general anesthetic and sedation drugs during surgeries or procedures in children younger than 3 years or in pregnant women during their third trimester may affect the development of children's brains."[31] This announcement took many in the sedation and anesthesia communities by surprise as it came without consultation with respective pediatric professional societies.

At least one major pediatric anesthesia department[32] has provided written guidance for proceduralists, surgeons, sedationists, and anesthesiologists about neurotoxicity. A specific discussion about the FDA warning is recommended during the anesthesia or sedation consent process for any child <3 years old. Ideally, any discussion of neurotoxicity with parents would occur before scheduling a procedure and would allow the parents to speak with the clinician.

Questions about the possible neurotoxicity of anesthetics and sedatives are expected to stay with us for a while. SmartTots is a public–private partnership formed between the FDA and the International Anesthesia Research Society to coordinate and fund efforts looking at the safety of anesthetics and sedatives in young patients. Its consensus statement on the Use of Anesthetic and Sedative Drugs in Infants and Toddlers was published in October 2015 and has been endorsed by a number of professional organizations, including the Society for Pediatric Sedation and the American Academy for Pediatrics.[33] This came before the FDA warning but it is still relevant. Some key points are as follows:

- Animal studies have raised the concern that some anesthetics and sedatives, when given to infants and young children, may be associated with long-term learning or behavioral deficits.
- To this point in time, human studies have been inconclusive.
- The possible risk of neurotoxicity must be weighed against the risks of forgoing or cancelling the planned procedure.

Since that time, evidence has emerged that a single exposure is safe but the effects, if any, of multiple exposures remains unknown. Therefore, it would be prudent to include a discussion of the expected duration of the procedure and whether multiple procedures will be needed.

Conclusion

Risks of sedation range from frequent but distressing (e.g., nausea) to severe and even life-threatening if not promptly treated (e.g., upper airway obstruction). The sedationist must be able to discuss these risks with parents when obtaining consent.

The neurotoxicity of anesthetic and sedative agents is an area of great interest to the medical community and the public. Published human studies suggest that a single exposure is safe in an otherwise healthy child, but data on multiple exposures have been inconclusive and more studies are being conducted.

Suggested Reading

Hansen TG. Anesthesia-related neurotoxicity and the developing animal brain is not a significant problem in children. *Pediatr Anesth.* 2014;25(1):65–72.

http://smarttots.org/wp-content/uploads/2015/10/ConsensusStatementV910.5.2015.pdf. Accessed November 16, 2016.

von Ungern-Sternberg BS. Respiratory complications in the pediatric postanesthesia care unit. *Anesthesiol Clin.* 2014;32(1):45–61.

Zhou Z, Ma D. Anaesthetics-induced neurotoxicity in developing brain: an update on preclinical evidence. *Brain Sci.* 2014;4(1):136–149.

References

1. Pascarella MR, Walls JD, Liu R, Chen L. Anesthesia providers are obligated to give patients the alternatives to general anesthesia when obtaining informed consent. *Trans Perioper Pain Med.* 2014;1(2):5–8.
2. Sanford SR. Informed consent: the verdict is in. *ASA Newsletter.* 2006;70/(7):15–16.
3. Cravero JP, Beach ML, Blike GT, et al. The incidence and nature of adverse events during pediatric sedation/anesthesia with propofol for procedures outside the operating room: a report from the Pediatric Sedation Research Consortium. *Anesth Analg.* 2009;108(3):795–804.
4. Ikonomidou C, Bosch F, Miksa M, Bittigau P, Vöckler J, Dikranian K, Tenkova TI, Stefovska V, Turski L, Olney JW. Blockade of NMDA receptors and Apoptotic Neurodegeneration in the developing brain. *Science.* 1999;283(5398):70–74.
5. Jevtovic-Todorovic V, Hartman RE, Izumi Yet al. Early exposure to common anesthetic agents causes widespread neurodegeneration in the developing rat brain and persistent learning deficits. *J Neurosci.* 2003;23(3):876–882.
6. Fredriksson A, Ponten E, Gordh T, Eriksson P. Neonatal exposure to a combination of N-Methyl-d-aspartate and gamma-Aminobutyric acid type A receptor anesthetic agents Potentiates Apoptotic Neurodegeneration and persistent behavioral deficits. *Anesthesiology.* 2007;107(3):427–436.
7. Brambrink AM, Evers AS, Avidan MS, et al. Isoflurane-induced neuroapoptosis in the neonatal Rhesus macaque brain. *Anesthesiology.* 2010;112(4):834–841.

8. Brambrink AM, Back SA, Riddle A, et al. Isoflurane-induced apoptosis of oligodendrocytes in the neonatal primate brain. *Ann Neurol.* 2012;72(4):525–535.
9. Dobbing J, Sands J. Comparative aspects of the brain growth spurt. *Early Hum Dev.* 1979;3(1):79–83.
10. Bayer SA, Altman J, Russo RJ, Zhang, X. Timetables of neurogenesis in the human brain based on experimentally determined patterns in the rat. *Neurotoxicology.* 1993;14(1):83–144.
11. Kodama M, Satoh Y, Otsubo Y, et al. Neonatal Desflurane exposure induces more robust Neuroapoptosis than do Isoflurane and Sevoflurane and Impairs working memory. *Anesthesiology.* 2011;115(5):979–991.
12. Yan J, Jiang H. Dual effects of ketamine. *J Neurosurg Anesthesiol.* 2014;26(2):155–160.
13. Xiong M, Zhang L, Li J, et al. Propofol-induced neurotoxicity in the fetal animal brain and developments in modifying these effects—an updated review of propofol fetal exposure in laboratory animal studies. *Brain Sci.* 2016;6(2):11.
14. Savage S, Ma D. The neurotoxicity of nitrous oxide: the facts and "putative" mechanisms. *Brain Sci.* 2014;4(1):73–90.
15. Sanders RD, Xu J, Shu Y, et al. Dexmedetomidine attenuates isoflurane-induced neurocognitive impairment in neonatal rats. *Anesthesiology.* 2009;110(5):1077–1085.
16. Li J, Xiong M, Nadavaluru PR, et al. Dexmedetomidine attenuates neurotoxicity induced by prenatal propofol exposure. *J Neurosurg Anesthesiol.* 2016;28(1):51–64.
17. Liu J-R, Yuki K, Baek C, et al. Dexmedetomidine-induced neuroapoptosis is dependent on its cumulative dose. *Anesth Analg.* 2016;123(4):1008–1017.
18. Rizzi S, Carter LB, Ori C, Jevtovic-Todorovic V. Clinical anesthesia causes permanent damage to the fetal guinea pig brain. *Brain Pathol.* 2008;18(2):198–210.
19. Young C, Jevtovic-Todorovic V, Qin Y-Q, et al. Potential of ketamine and midazolam, individually or in combination, to induce apoptotic neurodegeneration in the infant mouse brain. *Br J Pharmacol.* 2009;146(2):189–197.
20. Liu J-R, Liu Q, Li J, et al. Noxious stimulation Attenuates Ketamine-induced Neuroapoptosis in the developing rat brain. *Anesthesiology.* 2012;117(1):64–71.

21. Shu Y, Zhou Z, Wan Y, et al. Nociceptive stimuli enhance anesthetic-induced neuroapoptosis in the rat developing brain. *Neurobiology of Disease*. 2012;45(2):743–750. doi:10.1016/j.nbd.2011.10.021.
22. Flick RP, Katusic SK, Colligan RC et al. Cognitive and behavioral outcomes after early exposure to Anesthesia and surgery. *Pediatrics*. 2011;128(5):E1053–e1061.
23. DiMaggio C, Sun LS, Li G. Early childhood exposure to Anesthesia and risk of developmental and behavioral disorders in a sibling birth cohort. *Anesth Analg*. 2011;113(5):1143–1151.
24. Hansen TG, Pedersen JK, Henneberg SW, et al. Academic performance in adolescence after Inguinal Hernia repair in infancy. *Anesthesiology*. 2011;114(5):1076–1085.
25. Hansen TG, Pedersen JK, Henneberg SW, Morton NS, Christensen K. Educational outcome in adolescence following pyloric stenosis repair before 3 months of age: A nationwide cohort study. *Pediatr Anesth*. 2013;23(10):883–890.
26. Ing C, DiMaggio C, Whitehouse A et al. Long-term differences in language and cognitive function after childhood exposure to Anesthesia. *Pediatrics*. 2012;130(3):e476–85.
27. FAQ for health care professionals. http://smarttots.org/faq-for-health-care-professionals. Accessed November 16, 2016.
28. Davidson AJ, Disma N, de Graaff JC, et al. Neurodevelopmental outcome at 2 years of age after General Anaesthesia and Awake-Regional Anaesthesia in Infancy (GAS): an international multicentre, randomised controlled trial. *Lancet*. 2016;387(10015):239–250.
29. Sun LS, Li G, Miller TLK, et al. Association between a single general anesthesia exposure before age 36 months and neurocognitive outcomes in later childhood. *JAMA*. 2016;315(21):2312.
30. Gleich SJ, Flick R, Hu D, et al. Neurodevelopment of children exposed to anesthesia: design of the Mayo Anesthesia Safety in Kids (MASK) study. *Contemp Clin Trials*. 2015;41:45–54.
31. http://www.fda.gov/Drugs/DrugSafety/ucm532356.htm. Accessed February 16, 2017.
32. Andropoulos DB, Greene MF. Anesthesia and Developing Brains—Implications of the FDA Warning. *New England Journal of Medicine*. 2017;376(10):905–907. doi:10.1056/nejmp1700196.
33. http://smarttots.org/wp-content/uploads/2015/10/ConsensusStatementV910.5.2015.pdf. Accessed November 16, 2016.

9.6

Methods of Rescue/Response

CHRIS A. REES AND CORRIE E. CHUMPITAZI

Sedation in pediatric patients can lead to decreased muscle tone and subsequent tissue relaxation and airway narrowing. Thus, sedated children are at risk of respiratory depression, laryngospasm, airway obstruction, apnea, and loss of airway reflexes. Hypotension and cardiopulmonary arrest may also occur, although these complications usually result from failure to recognize and correct respiratory compromise. Despite careful presedation assessment, appropriate medication and dose selection, and appropriate cardiovascular monitoring during the procedure, the risks associated with sedation cannot be eliminated entirely. As it is common for children to pass from the intended level of sedation to deeper levels of sedation, providers should be capable of providing appropriate rescue interventions from one level of sedation deeper than what is intended.

The most common causes of upper airway obstruction during procedural sedation are apnea, pharyngeal obstruction, and laryngospasm. Apnea is the cessation or pause in ventilatory effort for a certain duration or that which requires intervention to stimulate the patient or assist in ventilation. Methods for alleviating apnea are depicted in Figure 9.6.1.[1]

The upper airway of children has several anatomic differences that affect its ability to maintain patency. Since the airway is more anterior and cephalad, the "sniffing" position is ideal for maintenance of a natural airway. Apnea can be obstructive in nature, in which

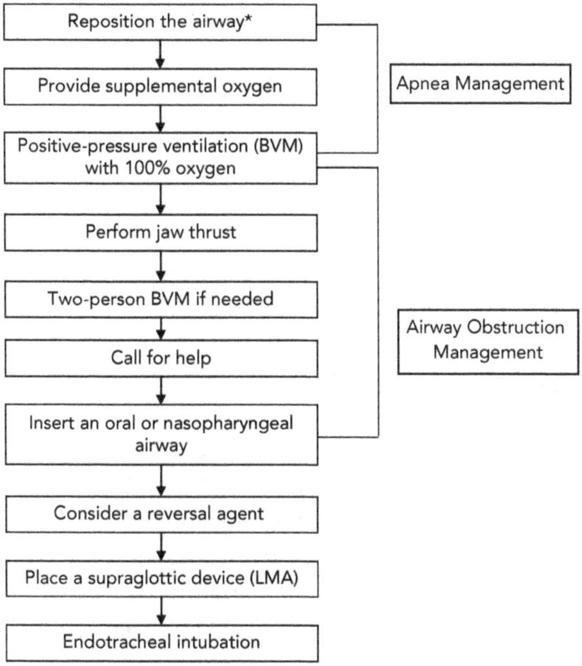

*Use chin lift or a shoulder roll to reposition the airway.

BVM: bag-valve-mask ventilation; LMA: laryngeal mask airway

FIGURE 9.6.1.

Airway response algorithm for apnea and airway obstruction.

case it is caused by pharyngeal obstruction resulting from displacement of the soft palate and epiglottis into the pharynx. The effort to breathe against an obstructed airway manifests as a paradoxical breathing pattern consisting of retraction of the sternal notch and exaggerated abdominal muscle activity that can be visualized by observing the patient and detected on end-tidal carbon dioxide tracing. Oxygen can be administered through end-tidal nasal cannula, so this may be turned up if not already used while evaluating the patient, but oxygen delivery alone will not rescue the child with symptoms of airway obstruction. Providers who provide procedural sedation must maintain proficiency in the ability to open the airway, suction secretions, perform successful bag-valve-mask ventilation, insert oral and nasopharyngeal airways, place laryngeal mask airways, and perform tracheal intubation. A second provider may be needed to perform an effective jaw thrust while performing two-person positive-pressure ventilation in older children in the case of suspected pharyngeal obstruction. Oral airways should be reserved for sedated patients, while nasopharyngeal airways may be used while patients are not fully sedated (see Figure 9.6.1).

Laryngospasm occurs when musculature at the glottis begins to spasm. It is an exaggeration of the normal glottic closure reflex that persists even after the stimulus has been removed and may result in partial or complete airway obstruction. Patients are at increased risk of laryngospasm if there are upper airway secretions present, if the airway has been manipulated, if they have had a recent upper respiratory tract infection, or if they have gastroesophageal reflux. A characteristic stridulous noise can be present if laryngospasm is partial, although it will be absent in complete laryngospasm. When suspected, follow the algorithm found in Figure 9.6.2. The suggested

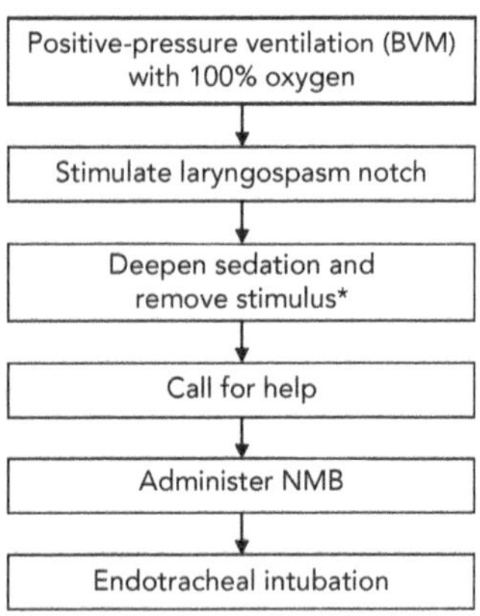

*if likely related to blood/secretions then gently suction

BMV: bag-mask-valve ventilation; NMB: neuromuscular blockade

FIGURE 9.6.2.

Airway response algorithm for laryngospasm.

management of laryngospasm resulting from procedural sedation begins with the initiation of positive-pressure ventilation with 100% oxygen. Any obvious secretions should be suctioned. While the depth of sedation lightens, the laryngospasm may resolve. However, if positive-pressure ventilation does not alleviate the laryngospasm and desaturation starts to occur, an increase in the depth of sedation is required; this can be achieved with the readily available intravenous sedative agent. If deepened sedation does not result in improved air entry (bag-valve-mask ventilation may be needed if central apnea has been produced by deepened sedation), providers should call for help and give the patient neuromuscular blocking agents such as succinylcholine (0.1–0.5 mg/kg), unless these medications are contraindicated in the patient undergoing sedation. Providers should be providing effective bag-valve-mask ventilation and actively preparing for endotracheal intubation.

Cardiovascular collapse may ensue if the airway obstruction is not immediately relieved. Providers should be prepared to follow standard advanced pediatric life support algorithms to manage bradycardia, hypotension, or arrhythmia. If continuous infusions of sedatives are being used, they obviously should be discontinued. Flumazenil is a useful, immediately active reversal agent for benzodiazepine-induced respiratory depression and hypotension, just as the more familiar naloxone will reverse the hypotension associated with opioids.

Reference

1. Coté CJ, Wilson S, American Academy of Pediatrics, American Academy of Pediatric Dentistry. Guidelines for monitoring and management of pediatric patients before, during, and after sedation for diagnostic and therapeutic procedures: update 2016. *Pediatrics*. 2016;138:220161212.

PART 2

PROCEDURAL SEDATION

10

Procedural Considerations

10.1

Procedural Aspects Affecting Sedation Care

Invasiveness and Duration

ANNE STORMORKEN

The goals of sedation for both diagnostic and therapeutic procedures are to manage preprocedural anxiety, minimize pain, and allow for successful completion of the procedure without adverse patient outcomes. To plan the appropriate way to achieve these goals, the sedationist must decide whether the procedure will cause the patient pain (invasiveness), the degree to which immobility is required for the procedure to be completed effectively, and the duration of time for which sedation is needed. If pharmacologic, systemic support is needed to manage the patient and meet procedural goals, medications should be selected based on the duration of sedation necessary. Pain control can often be effectively provided with local injectable or topical techniques. It is the responsibility of the sedationist to choose a medication, or combination of medications, that allows for administration of the lowest dose of drug(s) possible while maximizing the effective therapeutic effect.

Invasive Versus Noninvasive Procedures

Choosing the appropriate medication regimen is contingent on understanding the nature of the procedure. The sedationist should identify whether a procedure is invasive or noninvasive to determine the degree of analgesia and immobility required; however, it is pertinent to keep in mind that the pain intensity may vary during the course of the procedure (Table 10.1.1).

Noninvasive Procedures

Noninvasive procedures are those associated with minimal discomfort (e.g., CT, MRI, ECHO, and other imaging studies). and the purpose of sedation in these cases is to ensure immobility. Noninvasive procedures generally require anxiolytics and/or sedative–hypnotics, depending on the degree of immobility required. Medication options include midazolam, pentobarbital, propofol, dexmedetomidine, and etomidate.

Minimally Invasive Procedures

Minimally invasive procedures are associated with minimal to moderate pain; examples are peripheral intravenous catheter (PIV) placement, laceration repair, abscess incision and drainage, and voiding cystourethrography (VCUG). The purpose of sedation is to provide anxiolysis and immobility and to minimize discomfort. These procedures may require merely topical analgesics, but warrant sedation to achieve the level of immobility required to complete the procedure. Medication options include midazolam (Table 10.1.2), fentanyl, nitrous oxide, and ketamine. Topical anesthesia with distraction techniques may obviate the need for systemic analgesics.

TABLE 10.1.1 Diagnostic and therapeutic procedures

	Diagnostic and Therapeutic Procedures		
	Noninvasive	***Minimally Invasive***	***Invasive***
Indications	CT ECHO MRI Ultrasound	Intravenous line placement Phlebotomy Dental procedures Foreign body removal Voiding cystourethrography Laceration repair	Incision and draining Biopsies Lumbar punctures Bone marrow aspiration Fracture reduction Interventional radiology procedures Thoracostomy tube placement
Goals	Immobility	Analgesia Anxiolysis Immobility Hypnosis	Amnesia Analgesia Anxiolysis Hypnosis Immobility
Strategy	Nonpharmacologic ± Midazolam Pentobarbital Propofol Etomidate Dexmedetomidine	Nonpharmacologic ± Midazolam Fentanyl Nitrous oxide Ketamine	Ketamine Midazolam and fentanyl Propofol and fentanyl Propofol and ketamine

TABLE 10.1.2 Administration routes and doses of midazolam for anxiolysis

Route	*Dose (mg/kg)*	*Onset (min)*
Intranasal	0.2–0.5	5–7
Oral	0.3–0.5	10–20
Intravenous	0.05–0.1	3–5
Rectal	0.25–0.5	15–20

Invasive Procedures

During invasive procedures, tissues are instrumented and this often leads to significant pain. Examples include tissue biopsies, drainage tube placement, lumbar punctures, incision and drainage of larger abscesses, complex laceration repairs, and fracture reductions. The purpose of sedation is to provide analgesia as well as anxiolysis and sedation with immobility, therefore multiple drugs may be needed. For example, a patient undergoing CT-guided tissue biopsy may require greater immobility so that an adequate tissue sample can be obtained compared with a patient who is undergoing fracture reduction, in whom less immobility may be required. When two or more sedating medications are co-administered, particularly if the mechanism of action is similar, the potential for adverse outcomes increases due to synergy of adverse effects. Medication options include midazolam and fentanyl, propofol and fentanyl, and propofol and ketamine. Topical anesthetic techniques will be helpful with superficial skin penetration, but invasive procedures generally benefit from systemic analgesic use.

Nonpharmacologic Versus Pharmacologic Interventions

Nonpharmacologic Interventions

Every attempt should be made to provide non-pharmacologic support for the patient and their family whenever possible. Painful procedures often provoke anxiety for patients and their families, and addressing the patient's anxiety, before addressing the procedure's analgesia and mobility demands, can facilitate the appropriate degree of sedation. Anticipation of pain is often the greatest source of anxiety to patients and their families.

Age-appropriate distractions include blowing bubbles and movies (for younger children) or guided imagery, controlled breathing, and games (for older children). The patient should be made comfortable with parents nearby or sitting adjacent to the patient to facilitate patient cooperation. Patient anxiety can be managed with anxiolytics if age-appropriate distractions are insufficient.

Pharmacologic Interventions

When pain management is required, the regimen should reflect the severity and duration of pain to be experienced. See the Appendix for discussion of specific agents.

Local anesthetics should be used whenever possible. They can be administered topically, or by injection, for all invasive procedures and local anesthesia may reduce the sedative requirement.

In anticipation of more significant pain, systemic analgesics should be administered. In infants (<1 year old), oral sucrose solutions have been shown to decrease pain response to minor procedures. In older children, analgesia can be provided in oral, intranasal, and intravenous formulations that can be safely combined with anxiolytics and sedative–hypnotics. Medications can be administered intermittently or via continuous infusion. Nonopioid agents such as acetaminophen and nonsteroidal anti-inflammatories (e.g., ibuprofen, ketorolac) may provide sufficient analgesia with fewer adverse effects in combination with sedative agents (e.g., respiratory depression or hypotension). Acetaminophen, when administered intravenously, can provide analgesia within 5–10 minutes, while the oral formulation may take up to 1 hour to begin acting. Oxycodone (opioid agonist) as a single agent can provide analgesia for moderate pain and can be administered enterally with an onset of action of 10–15 minutes, time to peak effect of 60 minutes and a duration of action between 3 and 6 hours. Fentanyl and morphine (opioid agonists) can provide a dose-dependent sedation and analgesic effect. Fentanyl (synthetic opioid), which has a potency 100 times that of morphine, can provide analgesia within 2–3 minutes for procedures producing moderate to severe pain however it has a shorter duration of action (30–60 minutes). Synergistic sedative effects are observed when fentanyl is combined with midazolam or propofol. Ketamine, a dissociative sedative, blocks NMDA receptors and inhibits excitatory neurotransmission providing sedation, analgesia, amnesia, and a relative degree of immobility with preservation of upper airway muscle tone and airway protective reflexes. Hydromorphone, morphine, and ketamine can be administered intravenously and orally with increasing times to peak effect respectively.

Procedure Duration

Sedative pharmacokinetic properties such as time to peak effect, duration of action, and terminal half-life figure centrally in agent selection in the context of procedure duration.

Pharmacodynamics is defined as what the medication does to the body, is determined by drug-receptor interactions and tends to be similar amongst agents of the same class. Conversely, pharmacokinetics refers to the effect of the body on the drug and can be used to differentiate medications within a class. The pharmacokinetic properties of a medication vary according to the route of administration (e.g., intravenous, oral, intramuscular, intranasal; Table 10.1.3).

TABLE 10.1.3 Routes of administration for sedatives

Route	*Benefits*	*Limitations*	*Notes*
Intravenous (IV)	*Bolus*: Can achieve rapid clinical response as peak plasma concentrations can be reached within 1 minute due to rapid distribution to vessel-rich compartments such as the brain, which receive high blood flow. *Continuous*: Can be titrated to maintain appropriate plasma concentration and achieve clinical effect	Requires IV access	Fat solubility of the sedative influences the onset of action and duration of clinical effect. Higher lipid solubility means higher drug penetration and departure from the brain. Examples: propofol, midazolam, dexmedetomidine
Oral (PO)	No need for IV access; convenient	1st-pass hepatic metabolism resulting in "active" metabolites; unpredictable onset of action and potential for prolonged clinical effect; cannot titrate to effect	Examples: midazolam, ketamine

TABLE 10.1.3 Continued

Route	*Benefits*	*Limitations*	*Notes*
Intranasal (IN)	Absorption of medication directly into the systemic circulation, thereby avoiding 1st-pass hepatic metabolism; more rapid clinical effect than PO or rectal	Can burn when administered	Examples: midazolam, ketamine, dexmedetomidine
Inhalation (INH)	Rapid onset of action; tolerated well	Delivery is dependent on wearing mask, which may not always be tolerated by children	Example: nitrous oxide
Intramuscular (IM)	Can be used in an uncooperative child	Pain on administration; effect depends on blood flow to muscle	Common sites: deltoids, tricep, gluteus
Rectal	Can be used in patients with nausea and vomiting; no need for IV access; partial avoidance of 1st-pass hepatic metabolism: distal rectum allows for systemic absorption, while upper rectum and colon have blood flow and absorption via portal system	Difficult to administer in older patients	Examples: midazolam, ketamine

In deriving the appropriate sedative regimen, the sedationist must consider the desired clinical effect (analgesia, anxiolysis, immobility), onset of action, and duration of effect. Knowledge of the adverse effects of the medication is crucial. The medications should be administered such that their peak effect and duration of effect match the duration of the procedure. If more than one agent is to be administered, the relationship of each agent's mechanism of action, and the potential for synergism of adverse drug effects, must be evaluated.

If the procedure is predictably short (<10 minutes), then intermittent bolus dosing may be considered. Often a single medication may be sufficient, and an agent with a short half-life should be selected. For a procedure of medium duration (10–30 minutes), intermittent dosing may be sufficient, although if frequent boluses are necessary for example to address the invasive nature of a procedure, then an infusion may be more appropriate. The addition of a second agent may minimize the need for additional bolus dosing (e.g., using a combination of midazolam and ketamine for laceration repair). For a long procedure (>30 minutes), an infusion should be selected (e.g., dexmedetomidine or propofol).

If a procedure's duration is unpredictable, then an infusion will be more suitable, particularly if agents with short half-lives such as dexmedetomidine or propofol are selected. These agents can be titrated to effect with less risk of prolonged sedation during recovery after the procedure.

Suggested Reading

Coté CJ, Wilson S, American Academy of Pediatrics, American Academy of Pediatric Dentistry. Guidelines for monitoring and management of pediatric patients before, during, and after sedation for diagnostic and therapeutic procedures: update 2016. *Pediatrics.* 2016;138(1):e20161212.

Hsu DC, Cravero JP. Pharmacologic agents for pediatric procedural sedation outside of the operating room. *UpToDate.* Retrieved December 31, 2016, from https://www.uptodate.com/contents/pharmacologic-agents-for-pediatric-procedural-sedation-outside-of-the-operating-room.

Kazak AE, Penati B, Brophy P, Himelstein B. Pharmacologic and psychologic interventions for procedural pain. *Pediatrics*. 1998;102(1):59–66.

Krauss BS, Krauss BA, Green SM. Procedural sedation and analgesia in children. *N Engl J Med*. 2014;370:e23.

Yaster M, Easley RB, Brady KM. Chapter 12: Pain and sedation management in the critically ill child. In: Nichols DG, ed. *Rogers' Textbook of Pediatric Intensive Care*. 4th ed. Philadelphia: Wolters Kluwer, 2008:136–164.

10.2

Procedural Aspects Affecting Sedation Care

Skill Set and Location

KIMBERLY FUGOK AND SUSANNE KOST

Communication among sedationist, proceduralist, and other team members is key to carrying out a safe and successful procedure. A systematic approach should be implemented each time a sedated procedure occurs, allowing for proper checks and balances to ensure patient safety. Appropriate personnel, equipment, and space should be in place prior to the initiation of the sedated procedure. The preprocedure discussion among involved clinicians should review the anticipated level of discomfort, patient positioning, tolerance for patient motion, procedure duration, and any special procedural considerations. The need for preprocedural laboratory testing should be reviewed in advance, as should any chronic medication management (anticoagulants in particular).

Skills and Equipment

Thoughtful preparation serves as the foundation for successful procedural sedation. Checklists and timeouts, discussed in Chapter 6.3, have been shown to decrease morbidity and mortality. A team of qualified clinicians should be available to evaluate the patient, perform the procedure, monitor the patient, and supervise the patient's recovery appropriately. In some settings the proceduralist may be responsible for both the sedation and procedure, in which case the presence of a skilled clinician for monitoring and assisting in rescue is essential. Per the Centers for Medicare and Medicaid Services (CMS), "moderate sedation services provided by the same physician or other qualified healthcare professional performing the diagnostic or therapeutic service that the sedation supports, require the presence of an independent trained observer to assist in the monitoring of the patient's level of consciousness and physiological status."[1] This clinician should not be tasked with assisting the proceduralist. All team members should be present at the bedside prior to the induction of sedation. Sufficient number and type of staff should be determined based on the level of sedation, the nature of the procedure being performed, the rescue mechanisms available, and the assessment of risk presented by the particular patient's condition.

Necessary supplies, including medications, reversal agents, age- and size-appropriate resuscitation equipment, and appropriate procedural equipment, should be readily available prior to the induction of sedation. The use of procedural carts or kits for commonly performed procedures increases efficiency and safety, especially in the event of an unexpected break in sterility or procedural event. Supplies can be returned; however, team members leaving a sedated procedure to gather missing materials can lead to inability to rescue from a complication, prolongation of sedation time, and additional medication usage and necessitates increased handoff communication. In the medical imaging environment, scanning protocols and need for contrast agents should be set in advance when possible in order to avoid extending sedation time.

In addition to sedation- and procedure-specific medications and equipment, other aspects of patient procedural safety should be considered. Devices to minimize skin breakdown, such as gel pads and egg-crate foam, should be employed, especially for longer procedures. Care should be taken to protect the patient's eyes with tape or gel to prevent corneal injury. In certain loud environments such as the MRI scanner or the casting room, hearing protection should be provided (for both the patient and the staff).

The level of sedation should be appropriate for the procedure, taking into account pain, duration, access to the patient during the procedure, and intrinsic risk due to the patient's medical condition. Minimal, moderate, or deep sedation should be chosen carefully, with the understanding that not every procedural situation is predictable. The level of sedation is not uniformly correlated to a particular medication or specific dose, but rather to the patient's individual response. The level of sedation planned should be discussed with the family as part of the informed consent process, and patients who are of age should grant assent to the plan. Failure to meet expectations ("Don't worry, you won't feel or remember a thing") can lead to dissatisfaction and distrust for future procedural encounters. Backup plans should be in place prior to induction of sedation. If the sedation is not going as planned or the procedure cannot be performed as desired due to patient motion or distress, the procedure should be postponed, reassigned to a higher level of provider, or performed in a more controlled environment such as the operating room.

The intended level of sedation should be matched to the appropriate personnel. Sedation service efficiency can be improved when the credentials of the sedation provider align well with patient needs. For example, assigning a nurse practitioner to procedures where minimal to moderate sedation is anticipated and a physician to procedures where deep sedation is required may serve as a cost-effective model. Certain patients (due to airway concerns or medical complexity) and certain longer or more invasive procedures may warrant the care of an anesthesiologist; again, a conversation between the proceduralist and the sedationist well in advance of the patient's presence will avoid last-minute scrambling for coverage or cancellation of the procedure. Sedationists should be competent to manage patients from a level of sedation one level deeper than that which is intended.

Location

Procedural geography varies considerably from hospital to office settings, to clinics, and even freestanding imaging centers. Large facilities may have the luxury of a dedicated procedural suite, while some sedation services may travel to different locations within an institution with a mobile cart. Pediatric sedation teams operating in an adult-focused facility should be more vigilant to the availability of pediatric resources in the areas in which they provide service.

Procedural location within a large institution is often limited by fixed equipment. Common examples include large imaging devices such as MRI scanners and nuclear medicine cameras, dental or ophthalmology equipment, and special orthopedic tables or devices. Both the sedationist and proceduralist must be familiar with their surroundings and comfortable with the available supplies and space. Monitoring ability and rescue response is different when the seditionist is separated physically from the patient (e.g., observing through a window in the MRI suite) when compared to actively managing the airway when standing right next to the patient during a suturing event.

Although the location may vary, the attention to safety and necessary supplies should not. Supplemental oxygen, suction, and positive-pressure ventilation must be available at all times. Ideally oxygen and suction should come from headwalls; portable suction is not as consistently effective. In institutions with multiple layers of safety-net response (e.g., pediatric "code blue" teams, rapid response teams, emergent anesthesiology or critical care response), the need for help with sedation emergency rescue should be able to be communicated clearly and quickly. If pediatric procedural sedation care is taking place outside of a hospital environment, there is likely to be limited expertise available for immediate backup and rescue in the case of sedation-related patient emergencies. In clinic and office settings, proper risk assessment is key, practice with rarely used equipment should be scheduled for all team members, and arrangements with local healthcare facilities for immediate support may be available rather than simply relying on local 911 response calls and personnel.

Efficient organization of the procedural space expedites care. Spending time prior to sedation to prepare and organize the sedation/procedure room, maximizing flow for the scheduled event, will improve the process. Having the needed supplies within arm's reach for airway support, medication administration, and procedural tasks aids in the ease of sedation. Placing monitors in a location visible to both the sedationist and other monitoring team members allows easier tracking of the patient's status. Creating the desired environment takes time and discussion. Distractions should be minimized: turn down the television volume and discourage unnecessary conversation and people at the bedside during the event. If family members are present, ideally staff should be available to explain and interpret their experience.

The personal safety of the sedation staff and observing family members should be considered during the procedural event. Exposure to unscavenged nitrous oxide or anesthetic gas is a possible hazard. Standard infectious precautions should be employed routinely, and the need for special precautions must be communicated by the primary service when the sedation provider and proceduralist are consulted. The procedural sedation area should be designed for easy access to appropriate disposal of hazards, including sharps, chemotherapeutic agents, and radioactive materials. For those who frequently provide sedation for medical imaging procedures, radiation exposure should be measured with badges and risk should be minimized with lead glasses, aprons, and shields. Working within the magnetic field of the MRI scanner mandates an understanding of materials and processes for safety in that environment. Women of childbearing age should be questioned about pregnancy to prevent fetal exposure to inhaled gases and radiation. Staff safety should also be considered when providing procedural sedation for violent or aggressive patients, as significant harm can result if the team is unprepared. Moving large children or teenagers into required procedural positions while sedated can result in staff muscle strain or back injury.

Summary

Communication among personnel and advance preparation of available resources are the keys to successful procedural sedation.

Having appropriately skilled personnel, readily available supplies and equipment, and effective backup and rescue plans allows for safe, effective, and efficient procedural sedation in any scenario or location.

Suggested Reading

Coté CJ, Wilson S. Guidelines for monitoring and management of pediatric patients during and after sedation for diagnostic and therapeutic procedures: an update. *Pediatrics.* 2006;118:2587.

Coté CJ, Wilson S, American Academy of Pediatrics, American Academy of Pediatric Dentistry. Guidelines for monitoring and management of pediatrics patients before, during, and after sedation for diagnostic and therapeutic procedures: update 2016. *Pediatrics.* 2016;138(1):20161212.

Cravero JP, Beach ML, Blike GT et al. The incidence and nature of adverse events during pediatric sedation/anesthesia with propofol for procedures outside the operating room: a report from the Pediatric Sedation Research Consortium. *Anesth Analg.* 2009;108(3):795–804.

Evered LM. Procedural sedation and analgesia for paediatric patients in the emergency department. *Paediatr Child Health.* 2003;8(8):503–507.

Fenik Y, Celebi N, Wagner R, et al. Prepackaged central line kits reduce procedural mistakes during central line insertion: a randomized controlled prospective trial. *BMC Med Educ.* 2013; 13:60.

Fortier MA, Del Rosario AM, Martin SR, Kain ZN. Perioperative anxiety in children. *Paediatr Anaesth.* 2010; 20:318–322.

Kahlenberg L, Harsey L, Patterson M, et al. Implementation of a modified WHO pediatric procedural sedation safety checklist and its impact on risk reduction. *Hosp Pediatr.* 2017;7(4):225–229.

Rissavi BL, Sabotchick KJ, Heilie CJ. Portable suction unit failure in a rural EMS system. *Prehosp Disaster Med.* 2013;28(4):388–390.

Reference

1. Department of Health and Human Services. Centers for Medicare & Medicaid Services Manual System: Medicare claims processing. 2007; Pub. 100-04.

10.3

Urgent Sedation (Unscheduled Procedural Sedation) in the Emergency Department

BENJAMIN F. JACKSON AND ELYSHA PIFKO

The emergency department (ED) exists to facilitate acute, unscheduled care for patients with urgent/emergent needs related to injury and illness. The ED commonly manages patients who require performance of urgent/emergent painful or anxiety-provoking, diagnostic or therapeutic procedures such as the following:

- Reduction of fracture or joint dislocation
- Laceration repair
- Abscess incision and drainage
- Burn debridement
- Foreign body removal
- Lumbar puncture
- Arthrocentesis
- Thoracostomy tube placement
- Electrical cardioversion.

The developmental and psychological attributes of children render procedural care in this clinical context especially challenging, may have a negative impact on procedural accomplishment, and may translate into increased challenges with future pain and procedural needs. Safe, high-quality procedural sedation/analgesia (PSA) is an essential aspect of ED care for children, increasing the likelihood of procedural success and improving overall patient satisfaction.

Core competencies of Emergency Medicine include the ability to perform cardiovascular resuscitation for pediatric patients, to manage airway emergencies invasively and noninvasively, and to provide PSA. Under the care of clinicians trained to stratify the risks and benefits of PSA, pediatric patients in the ED are in an appropriate setting for PSA when needed to facilitate acute procedural care.

Patient Selection

Attention to management of acute pain and anxiety (whether procedurally induced or not) in conscious children is always indicated. The ED may not be the most suitable place or may lack or be unable to expend resources to manage PSA if the procedure is not required for an acute, urgent or emergent situation. In the absence of a life- or limb-threatening emergency situation, risk stratification of the patient and determination of appropriateness for PSA should proceed in the manner presented in the rest of this handbook.

In general, patients appropriate for ED PSA are American Society of Anesthesiologists (ASA) class I or II with favorable cardiorespiratory anatomy and physiology. In children with traumatic injury warranting procedural care, consideration should be given to the possibility of additional injury (e.g., brain, spinal cord, abdominal, pulmonary) and the potential implications of PSA on the patient. For instance, a child with a long bone fracture sustained from being struck by a car is more likely than an adult patient to have also suffered blunt force abdominal trauma that may become apparent only as hypotension during sedation for fracture reduction maneuvers.

Children presenting with hemodynamic or central nervous system compromise warrant careful scrutiny prior to proceeding with PSA. For instance the febrile, tachycardic child with pneumonia and pleural effusion may become more unstable with PSA for pleural drainage.

Procedural Complexity

Brief, simple procedures unlikely to involve complex procedural skills are ideal for ED PSA. These procedures may be performed by either ED physicians or consultants. Consideration for PSA should also be given to simple procedures that are very anxiety-provoking in young children, such as laceration repairs; for these procedures, distraction techniques, pharmacologic anxiolysis (minimal sedation), and local analgesia are insufficient.

Complex procedures that involve a large amount of resources (equipment, personnel, space) may be more appropriate for the operating room or other controlled venue. Procedures estimated to exceed 30–45 minutes in duration may not be appropriate for the ED. ED clinician presence during the procedure and PSA recovery time may exceed a reasonable timeframe, which will have an adverse impact on ED flow, triage, and capacity.

Procedural Urgency

Emergent procedures may require PSA for patients with a higher ASA class, but monitoring standards (personnel, equipment, time) should never be compromised. The American College of Emergency Physicians (ACEP) proposes the following classification:

- *Emergent*—cardioversion for life-threatening dysrhythmia, reduction of markedly angulated fracture or dislocation with soft tissue or vascular compromise, intractable pain or suffering
- *Urgent*—care of dirty wounds/lacerations, animal and human bites, abscess incision and drainage, fracture reduction, hip reduction, lumbar puncture for suspect meningitis, arthrocentesis, neuroimaging for trauma

- *Semi-urgent*—care of clear wounds/lacerations, shoulder reduction, neuroimaging for new-onset seizure, foreign body removal, sexual assault examination
- *Nonurgent or elective*—non-vegetable foreign body in external auditory canal, chronic embedded soft tissue foreign body removal, ingrown toenail management

The urgency of PSA for necessary management of less imminently threatening conditions should be determined via risk–benefit assessment. Procedures to remedy/markedly improve painful conditions requiring significant yet insufficient analgesic dosing should not be delayed. The risk to the healthy ASA class I or II patient for a significant PSA complication associated with preprocedural fasting/NPO status (see Chapter 6.4) is fairly low. Preprocedural fasting/NPO status should be considered but should not be the sole reason to delay PSA for emergent/urgent procedures when timely completion of the procedure is judged to be of more benefit to the patient.

Personnel

Necessary personnel are the sedationist (typically ED physician), proceduralist (ED physician, advanced practice provider, or consultant), registered nurse, patient care tech, and other ancillary staff (child life personnel may be particularly helpful). All should be trained and skilled in their assigned responsibilities:

- *Sedationist*—pharmacology, adverse event recognition/management, positioned to address airway needs rapidly, familiar with procedure for which PSA is being provided
- *Proceduralist*—competent to complete procedure; if also serving as the sedationist, must be able to safely and rapidly abandon the procedure to address the patient's sedation needs and attend to adverse events

- *Nurse*—familiar with pharmacology; must appropriately document, assess, and respond to monitored vital signs and sedation-related events; provides skilled assistance in possible rescue situations

While many professional society and regulatory guidelines mandate the presence of a separate sedationist and proceduralist during deep PSA, ACEP guidelines state that "there is no evidence that specifically identifies which cases, if any, require dual-physician involvement to prevent adverse outcome."[1]

Because of the unpredictable nature of ED census and acuity, effective ED personnel management requires that PSA personnel time commitment for a single patient must not represent a barrier to overall ED flow, triage, and capacity.

Pharmacologic Options and Depth of Sedation

Both the preprocedural state of the patient and the nature of the procedure to be performed should factor into the decision as to which PSA regimen is selected. In the ED, patients present with injury and illness associated with a generally higher level of anxiety, acute pain, and physiologic derangements than patients presenting for scheduled procedures. In addition, the younger the patient or the more painful the procedure, the deeper the state of sedation that will be needed to accomplish the procedure successfully.

Midazolam via the oral or intranasal route is a common preprocedural anxiolytic option. Inhaled nitrous oxide is emerging as a promising option for minimal to moderate PSA cases. Dissociative PSA with parenteral ketamine remains the most frequently employed strategy for children in the ED setting. Propofol is often used in conjunction with ketamine or after analgesic optimization.

The synergistic effects of medications must be taken into account, especially when opioids are being combined with benzodiazepines or propofol, due to the possibility of synergistic respiratory and cardiovascular depression.

Certified child life specialists and/or distraction and diversion techniques, including the use of digital interactive tablet devices, may dramatically increase procedural compliance of pediatric patients and may diminish dosing needs for PSA medications.

Suggested Reading

ACGME Program Requirements for Graduate Medical Education in Pediatric Emergency Medicine. Accreditation Council for Graduate Medical Education, 2007.

American Society of Anesthesiologists Task Force on Sedation and Analgesia by Non-anesthesiologists. Practice guidelines for sedation and analgesia by non-anesthesiologists. *Anethesiology*. 2002;96:1004–1017.

Coté CJ, Wilson S, American Academy of Pediatrics, American Academy of Pediatric Dentistry. Guidelines for monitoring and management of pediatric patients before, during, and after sedation for diagnostic and therapeutic procedures: update 2016. *Pediatrics*. 2016;138 (1):20161212.

Downey LV, Zun LS. Pain management in the emergency department and its relationship to patient satisfaction. *J Emerg Trauma Shock*. 2010;3(4):326–330.

Godwin SA, Caro DA, Wolf SJ, et al. Clinical policy: procedural sedation and analgesia in the emergency department. *Ann Emerg Med*. 2005;45(2):177–196.

Green SM, Roback MG, Kennedy RM, Krauss B. Clinical practice guideline for emergency department ketamine dissociative sedation: 2011 update. *Ann Emerg Med*. 2011;57(5):449–461.

Green SM, Roback MG, Miner JR, et al. Fasting and emergency department procedural sedation and analgesia: a consensus-based clinical practice advisory. *Ann Emerg Med*. 2007;49(4):454–461.

Mace SE, Brown LA, Francis L, et al. Clinical policy: critical issues in the sedation of pediatric patients in the emergency department. *Ann Emerg Med*. 2008;51(4): 378–399.

Sacchetti A, Baren J, Carraccio C. Total procedural requirements as indication for emergency department sedation. *Pediatr Emerg Care*. 2010;26(3):209–211.

Reference

1. Godwin SA, Burton JH, Gerardo CJ, et al. Clinical policy: procedural sedation and analgesia in the emergency department. *Ann Emerg Med.* 2014;63(2):247–258. [Erratum *Ann Emerg Med.* 2017;70(5):758.]

11

Special Patient Considerations

11.1

The Obese Child

JAMES H. HERTZOG

The incidence of obesity is increasing worldwide for both adults and children. In adults, obesity is defined as a body mass index (BMI) of 30 kg/m^2 or greater. Since children grow in both height and weight, norms for BMI will vary. Therefore, obesity in children between 2 and 20 years of age is defined as a BMI greater than the 95th percentile for age and gender (https://www.cdc.gov/growthcharts/cdc_charts.htm). Furthermore, multiple comorbidities are associated with obesity that may require diagnostic and therapeutic interventions facilitated by sedation and analgesia. Therefore, it is likely that the practitioner of pediatric procedural sedation (PPS) will encounter obese children. Understanding the obesity-related risks of PPS will assist the sedationist in managing and mitigating these risks.

Discussion

The incidence of adverse events in obese children during general anesthesia provides a starting point in understanding the impact of obesity on adverse events during PPS. During general anesthesia, obese children have a higher incidence of oxygen desaturation, difficult mask ventilation and direct laryngoscopy/airway management, upper airway obstruction, bronchospasm, failed peripheral intravenous catheter placement, and prolonged recovery time. While these insights are valuable, important differences between general anesthesia and PPS exist that may affect the applicability of these results to sedation practice. A study from the Pediatric Sedation Research Consortium that examines pediatric obesity suggests that there is a higher incidence of airway adverse events among obese children versus nonobese children during procedural sedation (see Chapter 9 for a general discussion of airway adverse events and their management).

More specifically in the obese child, oxygen desaturation is the result of multiple anatomic and physiologic interactions. The presence of additional pretracheal adipose tissue, with a resultant decrease in the cricomental space, may lead to airway obstruction. Respiratory system compliance is decreased by increased chest wall resistance. Functional residual capacity is decreased as well. These factors are exacerbated when the patient is in the recumbent position and abdominal pressure on the diaphragm is greatest.

While upper airway obstruction may occur in any child due to the effects of sedative medications on pharyngeal muscle tone, children with obstructive sleep apnea (OSA) are at a much higher risk for developing upper airway obstruction when sedated. When possible, the use of nonopioid analgesics is advised for these patients. OSA is a frequently occurring comorbidity in obese children. An evaluation for OSA should be considered prior to a sedation encounter.

Other comorbidities associated with obesity that may require management during PPS include asthma, hypertension, type 2 diabetes and metabolic syndrome, gastroesophageal reflux disease, and pseudotumor cerebri.

Identifying a patient as obese prior to the scheduled sedation encounter may optimize resource utilization and preparation. However, identifying obesity during a screening call may be difficult: the patient's weight alone may be inadequate for determining obesity, and calculating BMI requires knowledge of the patient's height, which may not be routinely asked.

Given the increased incidence of airway-related complications and the need for airway interventions in obese patients undergoing PPS, the following points should be considered:

- Ready access to the airway
- Establishing reliable intravenous access
- Patient positioning that minimizes airway obstruction
- Easy access to airway supplies
- Potential need for two-person bag-valve-mask ventilation
- Continuous capnography use (encouraged)
- Sufficient staff for an emergent change of patient position.

In general, the least effective medication dose to achieve the desired level of sedation should be provided, and opportunities to use nonpharmacologic intervention with the assistance of a child life specialist should be sought. There is little pharmacokinetic information available on children, and even less on obese children. Drug administration based on total body weight may result in an overdose; conversely, a dose based on ideal body weight may result in suboptimal effect. Changes in cardiac output and body composition (as seen in obesity) affect the distribution of drugs. Obesity will increase the volume of distribution (V_D) for lipophilic drugs, although this may be unpredictable, and total body weight is commonly used for dosing purposes. Typically, hydrophilic drugs are dosed based on ideal body weight. Induction times and recovery times may be prolonged in obese children versus nonobese children.

Summary

With proper screening and preparation, obese patients may be safely and successful sedated for diagnostic and therapeutic interventions. Given the increased incidence of adverse airway-related events and the need for airway interventions in obese patients undergoing PPS, timely recognition of these adverse events and the rapid availability of rescue interventions are essential. Collaboration with pediatric anesthesiology colleagues is extremely useful. Reasons for referring obese patients for general anesthesia may include significant obesity, severe OSA, procedures that require prone positioning, and a situation where the patient's airway has been identified as difficult.

Suggested Reading

El-Metainy S, Ghoneim T, Aridae E, et al. Incidence of perioperative adverse events in obese children undergoing elective general surgery. *Br J Anaesth.* 2011;106:359–363.

Grunwell JR, McCracken C, Fortenberry J, et al. Risk factors leading to failed procedural sedation in children outside the operating room. *Pediatr Emerg Care.* 2014;30:381–387.

Scherrer PD, Mallory MD, Cravero JP, et al. The impact of obesity on pediatric procedural sedation-related outcomes: results from the Pediatric Sedation Research Consortium. *Pediatr Anesth.* 2015;25:689–697.

Tait AR, Voelpel-Lewis T, Burke C, et al. Incidence and risk factors for perioperative adverse respiratory events in children who are obese. *Anesthesiology.* 2008;108:375–380.

11.2

The Child with Autism Spectrum Disorder

LAURIE J. BURTON AND PRADIP P. KAMAT

Autism spectrum disorder (ASD) is a general term that encompasses a group of complex developmental brain disorders caused by a combination of genetic and environmental interactions. ASDs now include a variety of conditions that were previously separate diagnostic entities, such as autistic disorder, pervasive developmental disorder not otherwise specified, and Asperger syndrome. In the United States the prevalence of ASD is 1 in 68 children, and it is now the fastest-growing developmental disability.[1]

Children with ASD are more likely to be hospitalized with prolonged length of stay and to be admitted due to injury compared to children without ASD.[2] Children with ASD may present to the sedationist for a variety of medical problems not seen in children without ASD. These include various diagnostic and therapeutic procedures and ongoing monitoring of drug therapy requiring sampling of blood, echocardiography, and electrocardiography to evaluate the effect of therapy on the heart.

Presedation Considerations

The following are common comorbidities in patients with ASD:

- Seizure disorder is seen in 30% of children with ASD, usually with an increased prevalence of treatment-resistant epilepsy.[3]
- Sleep issues: Children with ASD have problems with sleep duration and quality of sleep. There is a higher incidence of obstructive sleep apnea in preschoolers with ASD compared to preschoolers without ASD.[4]
- Metabolic and autoimmune disorders: Autoimmune disorders are more common in the autism population than in the general population. Perhaps the associated disorder of most concern in the autism population is mitochondrial disease (7.2% vs. 0.01% in general population).[5] The presence of mitochondrial disease may necessitate the need for special fasting instructions, laboratory evaluation before and after sedation, and changes in drug choice.
- Oral health: ASD patients have a higher incidence of caries and gingivitis (hence the potential for loose teeth) due to poor oral hygiene (partly because access to the mouth is difficult due to the child's behavior).[6]
- Sensory defensiveness and sensory dysfunction: Most children with ASD dislike unfamiliar sounds, textures, and odors and being touched. Conducting a detailed physical exam, especially of the upper airway, may be very difficult or impossible. When placed in an unfamiliar setting, children with ASD may comfort themselves by repetitive movements (twisting of hands or blinking), making sounds, and even biting.
- Noncompliance: Children with ASD can become uncooperative in unfamiliar environments such as the sedation unit or hospital. Noncompliance can manifest as emotional outbursts and aggression with self-destructive behavior or potential to cause harm to the caregiver (e.g., slapping, kicking, or punching).
- Difficulty in assessing pain: Due to their inability to communicate, children with ASD may be unable to let caregivers know about pain and the need for analgesia. The child with ASD may manifest pain as tantrums or emotional outbursts.

- Uncooperative and ritualistic behavior: Children with ASD like routines and are "creatures of habit." Breaking away from ritualistic behavior can result in behavioral problems or agitation.

Prior to the Day of Sedation

Children with ASD can be effectively sedated with the same medications commonly used for pediatric procedural sedation. It is the administration of these medications that becomes problematic due to the associated comorbidities in these patients, increasing the importance of preplanning and advance preparation. A team approach involving the child's parents/primary caregivers, child life specialists, sedation nurses, and sedationists is required (Box 11.2.1).

Probing for a detailed history from the parents regarding the severity of the disorder (mild, moderate, or severe with complete inability to communicate) and any violent behavior is required for best care. Many sedation programs now have an "autism coping plan" detailing the child's behavior, sensory cues, and triggers for tantrums, agitation, and violent behaviors. The plan can outline the specifics of what best calms the child (e.g., a favorite toy or game) so that the parents and staff can ensure it is provided. The plan can also include how the child expresses pain. Parents should be given clear instructions about fasting times and what to expect on the day of sedation, such as the need for their help to administer an oral or intranasal premedication before intravenous access.

Children with ASD should be scheduled as the first case in the morning since preparation and sedation will take longer than the non-ASD child. Another reason to schedule early in the day is that the ASD patient may have anxiety and agitation if kept fasting longer than necessary or if the sedation is delayed.

Prescreening for ASD children is similar to that of non-ASD children. A referral to an anesthesiologist should be made for the same anatomic, physiologic, or comorbid reasons that any child would be referred.

BOX 11.2.1. Pre-Visit Information from Parent/Caregiver for a Child with ASD

From professional sources:

Referral information
Information from child's autism treatment team

From family:

Severity of ASD and baseline behavioral profile
Triggers of anxiety and stress
History of violent behavior and need for additional personnel to restrain
Identifying the "go-to person" for comfort and calming down
Comfort factors: favorite toys, electronic devices/videos, music, and food/beverage items
Previous experience/difficulty with sedation or anesthesia
Recent illness

Encourage early involvement of child life specialist:

To make a plan with family for the child prior to arrival
Recovery and discharge planning

Facilities that sedate a lot of children with ASD may designate a particular room within the sedation suite or radiology department for these patients that is far away from general noise and environmental stimulation. Such a room should have minimal furniture, a closable door, and even a "Do not disturb" sign. Nurses should be trained on how to approach these children, including spot-checking vital signs, clustering care, and including parents in the care of the child (Box 11.2.2).

BOX 11.2.2. Presedation and Sedation Considerations for a Child with ASD

Schedule as the first case in the morning.

Preregister or skip registration and bring patient straight to the "prepared" sedation room.

Decrease patient stimulation by decreasing noise, bright lights, etc.

Cluster care using same nurse and with help of family/caregiver.

Involve child life specialists early during waiting period and until patient is sedated and also at recovery.

Limit fasting time.

Avoid stress/agitation triggers.

Provide comfort factors (toys, blankets, etc.) right from the beginning.

Premedicate prior to obtaining intravenous access if possible.

Recognize and manage pain early during procedure.

On the Day of Sedation

A complete focused presedation assessment needs to be performed on the day of sedation; however, the child may be uncooperative and the sedation physician may not be able to perform a detailed physical exam, especially of the airway. In light of this limitation, if the patient has grossly normal craniofacial and neck anatomy, the sedationist may have to assume the patient's airway is normal and sedate the child, provided the history does not suggest a contraindication. Forcing a physical examination using a tongue blade or physical restraint in a child with ASD may increase anxiety and agitation and could be dangerous to the patient and staff.

Child life specialists should establish rapport with the patient before the physical exam. They can use pictorial boards to prepare the child or toolkits containing toys geared toward the child with ASD or help to implement soothing sensory input.

Additional help, including nurses, security personnel, or even a behavioral therapist from an autism center specifically trained in restraining violent teenagers with ASD, may be required. It is important not to separate the child from an attachment figure such as the mother or other caregiver. Electronic tablets, music therapy, and so forth can be used during placement of an intravenous line in children with less severe forms of ASD.

Drugs for Use in Patients with ASD

Premedication before intravenous access should be considered, especially in patient with milder forms of ASD. Nitrous oxide, midazolam, and dexmedetomidine are options. Intramuscular ketamine may be used for patients with moderate or severe forms of ASD. Premedication may be difficult or impossible to administer in a child with severe autism.

A variety of sedative agents and regimens have been used in patients with ASD; the choice is made based on patient characteristics (e.g., anxiety, agitation, allergy, anatomy, comorbidity profile) and properties required for successful procedural completion (e.g., degree of motion tolerated, procedural pain). In some instances, higher doses may be needed, so it is vital for the sedation team to be prepared for rescue intervention.

Recovery/Discharge from Sedation

For the ASD patient in recovery, emerging from sedation in an unfamiliar environment can be particularly traumatic and can trigger a state of agitation that causes harm to the patient or others. Parents or familiar caregivers must be present during the recovery process

BOX 11.2.3. Postsedation Recovery Process in Child with ASD

Maintain a quiet environment.
Keep family/caregiver at bedside during recovery.
Provide beverage/food of comfort when awake and ready.
Keep same nurse who had helped with presedation and during the sedation process.
Treat any postprocedure nausea vomiting prophylactically.
Recognize and manage pain early during recovery process.

(Box 11.2.3). If the patient is allowed to eat or drink, then the child's favorite beverage or food item should be immediately available. Vigilance about the need for analgesia, especially for non-radiology procedural sedation, is key to preventing stress or agitation.

Conclusion

A multidisciplinary team approach is needed for procedural sedation of children with ASD. From the time of scheduling to entry into the sedation unit, the involvement of the family, child life specialists, and experienced nurses and sedation providers is pivotal to a successful outcome. It is important to gather enough information about the triggers of the child's stress as well as factors that help calm the child in an unfamiliar environment and work toward maintaining consistency of care. Such an approach decreases anxiety and prevents agitation/tantrums in this patient population. Hospitals are now developing coping plans with the help of child life specialists; research is needed to evaluate the success of such plans.

Suggested Reading

Kamat PP, Bryan LN, McCracken CE, Simon HK, Berkenbosch JW, Grunwell JR. Procedural sedation in children with autism spectrum disorders: A survey of current practice patterns of the society for pediatric sedation members. *Paediatr Anaesth.* 2018 Jun;28(6):552–557. doi: 10.1111/pan.13387. Epub 2018 May 6.

Kamat PP, Karaga MK, Wisniewski BL, McCracken CE, Simon HK, Sidhu R, Grunwell JR. Outpatient Procedural Sedation of Patients With Autism Spectrum Disorders for Magnetic Resonance Imaging of the Brain Using Propofol. *J Child Neurol.* 2018 Apr;33(5):313–319. doi: 10.1177/0883073817753908. Epub 2018 Feb 14.

Lai MC, Lombardo MV, Baron-Cohen S. Autism. *Lancet.* 2014;383:896–910.

Taghizadeh N, Davidson A, Williams K, Story D. Autism spectrum disorder (ASD) and its perioperative management. *Paediatr Anaesth.* 2015;25:1076–1084.

Vlassakova BG, Emmanouil DE. Perioperative considerations in children with autism spectrum disorder. *Curr Opin Anaesthesiol.* 2016;29:359–366.

References

1. Christensen DL, Baio J, Van Naarden Braun K, et al. Prevalence and characteristics of autism spectrum disorder among children aged 8 years—autism and developmental disabilities monitoring network, 11 sites, United States, 2012. *MMWR Surveill Summ.* 2016;65:1–23.
2. Carbone PS, Young PC, Stoddard GJ, et al. A comparison of ambulatory care sensitive hospitalizations among children with and without autism spectrum disorder. *Acad Pediatr.* 2015;15:626–635.
3. Cooper AS, Friedlaender E, Levy SE, et al. The implications of brain MRI in autism spectrum disorder. *J Child Neurol.* 2016;31:1611–1616.
4. Hirata I, Mohri I, Kato-Nishimura K, et al. Sleep problems are more frequent and associated with problematic behaviors in preschoolers with autism spectrum disorder. *Res Dev Disabil.* 2016;49–50:86–99.
5. Oliveira G, Diogo L, Grazina M, et al. Mitochondrial dysfunction in autism spectrum disorders: a population-based study. *Dev Med Child Neurol.* 2005;47:185–189.
6. Loo CY, Graham RM, Hughes CV. The caries experience and behavior of dental patients with autism spectrum disorder. *J Am Dent Assoc.* 2008;139:1518–1524.

11.3

The Child with Cerebral Palsy

JENNIFER K. GILLEN AND JOANNE M. HOJSAK

Cerebral palsy (CP) is a nonprogressive disorder resulting from an injury to the brain before, during, or slightly after birth that affects motor function. This disorder is a leading cause of childhood motor disability, affecting between 2 and 2.5 per 1,000 live births in developed countries.[1,2,3,4] While the lesion causing CP is static, the clinical picture is variable and evolves over time. Patients may have only minor motor symptoms in one limb; at the other extreme, they may be unable to control their arms, legs, and oropharyngeal and airway muscles and have poor gut motility.

Attempts to classify the variation in order to guide management are imperfect, but the most popular system is the Swedish classification, which is based on the type of motor symptoms. The approach to a person with CP needs to be specific to each individual patient's symptoms and needs.

All CP patients have motor disability, but many also have additional nonmotor comorbidities. The likelihood of nonmotor symptoms increases with the involvement of more limbs and a greater degree of spasticity.[1] Those with spastic quadriplegia may have bulbar muscle involvement, causing problems with swallowing and creating the potential for malnutrition and aspiration.[1] Recurrent pneumonia from aspiration, with inability to clear the airway, is often the cause of death in CP patients.[2] In addition, a patient may have cognitive impairment, communication and behavior issues, vision or hearing loss, seizures, gastrointestinal motility problems, respiratory insufficiency, and orthopedic concerns that develop as the child grows in the setting of muscle spasticity.[1] Management of these comorbidities often requires procedural intervention with sedation, and in general, the more severe the CP symptoms, the greater the risk of complications during a procedure.[3]

Discussion

The considerations for sedating a patient with CP can be broken down into three categories: preprocedural assessment, procedural concerns, and postprocedural management. The intelligence of patients with CP can be underestimated because of their motor and communication difficulties.[1] Also, they often have multiple prior experiences with procedures, leading to potential increase in anxiety, as well as a higher likelihood of latex allergy.[4] In addition, the comorbidities discussed earlier often require chronic pharmacologic management, which may affect the procedure. For these reasons, the family or caretakers should be partners in the patient's care.

Preprocedural assessment for CP patients should focus on deficits and comorbidities. Epilepsy occurs in about 30% of CP patients.[1,2] Careful management of antiepileptic drugs surrounding and during a procedure is important to efficient return to baseline health. Airway and breathing problems are of significant concern. Aspiration is common and can lead to chronic lung disease. Impaired coughing mechanisms may result in recurrent pulmonary infection, as well as prolonged recovery following procedures requiring sedation. In turn, management of aspiration and pulmonary infections can be complicated by restrictive lung disease due to scoliosis.[1] A thorough assessment of baseline respiratory health and airway tone is imperative. Gastrointestinal issues may complicate the airway concerns as well, as patients often have increased salivary gland activity and impaired swallowing. Esophageal dysmotility and sphincter dysfunction also contribute to gastroesophageal reflux.[1] Gastrostomy tubes are common in this population; the presence of a gastrostomy tube should alert the provider to preexisting concerns about swallowing, aspiration, or both.

Sedation plans for a patient with CP may differ from the standard management. Positioning may not be optimal, due to scoliosis and contractures, which are present in many patients with CP.[1] Patients with cerebral palsy also have a lower bispectral index score compared to unaffected patients at the same concentration of anesthetic agents.[2] This means they may achieve a higher level of sedation than expected for a given dose of medication, especially propofol. Weakness of the airway muscles may be present,[2] resulting in a lower threshold for referral to anesthesiologists, who may manage patients with an endotracheal device during a procedure. Oral secretions and reflux can be managed with premedications. Common pharmacologic treatments for CP patients, such as antiepileptic medications and those used for spasticity such as baclofen, can affect the response to sedatives. Benzodiazepine and barbiturate drugs potentiate the effects of baclofen, increasing the risk of toxicity. Baclofen is more effective when delivered via the intrathecal route, so patients with CP often have an internal baclofen pump. Baclofen withdrawal resulting in seizures or hallucinations can be precipitated by pump malfunction during the procedure.[1] In addition, spasticity often is treated with local injections of botulinum toxin. Overall, patients with CP may have unexpected differences in their response to standard medications used for sedation. These response variations, in combination with a greater likelihood of a hypotonic airway, increase the risk associated with sedation and airway control.

Postprocedural management of CP patients can be challenging, as they are more likely to have complications during this period and may be more difficult to assess due to communication difficulties. Wass et al.[3] found that 63% of CP patients experienced some type of perioperative complication. Most of these (80%) were hypothermia or hypotension, which were not found to be life-threatening. Other complications included delayed emergence from anesthesia, seizure, pneumonia, neuropathy, and airway compromise. Risk factors found to be associated with these complications in multivariate analysis include older age, a general surgery procedure, American Society of Anesthesiologists (ASA) class higher than II, history of seizures, and upper airway hypotonia.[3] Orthopedic procedures are often more extensive in CP patients and typically should be performed under general anesthesia due to concerns about lengthy procedures and concomitant complications of respiratory insufficiency, secretion clearance, and prolonged sedation. There is a greater risk of compartment syndrome due to the risk of repeat procedures and an inability to accurately assess pain. [1,4] Pain management in CP patients is critical, as undertreatment of postprocedural pain can result in worsened spasticity, which in turn can worsen pain. Many experts recommend regional pain control strategies when available. [1,4] In addition, clonidine has been used to help control postoperative spasticity.[1,4] Opiates have also shown greater potency in CP patients, leading to an increased risk of side effects, such as respiratory depression and constipation, at standard doses.[2] This makes the use of alternative pain control modalities even more important.

Conclusion

CP is a highly variable disorder. Patients are at increased risk of complications during sedation, but the significance of this risk depends on the individual patient's symptoms. Patients often present for procedural sedation despite these risks, as these procedures help to increase the independence of the child or improve the family's ability to care for the child.[4] Understanding what to look for and how to manage patients with CP will help to decrease these risks.

References

1. Nolan J, Chalkiadis GA, Low J, et al. Anaesthesia and pain management in cerebral palsy. *Anaesthesia*. 2000;55(1):32–41.

2. Theroux MC, Akins RE. Surgery and anesthesia for children who have cerebral palsy. *Anesthesiol Clin North Am.* 2005;23(4):733–743.
3. Wass CT, Warner ME, Worrell GA, et al. Effect of general anesthesia in patients with cerebral palsy at the turn of the new millennium: a population-based study evaluating perioperative outcome and brief overview of anesthetic implications of this coexisting disease. *J Child Neurol.* 2012;27(7):859–866.
4. Wongprasartsuk P, Stevens J. Cerebral palsy and anesthesia. *Pediatr Anesth.* 2002;12(4):296–303.

11.4

The Premature Infant

JEANA E. HAVIDICH AND REBECCA H. EVANS

Preterm and ex-preterm infants are a heterogeneous, high-risk population that provides unique challenges to sedation providers. Prematurity is associated with an increased risk for sedation adverse events, including death. Extremely preterm infants (<28 weeks postgestational age [PGA]) are at the highest risk, but recent studies have shown even "late" preterm infants have significant comorbidities compared to term infants.[1]

There are several aspects to consider when developing a sedation plan in a preterm infant:

- Take a careful history, including maternal history, and perform a physical examination. The cause(s) of prematurity may alter the management of sedation and should be determined before initiating a sedation plan.
- Be aware of the differences in the anatomy and physiology of preterm infants, including their limited physiologic reserve, which contribute to the development of adverse events in this population (Table 11.4.1).
- Keep in mind the hazards associated with transportation of preterm infants. The immediate presence of personnel with

TABLE 11.4.1 Anatomic and physiologic differences in preterm children

System	*Anatomic Differences*	*Physiologic Effect*	*Considerations*
Airway/Respiratory			
	Smaller airways Decreased functional residual capacity (FRC)	Alveolar collapse	Predisposed to hypoxia Increased work of breathing
	Subglottic stenosis	Increased work of breathing	Airway obstruction/hypoxia Smaller endotracheal tube required Development of croup if intubated
	Decreased surfactant	V/Q mismatch	Hypoxia Bronchopulmonary dysplasia Reactive airways
	Tracheobronchomalacia, laryngomalacia	Airway obstruction	Hypoxia Difficult to extubate
	Immature diaphragmatic muscles	Increased work of breathing	Hypoxia Hypercapnia

	Decreased number of type 1 diaphragmatic muscle fibers; ineffective accessory respiratory muscles; noncalcified rib cartilage	Increased work of breathing	Hypercapnia Hypoxia Apnea
Cardiovascular	Unorganized myocardial tissue Decreased myocardial tissue	Decreased compliance	Cardiac output dependent on heart rate Increased dependence on calcium
	Open patent ductus arteriosus (PDA)	Pulmonary hypertension Congestive heart failure	Sedatives can worsen pulmonary hypertension. Congestive heart failure resulting in cardiac arrest
Neurologic			
	Immature central nervous system	Central apnea Biphasic response to hypoxia Hypoventilation	Hypoventilation Apnea (procedural and postprocedural; reduced with use of methylxanthines) Hypercarbia Increased risk of intraventricular hemorrhage

(Continued)

TABLE 14.1.1 Continued

System	*Anatomic Differences*	*Physiologic Effect*	*Considerations*
	Autoregulation not well developed	Abnormal baroreceptor responses	Sensitive to hypovolemia
	Retinopathy of prematurity	Decreased vision	Use lowest oxygen level acceptable to maintain acceptable oxygenation
	Impaired thermoregulation	Stress response activated	Increased oxygen requirements Acidosis Apnea Hypoglycemia
Hepatic	Decreased metabolic proteins and glycogen storage	Immature function	Prolonged drug effects Bleeding Hypoglycemia Cholestasis Altered sedative drug binding
Renal	Decreased size and number of nephrons	Reduced creatinine clearance	Electrolyte abnormalities Prolonged effect of renally excreted drugs

appropriate equipment to care for the infant and manage any adverse events is vital.

- Make sure the procedural site is ready and able to maintain patient stability and manage emergency situations.
- Review procedural aspects such as invasiveness, necessity for immobility, location, and experience of the proceduralist.
- Determine whether performance of a safe, successful procedure requires sedation.

Scientific evidence regarding the care of these children during sedation is limited. Consultation with a neonatologist and/or pediatric anesthesiologist is advised before caring for complex children.

Is Sedation Required?

Reports of adverse neurodevelopmental outcomes have prompted sedation and anesthesia providers to explore nonpharmacologic methods for noninvasive or mildly painful procedures (see Chapter 9.5).[2–5] However, frequent exposure to painful stimuli has been associated with adverse outcomes; therefore, the impact of chronic pain/stress versus the administration of sedatives or analgesia should be determined for each patient. Discussions with providers involved in the care of the patient may help determine what level of sedation is required. Nonpharmacologic techniques (e.g., administration of sucrose, feeding and swaddling, and the use of immobilizers) may be attempted in nonurgent nonpainful studies to minimize the patient's exposure to sedatives. If a "feed and swaddle" technique is used, it should be made clear that if the sedation fails, the procedure would be delayed until deemed safe by the sedation provider. For minimally painful procedures, the use of acetaminophen and local anesthesia has been shown to be effective.

Anatomic and Physiologic Differences

Anatomic and physiologic differences in preterm infants may contribute to the development of adverse events. One of the most important differences pertains to the airway and respiratory system, so airway management is a critical component of the sedation plan (see Table 11.4.1).

Medications

Because preterm neonates have altered pharmacokinetics and pharmacodynamics, titration of sedative drugs is recommended. Prolonged clearance times have been reported with propofol, neuromuscular blockers, and narcotics. Medications that are frequently used to provide sedation in preterm patients may include fentanyl, morphine, remifentanil, propofol, midazolam, dexmedetomidine, and ketamine. Please see the Appendix for details on the dose and routes for administration of these medications.

Assessment Tools for Sedation

The Neonatal Pain, Agitation and Sedation Scale (N-PASS) is a validated and reliable tool for assessing pediatric patients <1 year old, including premature infants and mechanically ventilated infants.[6] The scale assesses five noninvasive domains to determine the level of sedation of a neonate: crying or irritability, behavior state, facial expression, extremity tone, and vital signs. Each domain's score ranges from -2 to $+2$, with a summative negative score associated with a deeper level of sedation. The score is also adjusted based on the corrected gestational age for prematurity. The sedation tool can be downloaded from the developer's website (http://www.anestesiarianimazione.com/2004/06c.asp).

Special Considerations

Apnea

Apnea (mixed, central, and obstructive) is more common in preterm infants than term infants. In general, the more preterm the patient, the higher risk of apnea after administration of sedation, as is also the situation with anesthesia. Risk factors that increase the development of apnea include postconceptual age (lesser PCA = higher risk), history of apnea, type of procedure, and anemia (defined as a hematocrit <30%).[7–9] Apnea may occur even if the patient does not have a history of apnea. Most apneic events occur within the first 24 hours; however, apnea has been reported as long as 48 hours after procedures in extremely premature infants. Intravenous caffeine has been reported to decrease the occurrence of apnea but should not be considered a substitute for close monitoring.[9] Policy on admission for monitoring preterm infants after administration of sedation varies, so consultation with institutional policies is suggested. A longstanding recommendation for preterm infants has included admission with postsedation monitoring for at least 12 hours.

Hypothermia

Premature infants are more susceptible to hypothermia since thermoregulation is not well developed until 6 months of age. These children are dependent in part on non-shivering thermogenesis. Also, their thin underdeveloped skin, decreased subcutaneous fat, and large mass-to-surface ratio contribute to the rapid development of hypothermia. Measures to decrease hypothermia include transporting infants in warmed incubators, blankets, wrapping in plastic covering, forced air warmer, chemical gel-filled warming pads, warming intravenous fluids, and warmed humidifiers. Complications of hypothermia include acidosis, apnea, impaired immune function, pulmonary hypertension, delayed metabolism of drugs, bradycardia, somnolence, and death.[10,11]

Glucose Metabolism

Preterm infants are predisposed to hyperglycemic and hypoglycemic events. The stress of the procedure may contribute to the development of hyperglycemia in patients receiving glucose-containing solutions. However, hypoglycemia may occur in preterm infants due to their decreased glycogen stores and low body fat. Glucose levels should be carefully monitored and adjustments made accordingly.

Neurotoxicity/Apoptosis

The human brain completes development of neurocognitive pathways up through the 3rd year of life. With the increasing prevalence of neurocognitive disease in young children, researchers are exploring the role of sedation and anesthetic agents in regards to cell growth and development.[12] At the time of this publication, there are no recommendations for which medications should or should not be used for sedation, although the need for a procedure requiring sedation should be carefully considered.

Suggested Reading

Anderson BJ, Allegaert K. The pharmacology of anaesthetics in the neonate. *Best Pract Res Clin Anaesthesiol.* 2010;24(3):419–431.

Bayley G. Special considerations in the premature and ex-premature infant. Anaesth Intensive Care Med. 2014;15(3):107–110. doi:10.1016/j.mpaic.2014.01.001.

Coté CJ, Wilson S, American Academy of Pediatrics, American Academy of Pediatric Dentistry. Guidelines for monitoring and management of pediatric patients before, during, and after sedation for diagnostic and therapeutic procedures: update 2016. *Pediatrics.* 2016;45(2):20161212.

Hall RW. Anesthesia and analgesia in the NICU. *Clin Perinatol.* 2012;39(1):239–254.

Haney B, Reavey D, Atchison L, et al. Magnetic resonance imaging studies without sedation in the neonatal intensive care unit: safe and efficient. *J Perinat Neonat Nurs.* 2010;24(3):256–266.

Harris J, Ramelet AS, van Dijk M, et al. Clinical recommendations for pain, sedation, withdrawal and delirium assessment in critically ill infants and children: an ESPNIC position statement for healthcare professionals. *Intensive Care Med.* 2016;42(6):972–986.

Havidich JE, Beach M, Dierdorf SF, et al. Preterm versus term children: analysis of sedation/anesthesia adverse events and longitudinal risk. *Pediatrics.* 2016;137(3):e2015–0463.

References

1. McLaurin KK, Hall CB, Jackson EA, et al. Persistence of morbidity and cost differences between late-preterm and term infants during the first year of life. *Pediatrics.* 2009;23(2):653–659.
2. Gano D, Andersen SK, Glass HC, et al. Impaired cognitive performance in premature newborns with two or more surgeries prior to term-equivalent age. *Pediatr Res.* 2015;78(3):323–329.
3. McPherson C, Grunau RE. Neonatal pain control and neurologic effects of anesthetics and sedatives in preterm infants. *Clin Perinatol.* 2014;41(1):209–227.
4. Rappaport BA, Suresh S, Hertz S, et al. Anesthetic neurotoxicity—clinical implications of animal models. *N Engl J Med.* 2015;372(9):796–797.
5. FDA Drug Safety Communication: FDA review results in new warnings about using general anesthetics and sedation drugs in young children and pregnant women. U.S. Food and Drug Administration. https://www.fda.gov/Drugs/DrugSafety/ucm532356.htm. Published 2016. Accessed March 6, 2017.
6. Hummel P, Puchalski M, Creech SD, Weiss MG. Clinical reliability and validity of the N-PASS: neonatal pain, agitation and sedation scale with prolonged pain. *J Perinatol.* 2007;28(1):55–60.
7. Walther-Larsen S, Rasmussen LS. The former preterm infant and risk of post-operative apnoea: recommendations for management. *Acta Anaesthesiol Scand.* 2006;50(7):888–893.
8. Kurth CD, Coté CJ. Postoperative apnea in former preterm infants. *Anesthesiology.* 2015;123(1):15–17.

9. Henderson-Smart DJ, Steer P. Caffeine versus theophylline for apnea in preterm infants. *Cochrane Database Syst Rev*. 2010;(1):CD000273.
10. Reynolds L, Beckmann J, Kurz A. Perioperative complications of hypothermia. *Best Pract Res Clin Anaesthesiol*. 2008;22(4):645–657.
11. Doufas AG. Consequences of inadvertent perioperative hypothermia. *Best Pract Res Clin Anaesthesiol*. 2003;17(4):535–549.
12. Stratmann G. Review article: neurotoxicity of anesthetic drugs in the developing brain. *Anesth Analg*. 2011;113(5):1170–1179.

12

Diagnostic and Therapeutic Procedures

12.1

Magnetic Resonance Imaging and Computed Tomography Imaging Sedation

AMBER ROGERS

Magnetic resonance imaging (MRI) and computed tomography (CT) are among the most common procedures to require some level of pediatric sedation. These procedures are painless but necessitate immobility for adequate imaging quality. This section will review the aspects of sedation that are particularly important to consider during these procedures and will describe techniques to optimize safety, efficacy, and efficiency.

MRI

MRI Sedation—Who Needs It?

MRI scans are ordered with increasing frequency in pediatrics for diagnosis and monitoring of many different conditions. While the MRI scan is not painful, the small confined space of the magnet bore, loud noises emitted, need for complete immobility, and relatively long duration make sedation frequently necessary for successful completion of this procedure. Despite efforts to make sedation as safe as possible, every sedation encounter carries some level of risk to the patient. Thus, facilitating successful completion of the MRI without sedation is in the best interest of the patient and often within the scope of practice of the sedation provider. Many children are able to successfully complete the MRI without sedation, but accurately predicting who can and who cannot is often challenging.

Developmentally normal children at least 7–8 years old frequently do not require sedation for a typical 30- to 60-minute MRI, although significant anxiety and attention-deficit/hyperactivity disorder comorbidities may make sedation necessary even in older children. Some centers will schedule "borderline sedation" patients with sedation but allow a few minutes for the patients to attempt the MRI without sedation first with sedation as a backup, while others will initially schedule these patients without sedation and then reschedule them for a sedation appointment if needed. The use of MRI-safe video goggle systems that play movies or MRI-safe headphones for music can greatly facilitate completing the MRI without sedation; although expensive, patients and parents very much appreciate these tools. Sedation may also be avoided in young infants (<3 months old) via the "feed and wrap" technique that facilitates natural sleep.

Considerations Due to the Magnet Effects

Given that the MRI magnet is always on, sedation administration and monitoring must be tailored to the MRI environment to minimize the risk of ferrous objects becoming projectiles via the pull of the magnet. MRI-compatible patient monitors and infusion pumps maintain the same level of safety in the scanner as in other sedation locations. Most MRI suites have a monitoring area immediately outside the MRI room where the MRI technologist controls the MRI and the sedation provider can monitor the patient. A window between the two areas and/or a video camera system aimed at the patient will enable the patient to be visualized despite the physical separation.

Capnography for monitoring ventilation is particularly important due to the impaired ability to directly visualize chest rise and assess for airway complications. Rescue equipment (e.g., bag-valve-mask or anesthesia circuit connected to the oxygen source, suction, oral/nasal airways) must always be immediately available.

Medication Regimens

Medication selection for MRI sedation varies greatly based upon institutional policies and sedation provider training. Table 12.1.1 describes advantages and disadvantages of different medications and some key points.

Nuclear Medicine Procedures (MIBG, Bone Scan, SPECT Scan)

The sedation requirements for these scans are similar to MRIs within a generally more forgiving environment. They are painless but require the patient to be motionless for a relatively long duration. Nuclear medicine procedures are quieter (no loud MRI banging noises) and involve less confining machines than in MRI. Many patients can complete the procedures without needing sedation at a younger age. If sedation is needed, generally lower doses of medications may be used. Sedation providers may monitor the patient directly instead of from a separate room.

CT

CT Sedation—Who Needs It?

CT scans typically last between seconds to a few minutes, so many patients can be successfully scanned without needing sedation with good child life and behavioral interventions. However, some patients cannot cooperate with the scan without great distress (e.g.,

TABLE 12.1.1 MRI medication regimen options

Medication	*Key Points to Consider*
Propofol	+ Rapid induction of deep sedation
	+ Rapid recovery
	– Significant airway side effects (upper airway obstruction, respiratory depression, laryngospasm)
	– Hypotension (be careful in hypovolemic patients and after long NPO times)
	– Requires infusion or repeated boluses to maintain sedation for long MRIs
	– Need rapid access to reliable backup/rescue system in case of airway emergency
	– Use may be restricted to only anesthesia-trained providers in some institutions
Dexmedetomidine	+ Very little effect on the airway
	– Bradycardia is common during intravenous induction, generally alleviated by slowing the rate of administration
	– Hypotension can occur during maintenance infusion
	– Typically longer induction and recovery times than propofol
	– Despite not causing airway obstruction, dexmedetomidine does not resolve it either; use with care in children with sleep apnea.
Propofol + dexmedetomidine	+ Can minimize side effects of both medications via lower doses of each (~50% of typical doses)
	+ Airway reflexes usually maintained, so airway obstruction or laryngospasm is less likely than with propofol alone
	+ Faster recovery than with dexmedetomidine alone
Pentobarbital	– High rates of emergence delirium and long recovery times

autistic children, "willful" toddlers), and the inclination to "just hold them down and get it done" should be avoided to deliver sensitive patient and family-centered care (see Chapter 11.2 for details on sedation for autistic children).

Medication Regimen

The duration of the sedation medication effect should match as closely as possible the procedure duration. CT scans are quite short, so fast-on/fast-off medications are well suited:

- Propofol—very effective and efficient; one bolus is usually all that is needed to sedate in seconds, complete the scan, and facilitate patient arousal within minutes
- Etomidate—effective and efficient with low rates of adverse events
- Nitrous oxide—fast induction and recovery with no intravenous access needed, but given the lighter level of sedation, the patient should be somewhat cooperative to tolerate mask placement
- Intranasal or intravenous dexmedetomidine—effective but requires longer induction and recovery times
- Oral or intranasal midazolam—slightly less effective, with higher adverse event rates than the aforementioned medications
- Pentobarbital—not ideal for CT sedation due to its long duration of action and higher likelihood of emergence delirium

Summary

MRI and CT scans frequently require sedation to obtain excellent imaging quality and to provide appropriate patient care. Multiple medication regimens may facilitate completion of the study, but consideration of safety, efficacy, and efficiency help guide appropriate care.

Suggested Reading

Antonov N, Ruzal-Shapiro C, Morel K, et al. Feed and wrap MRI technique in infants. *Clin Pediatr.* 2017;56(12):1095–1103.

Boriosi J, Eickhoff J, Klein K, Hollman G. A retrospective comparison of propofol alone to propofol in combination with dexmedetomidine for pediatric 3T MRI sedation. *Pediatr Anesth.* 2016;27(1):52–59.

Mallory M, Baxter A, Kost S. Propofol vs. pentobarbital for sedation of children undergoing magnetic resonance imaging: results from the Pediatric Sedation Research Consortium. *Pediatr Anesth.* 2009;19(6):601–611.

Mekitarian Filho E, Robinson F, de Carvalho W, Gilio A, Mason K. Intranasal dexmedetomidine for sedation for pediatric computed tomography imaging. *J Pediatr.* 2015;166(5):1313–1315.

Phelps J, Russell A, Lupa M et al. High-dose dexmedetomidine for noninvasive pediatric procedural sedation and discharge readiness. *Pediatr Anesth.* 2017;25:877–882.

12.2

Radiation Therapy

BRYAN P. MCKEE AND NICOLE M. JOHNSON

Radiation therapy involves the use of high-energy waves and/or matter to damage and kill cancer cells by altering their DNA. Multiple therapeutic modalities are available, and the treatment method is chosen by the patient's oncology team. When consulted, the goal of the sedationist is to maintain the optimal environment, in terms of patient safety and immobility, for the radiation oncology team to provide the most effective treatment. Several unique aspects of radiation therapy should be considered when evaluating a patient for concomitant procedural sedation.

Indications

Radiation therapy continues to expand as a therapeutic option in the treatment of many childhood cancers and is used to treat brain cancer, bone cancer, Hodgkin lymphoma, neuroblastoma, retinoblastoma, Wilms tumor, and sarcomas, among others.

Radiation therapy is delivered in three ways: external therapy, internal therapy (brachytherapy), and systemic therapy. External radiation therapy involves the delivery of photon, proton, or electron beams via a linear accelerator to the tumor to disrupt the tumor DNA and kill the tumor cells. It produces damage to all tissues to which the radioactive therapy is delivered, as well as those surrounding the treatment area. Proton beam therapy is gaining popularity as a treatment using external radiation therapy based on the Bragg peak, which is the depth point at which accelerated protons deposit most of their radioactive energy, thus decreasing the damage to normal tissues. Brachytherapy involves the implantation of radioactive implants within or near the tumor, which is often done under general anesthesia. Systemic therapy is the delivery of a radioactive drug parenterally or orally to treat certain types of cancers.

Procedural sedation is most frequently requested for external radiation therapy and is not commonly requested for brachytherapy or systemic radiation therapy. Regardless of the method of external radiation used, patient immobility contributes greatly to successful therapy. The use of procedural sedation minimizes mobility, thus allowing the external radiation beams to more effectively target the tumor cells and spare normal cells. This therapy is often performed 5 days a week for up to 7 weeks to damage tumor cells while allowing normal tissue recovery time.

Process

As the patient enters into a therapeutic relationship with the oncology team, a referral to the radiation oncology team will begin the process of planning radiation therapy. This process often begins before the patient meets the pediatric sedation team. We recommend that the sedationist and sedation team meet the patient early in this process, ideally during image-guided simulation, which occurs before the first treatment session. The radiation oncology team, including physicians, nurses, medical physicists, and dosimetrists, use image-guided simulation to develop the patient-specific treatment plan. Simulation involves the following:

- Imaging the target area (e.g., CT, MRI) to define the tumor and location for treatment
- Planning the radiation therapy path

- Marking the patient's body to provide an optimal landmark, ensuring treatment reproducibility.

Simulation can also serve as a time to introduce the patient and family to the entire staff and to familiarize the patient with the treatment suite.

During simulation the sedationist should prepare for the technical challenges of therapy by considering the anatomic location of the targeted therapy, as each affects the delivery of sedation in a different way. For example, delivery of external radiation therapy to the brain, head, and neck requires precise reproducible positioning and may be assisted by a custom-fitted head, face, and/or neck mask with the patient in supine position (Figure 12.2.1). The mask serves as a guide to help direct the external radiation beam to the same target area at every treatment. However, the mask, which often encompasses the

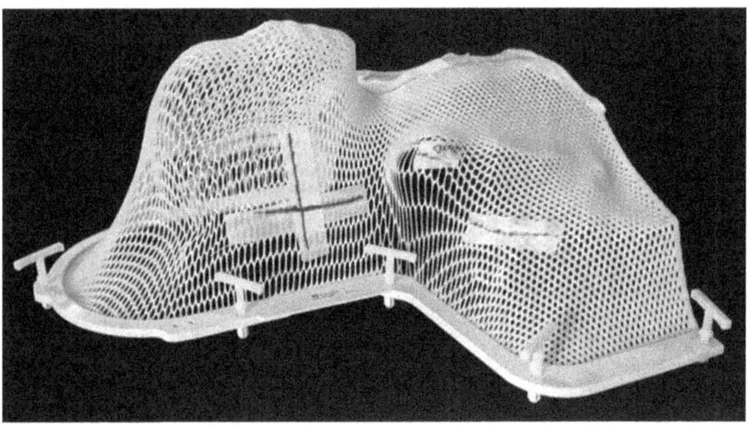

FIGURE 12.2.1.

Picture of a facial mask used for targeting beam therapy. Color markings are patient-specific for targeting beams. The mask may be customized to allow safe therapeutic delivery and monitoring. (Photo credit: Matt Sugerik, University Hospitals Cleveland Medical Center)

entire head, may pose difficulty with monitoring end-tidal CO_2, supplemental delivery of oxygen, and rescue maneuvers (see Chapter 9).

The sedationist should know the underlying diagnosis for the radiation therapy, the targeted area of radiation therapy, comorbid conditions, and any history of chemotherapy and its side effects. He or she should communicate with the radiation oncology team about sedation and monitoring needs.This will allow the sedationist to anticipate any technical challenges and potential sequelae affecting the sedation and recovery course. The information obtained from the simulation session and subsequent therapeutic sessions will provide the oncology and sedation teams with the required data for the safest and most effective treatment for the patient. As this process is ongoing, the sedationist and team must be willing to adapt to each individual patient and process.

In planning for the first radiation treatment session, the sedationist should know that the delivery of radiation therapy is acutely painless, so no tactile or painful stimulation is expected once optimal patient position has been achieved. The sedationist must be aware of the restrictions that positioning plays in the rescue of an apneic patient, a patient who needs airway clearance of secretions or emesis, or one who needs attention to the airway from anatomic obstructive hypoxia, should that include a head mask or not. Monitoring and therapeutic devices must not be placed in the treatment area (e.g., intravenous lines, blood pressure monitoring, pulse oximetry monitoring).

Medication Selection

To date no studies have found an absolute contradiction to sedative use during radiation therapy. Therefore, various medications are available to the sedationist, and the choice should be personalized to each patient. Our practice is to primarily use propofol if no patient-specific contraindications exist.

Sedation

The goal of the procedural sedation during radiation therapy is to maximize patient immobility to produce an optimal environment for therapy targeted to the tumor cells with maximal sparing of normal tissues. Induction typically occurs in the radiation therapy suite or in an adjacent room and the patient is then transferred to the radiation therapy suite. After induction the patient is positioned on the therapy table. Infusion pumps and monitoring equipment remain in the treatment room with the patient. Immediately after patient positioning, all monitoring devices must be checked to ensure they work adequately because the team is not present in the room during the sedation but is monitoring from a control room. Monitors are viewed from a control room with multiple cameras to view the patient, monitors, and therapy equipment. Delivery of radiation therapy typically takes 15–45 minutes.

External Radiation Therapy Side Effects

The side effects from external radiation therapy are not likely to impact the risk stratification for the procedural sedation itself but may contribute to the subtle management choices to optimize the outcomes, tolerance for the patient, and success of the therapy. All radiation therapy regardless of site of delivery may cause fatigue, which may impact the delivery of medication on a day-to-day basis. Both central nervous system radiation and abdominal radiation, more commonly, may cause nausea and emesis, which are often present in patients receiving chemotherapy for their malignancy. This may require the use of antiemetics prior to procedural sedation or after recovery. Radiation can cause blistering of skin, which should be considered during placement of monitors and the head mask if applicable.

Summary

Radiation therapy is essential to the treatment of many pediatric cancers. Procedural sedation provides an immobile target and optimizes the delivery of external radiation therapy to the tumor. Tumor location, patient positioning, and comorbidities should all be considered when planning the procedural sedation. Research shows that procedural sedation can be delivered safely to patients for radiotherapy and should be considered in all patients to optimize the delivery of external radiation therapy.

Suggested Reading

Anghelescu DL, Burgoyne LL, Liu W, et a. Safe anesthesia for radiotherapy in pediatric oncology: St. Jude Children's Research Hospital experience 2004–2006. *Int J Radiat Oncol Biol Phys.* 2008;71(2):491–497.

McFadyen JG, Pelly N, Orr RJ. Sedation and anesthesia for the pediatric patient undergoing radiation therapy. *Curr Opin Anaesthesiol.* 2011;24(4):433–438.

Verma V, Beethe AB, LeRiger M, et al. Anesthesia complications of pediatric radiation therapy. *Pract Radiat Oncol.* 2016;6(3):143–154.

12.3

Voiding Cystourethrography

PATRICIA SCHERRER AND LAURA BREDBENNER

Voiding cystourethrography (VCUG) is the "gold standard" procedure for the diagnosis of vesicoureteral reflux (VUR) in children. Performed in the fluoroscopy suite, it involves transurethral catheterization of the bladder and retrograde instillation and filling of the bladder with contrast medium while the patient is supine. Fluoroscopic imaging is performed during spontaneous voiding of the instilled contrast. The typical total procedure time is 45 minutes.

Sedation or No Sedation?

For many children, especially those who require repeated VCUGs over time to monitor the status of their VUR, these procedures can be associated with significant fear and distress for the entire procedure as well as discomfort associated with catheterization and bladder filling. More than 50% of patients and their families report that the catheterization part of the procedure is the most traumatic and uncomfortable, followed by bladder filling and voiding on the fluoroscopy table. It is challenging to adequately explain catheter placement to a preschooler or a child who has just been toilet trained. The majority of parents would request sedation of some sort for their child after their first VCUG experience. Many pediatric radiologists support procedural sedation as needed for patients undergoing VCUGs to minimize anxiety and trauma (especially during the catheterization process) and to improve tolerance and quality of imaging.

However, with robust preprocedural preparation and support by child life specialists, some children, especially older children, do not require sedation. Lidocaine gel provides significant analgesia for the catheterization. It should be used with all patients, and its use in older children may obviate the need for further sedation. Lidocaine gel's onset time is 1–4 minutes and the duration of action is ~15–30 minutes. The catheter tip is coated with gel prior to the catheterization attempt; the gel may also be applied to a cotton ball or gauze and used to coat the urethral meatus for (ideally) 2–3 minutes before catheterization is attempted.

There are concerns and conflicting evidence regarding the impact of deep sedation and general anesthesia on the VCUG findings. The spontaneous voiding portion of the study may be impaired. Patients are unable to void to completion, which could limit the ability to diagnose VUR. The assessment of the potential diagnostic impact often depends on the views of each hospital's pediatric radiology group.

Child Life Involvement

The presence of child life specialists during VCUGs can promote positive coping strategies in the child and can support family member's efforts as well. Performed well in advance, intervention and teaching, including an open discussion of the entire VCUG process, have been shown to significantly reduce child and family distress. Preprocedure preparation and the use of distraction and relaxation techniques during the study, when provided by expert child life specialists, can provide a very reassuring and comforting procedural environment. Some practical tips for success include:

- Engage the child, family, and sedation and procedure teams beforehand to ensure the child will be focused on the child life specialist or parent rather than the process using the ONE VOICE © technique or similar focused distraction.

- Practice the procedure steps beforehand, including deep-breathing techniques and butterfly-wing/frog-leg positioning for catheter placement.
- With the child, select several options beforehand for distraction during the procedure based on the child's age and developmental level.
- Position a tablet or toy in the child's line of sight during the preparation and catheter placement process.
- Gently redirect the child's hands with a game or activity ("Itsy Bitsy Spider").
- Encourage the child to take a deep breath and blow it out slowly while the catheter is being placed.

Procedural Sedation Options

Nitrous oxide's anxiolytic, amnestic, and analgesic properties, as well as its rapid onset and offset and ability to be titrated, are all well matched to this procedure. It is typically utilized for catheterization only, although it can be continued throughout the fluoroscopic portion of the procedure. In many programs, it may be administered by nurses.

Midazolam provides anxiolysis and amnesia and is easy to administer. The duration of action will last for the entire procedure.

Combining midazolam and nitrous oxide is another option. The administration of nitrous oxide during the catheterization can provide better analgesia and amnesia to patients who have already received midazolam. The combination generally produces anxiolysis and minimal sedation, although the patient is more likely to become more moderately sedated than with either agent alone. Neither agent is associated with significant alterations in the spontaneous voiding period of the procedure nor with documented alteration in the degree of VUR observed.

Deep sedation/anesthesia may be indicated for children who are not adequately sedated with midazolam and/or nitrous oxide, children with previous traumatic catheterization experiences, and children who will not tolerate application of a face mask for administration of nitrous oxide. If deeper sedation is needed, consider discussing the risks/benefits of deeper sedation/anesthesia versus test results with the family, the ordering provider, and the pediatric radiologist. There are conflicting data on the impact of propofol or sevoflurane on the detection/grading of VUR. Options include ketamine, propofol, and inhaled sevoflurane. These agents can be used for catheterization only or for both catheterization and bladder filling.

Summary

VCUGs remain the mainstay of diagnosis of VUR. Children can experience discomfort and significant distress during the procedure, most commonly but not exclusively during bladder catheterization. When possible, children and families should receive support from child life specialists before and during the procedure. All children and families should receive support from Child Life Specialists before and during the procedure, and all children should receive topical analgesia with lidocaine gel. Many children's experiences are improved with the anxiolytic and amnestic properties of midazolam or with nitrous oxide, which also offer additional mild analgesia. Patients who remain frightened and distressed despite these therapies will likely benefit from a deeper level of dissociation, sedation, and/or anesthesia for successful completion of the VCUG.

Suggested Reading

Frimberger D, Mercado-Dean M-G, AAP Section on Urology, AAP Section on Radiology. Establishing a standard protocol for the voiding cystourethrography. *Pediatrics*. 2016;138(5):e20162590.

Herd DW. Anxiety in children undergoing VCUG: sedation or no sedation? *Adv Urol.* 2008:498614.

Merguerian PA, Corbett ST, Cravero J. Voiding ability using propofol sedation in children undergoing voiding cystourethrograms: a retrospective analysis. *J Urol.* 2006;176:299–302.

Noga ML, Yarr JE, Chen PE. Evaluation of sevoflurane as an anesthetic agent for voiding cystourethrograms in pediatric patients. *Can Assoc Radiol J.* 2012;63:222–227.

Zier JL, Kvam KA, Kurachek SC, Finkelstein M. Sedation with nitrous oxide compared to no sedation during catheterization for urologic imaging in children. *Pediatr Radiol.* 2007; 37:678–684.

12.4

Endoscopy

Upper Endoscopy and Colonoscopy

BARBARA DILOS AND CHERYL K. GOODEN

Two of the more commonly performed gastrointestinal (GI) procedures in children are esophagogastroduodenoscopy (EGD) and colonoscopy. The diagnostic and/or therapeutic indications for these procedures include abdominal pain, failure to thrive, vomiting, dysphagia, gastroesophageal reflux, anemia (unexplained), caustic ingestion, foreign-body removal, dilation of esophageal and upper GI strictures, and esophageal variceal banding. The sedation practices for these procedures will be described collectively unless there is something unique to either of them. For the most part, EGD and colonoscopy can be performed with sedation; generally deeper levels are required for the younger, less cooperative child. There are clinical scenarios in which these procedures will require general anesthesia and artificial airway maintenance. A discussion of general anesthesia for these GI procedures is beyond the scope of this book.

Considerations and Goals of GI Sedation

The sedation provider plays a key role to ensure a safe and successful outcome from GI endoscopy. As with all intended deep sedation, the person who is performing the endoscopic procedure should not be responsible for sedation. A second provider (sedationist) should be responsible for observing the patient's vital signs, airway, and depth of sedation. This is good practice even if moderate sedation levels are intended. It is important that the sedationist and any other members of the sedation team have a thorough understanding of the considerations for these procedures, which include the following:

- Concurrent airway patency is required during EGD.
- There must be a GI bite-block in the mouth during EGD.
- Secretions may pool in the oropharynx.
- The depth of sedation must be appropriate for endoscope placement.
- The intestinal tract will be insufflated with air.
- Possibilities exist for airway obstruction, laryngospasm, and rapid desaturation.
- Patient may require a lateral decubitus position.

Presedation Evaluation and Selection

The presedation evaluation is fundamental to the management of patients. The sedation provider must perform a thorough evaluation of the child presenting for GI endoscopy (see Chapter 6). The selection of a patient who is deemed appropriate for GI sedation is as important as the evaluation process. Some children may present with complex medical conditions that increase their risk for sedation (see Chapter 6). Factors specific to GI procedures that may contribute to a child being considered "high risk" for procedural sedation (and thus may prompt referral for general anesthesia management) include the size of the child relative to the endoscope and the predicted difficulty of the procedure (e.g., prior difficulty reaching the terminal ileum, resulting in prolonged procedure/sedation time; known GI strictures).

Premedication

Depending on the child's age and psychological maturity, premedication may be required in order to have a cooperative patient. Oral agents such as midazolam or ketamine may be used. Intramuscular ketamine or intranasal or buccal dexmedetomidine may also be considered (see the Appendix for dosing information). Apart from the use of premedication, a few other measures can be taken to improve the overall experience of the patient between the arrival time to the facility and the start of the procedure:

- Use of topical pain control products for intravenous catheter insertion
- Child life distraction techniques
- Private bathroom facilities if the GI procedure requires a final bowel preparation
- Topical anesthetic oropharyngeal spray shortly before endoscope insertion (older children and adolescents).

Monitoring

For the most part, routine monitors used during procedural sedation include an electrocardiogram, pulse oximeter, and blood pressure cuff (see Chapter 7). Often respiratory rate and effectiveness are determined by observation. In the presence of a "shared airway," as is the case with EGD, the patient's respirations may not be as readily detected solely through observation, so the use of capnography should be strongly considered during all EGD procedures; it may also be helpful during prolonged colonoscopy procedures.

GI Procedural Sedation

Several medications may be considered for GI procedures. The choice depends upon the patient's history (past and current), the length of the anticipated procedure, and whether it is a diagnostic or therapeutic procedure.

One of the key moments of GI procedural sedation occurs at the beginning of the EGD, when the endoscope is passed through the oropharynx and into the esophagus. During this time a deeper plane of sedation as well as a good line of communication with the gastroenterologist is required. There is a narrow margin for error as the level of sedation progresses from moderate sedation to deep sedation and possibly general anesthesia (see Chapter 3). The pharyngeal and laryngeal stimulation of the scope may contribute to laryngospasm and significant airway obstruction.

Commonly used medications for GI procedures include midazolam, propofol, ketamine, dexmedetomidine, fentanyl, and remifentanil (this list is not exhaustive; dosages and side effects are detailed in the Appendix). It is likely that one or more of these medications will be used during GI procedural sedation. As discussed above, EGD may require rapidly altering the level of sedation achieved early on during scope introduction. Colonoscopy is less complex at induction, but air insufflation and scope manipulation during what may be a 45- to 60-minute procedure create acute episodes of cramping and pain for which the sedationist must be prepared.

Adverse Events

There is always the possibility of an adverse event occurring during procedural sedation, and GI procedures are no exception. Early recognition and management of them are crucial. The shared airway characteristics of EGD in particular are associated with respiratory-related adverse events such as airway obstruction, laryngospasm, desaturation, and cough. The prepared sedationist will be capable of managing these events safely and efficiently, resulting in a cost-effective service and a satisfied, treated patient.

Suggested Reading

Biber J, Allareddy V, Allareddy V, et al. Prevalence and predictors of adverse events during procedural sedation anesthesia outside the operating room for esophagogastroduodenoscopy and colonoscopy in children: age is an independent predictor of outcomes. *Pediatr Crit Care Med.* 2015;16:e251–e259.

Chung H, Lightdale J. Sedation and monitoring in the pediatric patient during gastrointestinal endoscopy. *Gastrointest Endoscopy Clin North Am.* 2016;26:507–525.

Orel R, Brecelj J, Dias J, et al. Review on sedation for gastrointestinal tract endoscopy in children by non-anesthesiologists. *World Gastrointest Endosc.* 2015;7:895–911.

van Beek E, Leroy P. Safe and effective procedural sedation for gastrointestinal endoscopy in children. *J Pediatr Gastroenterol Nutr.* 2012;54:171–185.

12.5

Solid Organ Biopsies

Kidney and Liver

JENNIFER BIBER AND JENNA WHEELER

It has been shown that pediatric sedation/anesthesia outside the operating room (PSA-OOR) is safe in institutions with highly motivated and organized sedation services for various procedures.[1] While solid organ biopsies (SOBs) are routinely done on adults with only local anesthesia or minimal sedation, children frequently require deep sedation or general anesthesia to achieve acceptable conditions (stillness, anxiolysis, analgesia) to facilitate these procedures.[1–3]

Discussion

After determining that the patient is an appropriate candidate for PSA-OOR, the next step is choosing a sedation plan. SOBs present unique challenges to performing PSA-OOR, largely due to the pain caused by the procedure, the need for relative immobility, and the patient positioning required during and after the procedure (e.g., native renal biopsies).

Pain control can often be provided with a choice of sedation medication. Many sedation services rely heavily on propofol, which works well as an anxiolytic but provides no analgesia. To that end, for painful procedures, the sedationist should provide analgesia in addition to the propofol. Several options for analgesia are (1) local anesthesia (typically provided by the proceduralist; the sedationist must frequently ask for it); (2) opioids and propofol; and (3) ketamine and propofol.

For dosage information about the medications discussed in this section, see the Appendix.

Another option for pain control and sedation is to use ketamine as a solo agent. Side effects often noted with ketamine include the emergence phenomenon, which is frequently seen in patients >5 years old. This is often mitigated by administering midazolam intravenously before ketamine. Midazolam has the side effect of depressing the respiratory drive, and ketamine may also increase secretions, so the sedationist must be prepared to deal with these consequences. These may be mitigated to a certain extent by administering glycopyrrolate with the initial ketamine bolus. Ketamine is a dissociative agent, and while it does provide sedation, the team must be aware that the patient may not appear to sleep and may continue to talk through the procedure.

Inhaled nitrous oxide is another option to provide adequate sedation and analgesia for PSA-OOR SOBs. This has the added benefit of not requiring intravenous line placement and is easily reversed by removing the gas. There are potential drawbacks, however, not the least of which is requiring scavenging capabilities for the gas and education on the use of inhaled anesthetics.

Ultimately, sedation and analgesia must be provided and the choice should be determined based on the patient, organizational capabilities, and the sedation team's comfort with the drugs.

Regardless of the choice of drugs, adequate monitoring should occur during the procedure as well as during the recovery period. Monitoring is key for any sedation, but it is arguably more important for SOBs where the patient is not necessarily in a supine position. Due to prone positioning for native renal biopsies and draping for all SOBs, monitoring becomes even more important as it is often difficult to see chest rise or note any obstruction that may occur. The monitoring should include continuous pulse oximetry, capnography, continuous heart rate and plethysmography, and frequent noninvasive blood pressure monitoring.

Ideally, the sedationist will also be able to directly observe the patient and should be positioned close to the airway to help with airway maneuvers if necessary. During the procedure, vital signs should be recorded at least every 5 minutes. The sedationist must also maintain good communication with the proceduralist and should feel confident to stop the procedure if necessary.

Depending on the facility, sedations may begin in a sedation suite, in the procedure room itself, or in an anteroom. If the sedation suite is far removed from the procedure room, transport of the patient with monitoring and tools for catastrophic events should be arranged. If the patient is sedated outside the procedure room, there may be more staff required to position the patient, especially when lying face down is needed. The sedationist (or another person qualified in airway management) should maintain the airway during patient movement. If sedation is done in the procedure room, it may be helpful to have the patient assume the required position himself or herself (if cooperative) by lying face down before the sedation medications are administered. The advantage is that the patient can actively control all of his or her movements while adjusting to the prone position.

Before starting the procedure, the sedation team needs to ensure that the patient's airway is maintained and remains hemodynamically stable with the sedation, as it becomes increasingly difficult to move the patient while the biopsy is taking place. While lying prone does have the benefit of allowing the airway to open up, obstruction is still possible and the sedationist should be ready to reposition the airway and use adjuvants if necessary (i.e., oral or nasal airways and suctioning). If resuscitation is emergently needed, staff should be ready to turn a prone patient supine quickly. Having a good sedation plan and contingency plans in place, good monitoring, and good communication with the proceduralist will make this less likely to occur. The sedationist should aim to keep the patient deeply sedated during the procedure, which will optimize the biopsy and ultimately decrease the procedure and sedation time.

After the procedure, SOB patients will need to stay supine or in the right lateral decubitus position for a prescribed amount of time to allow for clot formation to occur and minimize bleeding. This varies based on the proceduralist but will be likely 4–6 hours and may be as long as 12 hours.[2,3] Many of these patients will be scheduled for inpatient monitoring following a procedure, but they could conceivably go home. They should be monitored by the sedation team until their Aldrete scores return to baseline (or following the standard of the facility) with vital signs taken at least every 15 minutes. They will then need to be monitored in an observation unit for the duration. While most children can be redirected with a combination of child life specialists, family involvement, immobilization (with papoose or other device), and other redirection techniques, a few children may have problems staying still for that amount of time. If this is the case, sedation with a low dose of dexmedetomidine may help. This would require monitoring in an intensive care unit or suitable stepdown unit (based on the facility's capabilities) and would likely delay discharge, but it could conceivably help the patient who would otherwise not be able to stay still for the prescribed amount of time. .

References

1. Cravero J, Blike G, Gallagher S, et al. Incidence and nature of adverse events during pediatric sedation/anesthesia for procedures outside the operating room: Report from the Pediatric Sedation Research Consortium. *Pediatrics.* 2006;118:1087–1096.
2. Kamat P, Ayestaran F, Gillespie S, et al. Deep procedural sedation by sedationist team for outpatient pediatric renal biopsies. *Pediatr Transplant.* 2016;20:372–377.
3. Mason K, Padua H, Fontaine P, Zurakowski D. Radiologist-supervised ketamine sedation for solid organ biopsies in children and adolescents. *AJR Am J Roentgenol.* 2009;192:1261–1265.

12.6

Pulmonary

Bronchoscopy

PAUL G. SMITH

Pediatric sedation and fiberoptic airway endoscopy (FAE) share parallel histories. Following early controversy, both are now done frequently and are essential in the care of children. Their recognized risks intersect in the respiratory system as they "share the airway." These shared risks include suppression of respiratory drive, loss of upper airway tone, compromised function from the defects necessitating FAE, airway instrumentation, and the characteristics of the child (e.g., age, degree of cooperation). The sedationist must be able to recognize risk factors, perform rescue from adverse events of sedation or airway manipulation, and anticipate additional postprocedural complications.

While surgical suites should be used for FAE procedures in patients who have significant American Society of Anesthesiologists (ASA) classification risks, some pediatric centers perform sedated FAE in endoscopy suites or intensive care units. The goals of the sedationist remain the same regardless of the setting: (1) maintenance of adequate gas exchange while facilitating assessment of the upper and lower airways (in both dynamic and static states) (2) completion of interventions such as bronchoalveolar lavage (BAL) (3) patient comfort.

Standards for pediatric FAE and sedation have been published separately, although standards for sedation specific to FAE in children have not.[1]

Setting

The setting for sedated FAE requires equipment to administer medications and to monitor and respond to cardiopulmonary events, and adequate working space for sedating and procedural personnel. If emergent establishment of an airway or conversion to rigid bronchoscopy might be necessary, an operative suite and the presence of skilled surgical personnel should be planned.

Preprocedural Assessment

The presedation assessment specific to FAE includes (1) patency of the nares, (2) craniofacial abnormalities, (3) oral cavity size and stridor, and (4) signs of lower tract parenchymal disease and wheeze. Many upper airway anatomic abnormalities are accompanied by unrecognized abnormalities in other pulmonary sites; for instance, tracheal anomalies or gastroesophageal reflux coexist in a significant percentage of infants with laryngomalacia.

FAE Indications and Interventions

Stridor

Causes of stridor vary according to age. In the young infant, laryngomalacia is the most common cause of stridor, but it usually has a benign course, so FAE is done for atypical presentation. Any cause of stridor represents a reduced cross-sectional area of the airway. A depth of sedation that allows spontaneous respiration is important so that laryngeal structure motion and symmetrical vocal cord motion can be seen, thus eliminating vocal cord paralysis from consideration. The transnasal approach is ideal because laryngeal mask airway (LMA) or endotracheal tubes obscure the anatomy. "Getting past the nose" is the most distressing part of the exam; once passed, the sedation needs lessen until prolonged examination of lower airways is necessary. The glottis structures are first inspected without topical lidocaine that might alter glottis motion. After inspection of the upper airway, inspection of the lower airways will rule out accompanying secondary lesions such as tracheomalacia. This can be done by continuing the transnasal approach, though some prefer to convert to an LMA. In either case, inspection of the lower airways requires deeper levels of sedation, and lidocaine is applied to minimize cough (Table 12.6.1).

Persistent Infiltrates/Pneumonitis

Persistent pulmonary infiltrates, either diffuse or discrete, prompt FAE in order to rule out anatomic abnormalities, determine presence of foreign bodies or mucous plugs, and often to perform BAL for diagnostic purposes. A transnasal approach is sometimes feasible, but the naris needs to accommodate a bronchoscope with a sufficiently sized working channel for suctioning. FAE through an LMA will accommodate a larger bronchoscope and improve gas exchange. If there is significant disease or baseline hypoxia, endotracheal intubation is the safest approach, as sedation and airway obstruction by the bronchoscope will worsen gas exchange. Sedation depth during BAL needs to be sufficient to minimize cough, which will "break the wedge" of the scope in a lower airway and greatly reduce both the quantity and quality of the BAL return. With BAL, a 50% return of the instilled fluid is considered a "good yield." Anticipate that lavage fluid left behind migth further worsen oxygenation until it is absorbed.

TABLE 12.6.1 General indications for FAE

Indication/Differential Diagnosis	*Considerations*	*Specific Complications*
Stridor Laryngomalacia Subglottic stenosis Vocal cord paralysis/paresis Discrete lesions (webs, cysts, papilloma)	Transnasal approach Narrowed upper airway possibly present Documentation of dynamic glottic function Possible coexisting lower airway lesions	Worsening stridor/distress from procedural swelling Laryngospasm
Persistent infiltrates Focal: airway occlusion (mucous plug, foreign body, anatomic block) Diffuse: pneumonitis, interstitial lung disease	Impaired gas exchange/hypoxia Potential need for secured airway Large working channel for suctioning, BAL Deeper sedation level to inhibit cough	Worsening hypoxia Potential need of mechanical ventilation Postprocedural cough
Chronic cough Sinusitis, reflux, asthma Laryngeal lesions Foreign body Infection (airway or parenchymal)	Inspection of upper and lower airways Potential need for BAL Potential need to convert to rigid bronchoscopy if foreign body present	Postprocedural cough Laryngospasm Bronchospasm
Atypical wheeze Asthma Tracheomalacia Discrete lesions (masses, webs, vascular ring, extrinsic compression, foreign body)	Narrowed airways Impaired ventilation Hyperresponsiveness	Worsening wheeze Airway swelling Ventilation defects
Tracheostomy evaluation Airway granuloma Tracheomalacia Airway erosion Airway infection	Need for lower and upper airway inspection Brief decannulation for thorough inspection	Airway irritation Worsening distress Bleeding Difficult tube reinsertion

Chronic Cough

There is a wide differential for chronic cough that also varies with age group. Assessment of laryngeal structures as well as lower airways is important, so a transnasal approach is often used. Dynamic assessment of both upper and lower airways is of value, so moderate or deep sedation is often preferable to general anesthesia. The possibility of an unrecognized foreign body might prompt the need to convert to rigid bronchoscopy and general anesthesia. Pretreatment with beta agonists and/or inhaled lidocaine aerosols may help minimize coughing during the procedure.

Persistent Wheeze

Persistent wheeze atypical for asthma is an indication for FAE, and the goal is usually airway inspection. When accompanied by inspiratory stridor, the presence of fixed, large airway lesions should be anticipated. Maintaining spontaneous respiration allows for observation of dynamic airway motion and promotes gas exchange. If airway hyperresponsiveness is suspected, pretreatment with beta agonists is advisable and systemic glucocorticoids are useful. In cases of tracheobronchomalacia however, beta agonists can worsen wheezing in some patients. Manipulation of the airway can temporarily worsen respiratory function through irritation and airway swelling. A level of sedation that minimizes cough and trauma from the bronchoscope is desirable.

Foreign-Body Aspiration

FAE is indicated for airway inspection when the diagnosis of foreign-body aspiration is uncertain or after foreign-body removal by rigid bronchoscopy to inspect the airways distal to the obstruction. While there are numerous reports of foreign-body removal via FAE, such attempts are made only in specific situations and when conversion to rigid bronchoscopy and emergent tracheostomy is immediately available. In each of these cases, FAE is done through an artificial airway, so general anesthesia and equipment and personnel for conversion to rigid bronchoscopy are important.

Tracheostomy Evaluation

Evaluation of tracheostomy tubes is done at regular intervals, before decannulation or for evaluation of cause of bleeding, suctioning difficulty, new-onset wheezing, or distress. A common approach is FAE first through the tracheostomy tube followed by a transnasal approach to examine the glottis and subglottis. The tracheostomy tube may be removed near the end of the procedure to fully assess for any suprastomal granulation tissue. Sedation requirements vary during the procedure, starting with light to moderate needs during the initial stages and deeper levels during the transnasal portions of the exam. General anesthesia is rarely necessary unless surgical intervention is planned. Postprocedural complications include airway swelling, cough, and difficulty with recannulation.

Sedative Choice

Midazolam/Opioid

The most frequently reported sedation for FAE is the combination of fentanyl and midazolam. The availability of reversal agents is attractive should respiratory drive be compromised. Remifentanil, as an ultrashort-acting opioid, may be used instead of fentanyl, with the same analgesic and cough-diminishing properties and the added advantage of very rapid onset and recovery.

Propofol

Propofol may be used either alone or in combination with short-acting opioids and can provide sufficiently deep sedation for FAE while maintaining respiratory drive if titrated slowly to effect. Propofol alone can be effective in decreasing cough but often is supplemented with topical lidocaine and/or short-acting opioids. The combination of propofol and remifentanil is reported to allow smaller doses of either agent and to lessen cough; it offers the advantage of a rapid return to baseline.

Ketamine

Ketamine is an attractive option for FAE sedation because it causes minimal depression of respiratory drive and has a favorable cardiovascular profile (maintenance of cardiac output and blood pressure).[2]

Dexmedetomidine

A central alpha-2 agonist, dexmedetomidine has a place in the FAE sedation armamentarium because respiratory effort is maintained and side effects are minimal. Often combined with other agents such as short-acting opioids for increased pain management, its use has been reported even during airway foreign-body removal to maintain spontaneous respirations.[3]

Adjuncts

Lidocaine, administered topically or by aerosol, is frequently used to minimize cough and allow passage of the bronchoscope below the vocal cords. The maximum safe dose is 7 mg/kg, and overdoses can lead to seizures. Atropine/glycopyrrolate use to dry secretions prior to FAE has been discouraged as ineffective.[4] However, use of atropine to prevent ketamine-induced bronchorrhea is common practice.

References

1. Faro A, Wood R, Schechter M, et al. Official American Thoracic Society Technical Standards: flexible airway endoscopy in children. *Am J Resp Critical Care Med.* 2015:191(9):1066–1080.
2. Stark J, Graff G, Berkenbosch, J. Safety and efficacy of ketamine sedation for infant flexible fiberoptic bronchoscopy. *Chest.* 2004;125(3):1132–1137.
3. Cai Y, Li W, Chen K. Efficacy and safety of spontaneous ventilation technique using dexmedetomidine for rigid bronchoscopic airway foreign body removal in children. *Pediatr Anesth.* 2013;23(11):1048–1053.
4. Silvestri G, Lamb C, Barbour S, et al. American College of Chest Physicians consensus statement on the use of topical anesthesia, analgesia, and sedation during flexible bronchoscopy in adult patients. *Chest.* 2011;140(5):1342–1350.

12.7

Cardiology

Transthoracic and Transesophageal Echocardiography, Cardioversion

JANEY PHELPS

Congenital heart disease is the most common type of birth defect and is estimated to affect nearly 1% (~40,000) of all births each year in the United States.[1] Echocardiograms are necessary to fully evaluate these defects, and depending on the age of the child, sedation may be required to ensure optimal imaging. In this section we will discuss the sedation/anesthesia options for transthoracic echocardiography, transesophageal echocardiography, and cardioversion. For all of these procedures, high-risk patients should be triaged to a pediatric anesthesia provider and in some cases, a pediatric cardiac anesthesiologist. These patients include, among others, those with unrepaired cyanotic heart disease and pulmonary hypertension.

Transthoracic Echocardiography

Transthoracic echocardiograms (TTEs) are the most common way to study basic cardiac anatomy and function. Depending on the patient's age and the complexity of the cardiac anatomy, distraction

TABLE 12.7.1 Echocardiography: risk factors associated with a need for sedation

- Patients aged 6 months to <2 years old
- Higher anatomic complexity
- Kawasaki disease

or a natural sleep state may be all that is needed to complete the procedure. However, the need for unplanned repeat procedures with sedation is associated with several risk factors (Table 12.7.1).[2] Centers should consider offering sedation to children with these risk factors to improve image quality and to avoid making preventable diagnostic errors.

If distraction techniques, such as watching a movie or interventions by child life personnel, do not produce optimal conditions for the TTE, sedation should be considered. The most stimulating parts of a TTE should be saved for the end of the exam so as not to disrupt the sedation. Historically, a successful sedation option for TTE has included chloral hydrate, but due to its unpredictable safety profile it is no longer recommended; other than as a compounded agent, it is not available in the United States. Often oral or intranasal midazolam can be used to achieve minimal sedation (see Chapter 15). If moderate sedation is required, due to patient characteristics or previous history of failure with minimal sedation, then intranasal dexmedetomidine is a good option (Table 12.7.2). The use of propofol can also be considered in these patients. However, for the most part deep sedation is not necessary for patients undergoing a TTE. Concerns about the possible neurotoxicity of many agents and the U.S. Food and Drug Administration (FDA) warning make intranasal dexmedetomidine a good choice. Dexmedetomidine is one of the few agents that is not listed on the FDA warning list for children <3 years of age (see Chapter 9.5).

TABLE 12.7.2 Sedation options for TTE, TEE, and cardioversion

Study/Procedure	*Sedation Options*	
TTE	Distraction, child life, and/or oral/intranasal midazolam for minimal sedation	If complex anatomy, age 6 months to <2 years, or Kawasaki disease, consider moderate sedation with 2.5–3 mcg/kg intranasal dexmedetomidine.
TEE	For children <2 years old, recommend intubation and general anesthesia	In children >2 years old, propofol by highly skilled provider with advanced airway skills
Cardioversion	Propofol	

Patients with unrepaired cyanotic heart disease and pulmonary hypertension should be referred to a pediatric anesthesiologist for sedation/anesthesia.

Transesophageal Echocardiography

Transesophageal echocardiograms (TEEs) provide more detailed information since the impedance from the thoracic wall is avoided; however, this is an invasive procedure. In children these studies often require deep sedation or general anesthesia (see Table 12.7.2). It is generally accepted that children <2 years of age should be intubated for TEEs. Intubations are recommended in part because the TEE scope can compress the trachea and lead to difficulty in spontaneous ventilation in infants. Children >2 years of age can be safely sedated with a propofol infusion and a native airway but should be cared for in the hands of airway and sedation experts. These children are best cared for with a highly skilled sedation service. Not only is it more challenging to maintain a deeply sedated, spontaneously ventilated patient with a TEE probe in the pharynx, but patients requiring this exam will have complex cardiac disease.

Cardioversion

Cardioversion is used to restore sinus rhythm in patients with tachyarrhythmias and is most commonly performed in adults for atrial fibrillation. Atrial fibrillation is rare in the pediatric population. There is limited data on the prevalence or types of arrhythmias that exist in children.

Cardioversion is a brief but highly stimulating procedure that requires both a short and deep level of sedation to mitigate discomfort. Deep sedation with propofol is the best way to achieve these goals (see Table 12.7.2). Discretion should be used when deep sedation is provided based on NPO status and the urgency of the cardioversion. Midazolam and fentanyl have been successfully used as well. In the pediatric population, cardioversion would be most frequently used for unstable supraventricular tachycardia.

Suggested Reading

Hammer G, Drover D, Cao H, et al. The effects of dexmedetomidine on cardiac electrophysiology in children. *Anesth Analg.* 2008;106:79–83.

Tobias J, Gupta P, Naguib A, Yates A. Dexmedetomidine: applications for the pediatric patient with congenital heart disease. *Pediatr Cardiol.* 2011;32:1075–1087.

References

1. Hoffman JL, Kaplan S. The incidence of congenital heart disease. *J Am Coll Cardiol.* 2002;39:1890–1900.
2. Stern S, Chen C, Cohen, et al. Unplanned repeat echocardiography with sedation in children: patient risk factors. *Pediatr Cardiol.* 2016;37:1057–1063.

12.8

Oncology

Bone Marrow Biopsy and Aspiration, Lumbar Puncture

GORDON GALE

Infants and children often require procedural sedation to tolerate lumbar puncture (LP) or bone marrow aspiration or biopsy. These are painful procedures that require specific positioning and some degree of immobility for successful completion. While LP or bone marrow aspiration/biopsy performed to diagnose an infection, raised intracranial pressure, or certain blood dyscrasias is a one-time event, patients with oncologic or hematopoietic disorders often need repetitive procedures over the course of months to years. The most common malignancy in childhood is acute lymphoblastic leukemia, which can affect children of all ages but is most common in the toddler, preschool age group. Protocols of therapy for these children may include as many as 25 lumbar punctures with intrathecal chemotherapy over a 2- to 3-year course of treatment and at least 2 bone marrow aspirates. Children diagnosed with solid tumors may require bone marrow aspiration/biopsy as part of their initial evaluation. Children suspected of having aplastic anemia may need multiple bone marrow biopsies over the course of their treatment. The procedural sedation techniques described in this section are appropriate as an approach to an isolated procedure, and suggestions for approaches for repetitive procedures are included.

The initial approach to anxiety, pain control, and amnesia for newly diagnosed children with oncologic disorders may affect the child's and caretaker's behavior for all future procedures.

There is a distinction to be made regarding bone marrow aspirates (BMA) and bone marrow biopsies (BMB). The sample obtained during a BMA involves only the "liquid" part of the marrow, which is diagnostic in most leukemias. The BMB involves a core of "solid" marrow, which is used to assess cellularity and the presence or absence of solid tumor metastases and may dictate malignancy staging. Children with pancytopenia (myelodysplasias, aplastic anemia) or solid tumors (lymphoma, neuroblastoma, muscle tumors) are frequently subjected to both BMA and BMB.

During any procedure involving pain and/or immobility in specific positions, particularly in the unpleasant environment of a healthcare setting, controlling the negative aspects of the environment (parental presence, for instance) and providing distraction techniques, anxiolysis, and analgesia are of the utmost importance. While there is no known direct relationship between the number of painful procedures and subsequent anxiety, distress, or uncooperative behaviors, for children who are projected to require repetitive experiences of this kind, the more negative the initial experience, the greater the risk for subsequent anxiety, distress, and lack of cooperation.

Most childhood oncology treatment regimens are heavily protocolled and planned out over several years and include specific timing of screening or diagnostic LP and bone marrow aspirates and biopsies. Children in the midst of chemotherapy cycles are often thrombocytopenic, increasing the risk of bleeding complications with procedures. Site infection is always a risk during invasive procedures in immunocompromised patients. Having a calm, cooperative, or sedated child enhances the proceduralist's ability to provide appropriate site sterilization and lessens the risk of numerous procedural attempts that increase the risk of bleeding or infectious complications. Many oncology teams provide coordinated sedation care in the oncology clinic or infusion center themselves. Other programs have been able to arrange the care of the child with a first stop in the clinic setting to check blood cell counts and administer chemotherapy with a second stop in a sedation suite for sedationist-led deep sedation, with members of the oncology team acting as the proceduralist. This latter approach often allows a sedationist familiar with the child to be available for the frequent radiologic exams that are often part of oncology treatment protocols.

Lumbar Puncture

The keys to a successfully completed LP from the proceduralist's viewpoint are (1) a calm and immobile child who can be effectively positioned for successful introduction of the needle into the subdural space; (2) clear CSF removal; and (3) smooth and slow injection of intrathecal medication. The keys from the patient's viewpoint are (1) no pain during the procedure; (2) speedy completion of the procedure; and (3) no cerebrospinal fluid (CSF) leak or headache afterwards.

Local Anesthesia

The application of a topical lidocaine patch/cream at the site of needle insertion can help with the needle injection pain, but the painful aspect of local intradermal and subcutaneous anesthesia is frequently the actual injection of the deeper local anesthetic lidocaine. One should consider injecting slowly, deeply, and generously with a very-small-gauge (27 or 30) needle. The buffering of lidocaine with sodium bicarbonate (9 parts lidocaine and 1 part sodium bicarbonate) may also help minimize the pain of injection. Many times, for children who are cooperative and not fretful, an LP can be accomplished with just local anesthesia, which avoids the inherent risks of sedation.

Positioning During the Procedure

An LP performed simply to obtain a CSF sample may be most easily accomplished in the sitting position, with the patient instructed or helped to "push" the lower back outward toward the proceduralist. For safety, no more than minimal sedation or anxiolysis is appropriate. For children who cannot sit or who are too large to be held in a sitting position, the patient is in the lateral decubitus position with the knees drawn upward and the shoulders curled inward. (If an opening pressure measurement is needed, the lateral decubitus position with the knees straightened is necessary for accurate pressure readings.) Moderate or deep sedation may be needed to ensure maintenance of a curled, lateral decubitus position throughout the procedure. In infants and young children, it is quite easy to inadvertently create airway obstruction or difficult diaphragmatic excursion with this positioning, exacerbating the potential respiratory insufficiency inherent in moderate or deep sedation. End-tidal carbon dioxide monitoring is recommended.

Positioning After the Procedure

CSF drainage with or without replacement of the volume with intrathecal chemotherapy may result in postprocedure headache. Some proceduralists recommend that the patient remain supine for about 30 minutes after lumbar puncture to reduce the chance of headache and nausea. Moderate or deep sedation achieved during the procedure is usually sufficient to achieve this goal if the child is allowed to awaken naturally in a quiet, dim environment while closely monitored for respiratory sufficiency.

Sedation Regimens

Many sedationists approach the young infant or child by providing minimal or moderate sedation with midazolam (usually given intravenously through indwelling central lines or ports for oncology patients) or deeper sedation with additional ketamine or ketamine or propofol alone before positioning. Analgesia with a bolus dose of fentanyl may be added before lidocaine injection or the LP attempt. These regimens provide amnesia, sedation, and analgesia and provide predictable onset and recovery. It is important to consider the frequency with which the oncology patient will be undergoing procedural sedation not only for LP and bone marrow aspiration and biopsies, but also for nuclear medicine and CT and MRI screening or follow-up exams. Ketamine is a very commonly used, safe medication for short, painful, isolated procedures, but many children do not tolerate repeated procedures with ketamine, exhibiting diverse emotional responses upon awakening that can be very disturbing for staff and parents as well as prolonged recovery time. Anecdotal experience, particularly in teenagers undergoing repeated LP with propofol who then received ketamine instead when propofol was unavailable, reported more unpleasant dreams, dysphoria, and more nausea after the procedure when ketamine was used.

Bone Marrow Aspiration and Biopsy

Appropriate patient positioning and immobility will enhance the success of bone marrow aspiration/biopsy for the proceduralist. Procedural pain control is the most important measure of success for the patient.

Local Anesthesia

Pain occurs when the needle is introduced through the skin and the periosteum. A topical lidocaine patch or cream over the intended biopsy site can reduce the pain of the lidocaine injection into the skin, subcutaneous tissue, and periosteum. Lidocaine injection is painful, so buffering with 1 part sodium bicarbonate to 9 parts lidocaine may be helpful. Local anesthesia is crucial for tolerance of the bone marrow needle introduction through the skin and periosteum, but the actual marrow aspiration can also be very painful, and this pain is not obviated by local anesthetics. If a BMB is needed after the BMA, the procedure can be streamlined into a single needle insertion by placing the biopsy needle, obtaining the aspirate through the biopsy needle, and then taking a core of marrow. Local anesthesia alone is not very effective as pain control for BMB, which may require significant manipulation and rotation of the biopsy needle to acquire an adequate core sample.

Positioning

Most bone marrow aspirations/biopsies in small children and infants are obtained from the posterior superior iliac crest. The patient position may include (1) prone—often positioned with a small towel roll under the hips; (2) lateral decubitus—as for an LP, and in addition to the superior iliac crest, spinal processes may be an appropriate site for bone marrow aspirations/biopsies; and (3) supine—for the anterior iliac crest. While the semifetal positioning often used for LP is unnecessary, airway compromise may occur in either the prone or lateral decubitus position, exacerbating the potential respiratory insufficiency inherent in moderate or deep sedation. End-tidal carbon dioxide monitoring is recommended. Prone or lateral decubitus positioning does hamper the ability to rescue a patient with bag-valve-mask ventilation. The sedationist and proceduralist must practice good communication if there is a need to change the patient's position.

Sedation Regimens

Small children and infants will not tolerate the local lidocaine injection pain well without achieving at least a state of moderate sedation. While bone marrow aspirations/biopsies are quite painful, positioning is not as difficult to maintain and immobility is not as procedurally important compared to LP. Short-acting opioid medications followed by deep sedation achieved with propofol is a successful combination. Many sedationists use midazolam and generous doses of ketamine. Fentanyl with midazolam may be sufficient for the older child who can understand and tolerate the painfulness of the procedure. Because LP and bone marrow aspirations/biopsies are frequently performed at the same clinic visit in oncology patients, similar short procedural sedation regimens are often used.

Postprocedure Pain

Bone marrow aspirations/biopsies rarely produce more than an "ache" that may be relieved with acetaminophen. Some proceduralists recommend acetaminophen administration before the procedure. Difficult aspiration, many attempts needed to obtain the core sample, or soft tissue injury in larger muscular or obese children and teenagers may produce more significant pain, which is usually manageable with local heat or ice packs and outpatient opioid medications.

Suggested Reading

Christoph RA, Buchanan L, Begalla K, Schwartz S. Pain reduction in local anesthetic administration through pH buffering. *Ann Emerg Med.* 1988;17(2):117–120.

Dahlquist LM, Gil KM, Armstrong FD, et al. Preparing children for medical examinations: the importance of previous medical experience. *Health Psychol.* 1986;5(3):249–259.

Gottschling S, Meyer S, Krenn T, et al. Propofol versus midazolam/ketamine for procedural sedation in pediatric oncology. *J Pediatr Hematol Oncol.* 2005;27:471–476.

12.9

Intravascular Access

Intravascular Catheters, Intraosseous Needles, PICC Lines, Central Venous Catheters

JENNA FINE, NDIDI NWOKORIE, AND

LIA H. LOWRIE

Vascular access is necessary for routine and emergent care of patients for delivery of fluids and medications. Vascular access devices (VADs) discussed here include peripheral intravascular catheters, intraosseous needles, peripherally inserted central catheters (PICC lines), and centrally inserted venous catheters (CVCs) (Table 12.9.1). Insertion techniques for intra-arterial catheters peripherally and in more central arteries similar those for to intravascular catheters and CVCs, so potential procedural sedation issues are similar.

VADs require insertion through skin as well as connective tissues, muscle, and sometimes periosteum, resulting in at least momentary pain. VAD insertion is most safely performed in a cooperative patient who can follow commands and remain immobile. Infants and children pose challenges for placement of VADs because of the small size of their vessels, their inability to understand and maintain positioning requirements and to understand the momentary nature of a painful stimulus. The depth of sedation required for VAD placement in children will depend on the type of the device, the circumstances of placement (i.e., emergent or planned), and the child's age, developmental

TABLE 12.9.1 Comparison: PICC lines, CVCs, and intraosseous needles

	Pros	*Con*
PICC Line	Peripherally inserted via upper arm/saphenous vein in infants Can remain in place for weeks or months Can be used within the hospital setting or chronic care facility or as part of a home care treatment plan Indication: frequent needlesticks and/or prolonged intravenous medication/nutrition Low potential for complications during insertion Wide range of licensed clinicians able to insert Lower cost compared to CVC	Small peripheral vessels Require sterile technique for maintenance of patency and dressings Usually not adequate for dialysis Moderate skill acquisition for proceduralist High degree of patient immobility required during insertion
CVC	Inserted through internal jugular, subclavian, or femoral vein Indication: Rapid volume resuscitation and/or administration of life-saving drugs caustic to peripheral veins, pressure monitoring in critically ill children	Generally removed within 2 weeks Higher infection and complication rate than PICC High skill acquisition for proceduralist Increased risk of pneumothorax, hemothorax, and air embolism High degree of patient immobility required during insertion

TABLE 12.9.1 Continued

	Pros	*Con*
Intraosseous Needle	Rapid vascular bed access (within 30–60 seconds) Little skill acquisition required Access to noncollapsible vascular bed Life-saving when vascular access cannot be attained via other routes Can infuse all intravascular medications and fluids High percentage of successful first-attempt placement; less painful than multiple IVC attempts	Short duration of use Single attempt per bone

status, and previous experiences with painful medical procedures. Careful attention to local anesthesia techniques at the site of skin insertion and anxiolysis (whether medication-induced or through behavioral techniques) is good practice for patients of all ages and all VADs, and will result in less future "needle phobia" and greater first-time procedural success with VAD placement.

Intravascular Catheters

Pain control at the insertion site is best approached with the newer needleless skin-numbing techniques discussed in Chapter 15.4. Distraction techniques and other behavior-modification techniques are always indicated. Support from child life specialists should be encouraged to minimize the need for immobilization techniques (e.g., mummy wraps, papoose boards). Minimal to moderate sedation may be required to help manage anxiety and fear. Children may perceive the paresthesias associated with a tourniquet as painful and may be frightened by immobilization techniques. Midazolam and nitrous oxide are well studied in this setting, and have been found to be quite effective.

Intraosseous Needles

Intraosseous needles are traditionally used as an excellent way to achieve emergency access to the intravascular bed. Insertion requires less skill in small children than even intravascular catheter placement. Traditional intraosseous needles require blunt manual force for placement, whereas the newer power "drills" are safe and effective and enhance the chances of success on the first placement attempt.

Use of intraosseous needles is increasing in nonemergent situations. With attention to local anesthesia (see Chapter 15.4), an intraosseous needle can provide access for fluids and medications with less pain and anxiety than multiple attempts to insert an intravascular catheter.

The initial infusion through the intraosseous may be painful. Instillation of lidocaine prior to the infusion may ameliorate this discomfort.

PICC Lines

Despite the similarity of the insertion site to an IVC, the pain at that site during PICC insertion may be greater and more prolonged because of the techniques involved with vein locating, dilating, and wire and catheter exchange and threading. PICC lines are designed for prolonged use, necessitating attention to sterile technique during insertion and maintenance. Standard central line insertion techniques to prevent central line–associated bloodstream infection include sterile draping of approximately 80% of the patient. Children may be frightened by the perception of being blanketed by the sterile fields.

Children's small veins are difficult to access, and positioning of the PICC tip in the superior vena cava or inferior vena cava may require modification of the patient's position under the drapes.

Moderate to deep sedation is often necessary for young children to tolerate the 20–60 minutes of immobility often needed for successful PICC placement. Midazolam, dexmedetomidine, and propofol in conjunction with opioids or ketamine are commonly used.

CVCs

Centrally placed vascular access may be necessary emergently or in a more planned setting. Emergent cannulation of central veins in a young conscious patient without IVC access is an indication for intramuscular administration of sedatives and analgesia. Ketamine is a common choice. As with PICC lines, standard central line insertion techniques to prevent central line–associated bloodstream infection include sterile draping of approximately 80% of the patient. Young children may be frightened by the perception of being blanketed by the sterile field.

As always, attention to local anesthesia at the insertion site is important. Commonly used Seldinger techniques are associated with pain during the initial needle insertion but even more so with the use of serial dilation of the skin and vessel. Subclavian insertion techniques are commonly associated with needle puncture of the clavicular periosteum, which is quite painful. Cut-down techniques for CVC placement obviously involve skin incisions, for which local anesthesia is necessary even when opioid or ketamine sedatives are used systemically.

Anatomically small structures in infants and children are a challenge for the proceduralist even with ultrasound use and immobility. During CVC placement it is critical to avoid inadvertent arterial puncture or only partial cannulation of the internal jugular, subclavian, or femoral vessel.

Positioning during CVC placement also enhances procedural success. Trendelenburg positioning (supine and head 15–30 degrees below the feet) is used to improve venous flow to the superior vena cava and subclavian vein. The risk for hypoventilation during deep sedation may be increased if the diaphragm has also moved cephalad.

Deep sedation is often necessary for infants and young children. Midazolam, dexmedetomidine, and propofol in conjunction with opioids or ketamine are commonly used.

The proceduralist should be aware that a sedated patient cannot follow commands to avoid taking a breath during cannulation and manipulation of the superior vena cava or subclavian vein. Reduced intrathoracic pressure during thoracic cavity vein cannulation is associated with air embolism.

Suggested Reading

American Heart Association. 6 *Pediatric Advanced Life Support Provider Manual.* 2016.

Green SM, Denmark TK, Cline J, et al. Ketamine sedation for pediatric critical care procedures. *Pediatr Emerg Care.* 2001;17(4):244–248.

Heard CMB, Al Ibrahim O. Sedation and analgesia. In: *Pediatric Critical Care.* 5th ed. 2017:1827–1861.

Roberts JR.7 *Roberts and Hedges' Clinical Procedures in Emergency Medicine and Acute Care* [e-book]. Elsevier Health Sciences, 2017.

Scott-Warren VL, Morley RB. Paediatric vascular access. *BJA Education.* 2015;15(4):199–206.

12.10

Orthopedic

Fracture Reduction, Joint Injection, and Aspiration

MARY A. HEGENBARTH

Orthopedic procedures, including fracture reduction and muscle/joint injections, are common and are performed in a variety of settings, including emergency departments (EDs), clinics, sedation units, and radiology suites. When planning sedation, consider both patient factors (age, level of pain/anxiety, baseline health, sedation risk) and procedural aspects (anticipated length, painfulness, difficulty, need for immobility, operator experience and preferences). Briefer, less painful procedures may be accomplished with minimal sedation options such as nitrous oxide or midazolam; longer or more painful procedures often require deep sedation options such as ketamine or propofol (see Chapter 15 and the Appendix). Adequate analgesia is essential, whether provided systemically or with local/topical anesthesia.

Acute Orthopedic Injuries

Orthopedic injuries requiring sedation in the ED include fractures needing reduction and casting; joint dislocations; and complex lacerations (e.g., fingertip injuries). Most children with these injuries are healthy (American Society of Anesthesiologists [ASA] class I or II) and tolerate sedation well. Children presenting with acute injuries are seldom fasted, so the practitioner must balance the benefits of proceeding with sedation against possible increased risks (see Chapters 6 and 9).

Reduction and casting of angulated or displaced fractures usually requires at least moderate to deep sedation, unless analgesia can be accomplished with local or regional anesthesia. These injuries are often very painful, requiring analgesia with agents such as fentanyl or morphine upon presentation and as needed to control pain prior to the procedure. Intranasal fentanyl is an excellent initial option for children without intravenous (IV) access, allowing time for X-rays and obtaining subsequent IV access. Suspected fractures should be immobilized and elevated and ice packs should be applied to reduce swelling and pain. The patient's neurovascular status and whether the injury is open or closed are key factors in determining how quickly the procedure should be accomplished.

Ketamine is a very frequently used agent for fracture reduction/casting. Although usually given IV, intramuscular ketamine is effective and particularly useful in settings such as general EDs or in children with difficult IV access. IV ketamine is administered until signs of dissociation are seen (blank stare, nystagmus). Additional, smaller doses may be needed during longer procedures or during cast molding.

Propofol is another agent commonly used for deep sedation for orthopedic procedures. Although propofol alone may be adequate for brief procedures such as simple joint reduction, when used for fracture reduction it is usually combined with an analgesic such as fentanyl or sub-dissociative ketamine. Combining ketamine and propofol ("ketofol") is becoming increasingly common, as the two agents appear complementary in their effects. Regimens include 1:1 mixtures in the same syringe titrated to effect, or administration of a sub-dissociative dose of ketamine followed by propofol titration. While most young children tolerate ketamine well, older children and especially adolescents who have a higher risk of unpleasant recovery with ketamine monotherapy appear to benefit most from the addition of propofol.

Alternatives to ketamine or propofol include etomidate and combinations such as fentanyl and midazolam. Etomidate (often given with fentanyl) is not as widely used due to its short duration of action and myoclonus that can sometimes interfere with procedural success. Fentanyl with midazolam was commonly used in the past, but this combination is not as effective as ketamine or propofol and has little advantage if IV sedation is planned. However, for some minor procedures (e.g., minimally angulated distal radius needing "just a little push"), fentanyl plus midazolam may be adequate and may be given intranasally, sparing the child an IV. Alternatively, for minor procedures nitrous oxide with an analgesic such as intranasal fentanyl may suffice. Nitrous is particularly useful when local anesthetic techniques such as hematoma, Bier, or nerve blocks can be used for pain control.

Joint Injection and Aspiration

Intra-articular corticosteroid injections are commonly performed in children with rheumatologic conditions such as juvenile idiopathic arthritis. Joint fluid aspiration may be performed for diagnostic reasons (suspected infection) or for pain relief of large effusions. Ultrasound guidance may be used, especially for smaller/deeper joints that are more difficult to localize with external landmarks.

Analgesia is usually provided by local/topical anesthetic options such as EMLA (Eutectic Mixture of Local Anesthetics) alone or with injected lidocaine, cold sprays (e.g., ethyl chloride, Pain Ease®), or lidocaine iontophoresis. In clinical practice, EMLA alone has been found to be suboptimal due to the inability to reach the synovium. Minimal sedation options include nitrous oxide or midazolam, along with distraction techniques. Children who are younger, more anxious, or undergoing more technically difficult procedures (e.g., injection of smaller or multiple joints) often need deeper sedation.

Suggested Reading

Lee-Jayaram JJ, Green A, Siembieda J, et al. Ketamine/midazolam versus etomidate/fentanyl procedural sedation for pediatric orthopedic reductions. *Pediatr Emerg Care.* 2010;26(6):408–412.

Luhmann JD, Schootman M, Luhmann SJ, Kennedy RM. A randomized comparison of nitrous oxide plus hematoma block versus ketamine plus midazolam for emergency department forearm fracture reduction in children. *Pediatrics.* 2006;118(4):e1078–e1086.

Oren-Ziv A, Hoppenstein D, Shles A, Uziel Y. Sedation methods for intra-articular corticosteroid injections in juvenile idiopathic arthritis: a review. *Pediatr Rheumatol.* 2015;13:28.

Shah A, Mosdossy G, McLeod S, et al. A blinded, randomized controlled trial to evaluate ketamine/propofol versus ketamine alone for procedural sedation in children. *Ann Emerg Med.* 2011;57(5):425–433.

12.11

Neurology

Electroencephalography, Brainstem Auditory Evoked Response

DANIEL J. SEDILLO AND SAMUEL L. ZUCKERMAN

Children often require neurophysiologic testing such as an electroencephalogram (EEG) or a brainstem auditory evoked response (BAER) testing in the evaluation of neurologic disease or varying degrees of developmental delay. Most children >5 years of age who are cognitively intact can undergo an EEG or BAER without requiring sedation. Infants can often sleep through their study, especially if sleep-deprived. However, toddlers and children with autism or pervasive developmental disorder may not be capable of cooperating with the audiologist and thus will require sedation.

The EEG is a diagnostic study that is primarily used in children to assist in the diagnosis and treatment of epilepsy and other paroxysmal events. It may also be used to assess the cerebral activity status of a child with an acute or chronic neurologic condition. Up to 55% of epilepsy patients (adults and children) have epileptiform abnormalities on a single EEG outpatient study. The yield may improve with serial examinations and with longer studies. The American Clinical Neurophysiology Society recommends a minimum of 20 minutes of artifact-free study. Burkholder et al. demonstrated that extended EEGs (30–60 minutes long) improved the yield of interictal epileptiform discharges (IEDs) compared to 30-minute studies. These authors suggest performing an EEG for a minimum of 45 minutes to optimally detect IEDs, however with longer studies, the ability for patients to minimize movement becomes more difficult.

Auditory brainstem response (ABR) testing or BAER are electrophysiologic tests of hearing thresholds that do not require any behavioral responses by the child. In the BAER exam, click stimuli and tone bursts are presented into the external auditory canal, and the responses of the auditory pathway are recorded with standardized placement of skin recording electrodes. These responses are compared to normative data to determine if the child has either sensorineural or conductive hearing loss, or both. The testing equipment can be quite sensitive to interference and artifact from the patient and from the testing environment. The technology is evolving to minimize this type of interference, so more patients may be able to undergo BAER testing without sedation or anesthesia.

Keys to Successful Study Completion

Successful completion of a reliable, high-quality EEG or BAER depends on patient factors, environmental factors, and provider factors.

Patient factors include the level of patient cooperation, partial sleep deprivation, and the ability of the child to remain nearly motionless (to maintain lead integrity and minimize testing artifact). Many centers use behavioral training for uncooperative children so that both outpatient and extended inpatient EEG studies can be obtained without using sedation.

The environment must be quiet, not too hot or cold, and dimly lit. Activity in the immediate testing area should be minimized. The operating room or the intensive care unit may be a difficult testing environment due to electrical interference and excessive noise. An appropriate recovery area with the ability to monitor the patient until back at baseline is mandatory for the sedated or anesthetized child.

The audiologist or examination technician must be very patient, must have pediatric-specific experience, and must have the appropriate testing equipment and protocols.

Goals of Sedation

The goals of sedation for either EEG or BAER are as follows:

- Successful placement of the recording electrodes
- Successful data acquisition
- Minimal effect of sedative medication on examination interpretation
- Minimal invasiveness to avoid intubation or IV catheter placement
- Minimal patient discomfort or pain
- Use of sedative agents with predictable onset of action and minimal cardiopulmonary effects
- Maintenance of patient safety during and after the procedure.

Selection of Sedative Agent

Children who require sedation for either placement of the leads or completion of the study may present many diverse challenges. Many of these patients have complex medical conditions with impaired cardiopulmonary function, which can complicate sedation and airway management. Furthermore, many of the commonly used sedative agents may alter the reliability of the EEG interpretation because of direct central nervous system effects. Agents such as dexmedetomidine, ketamine, and clonidine have less deleterious effect on the EEG than other agents (Table 12.11.1).

There is a much larger selection of sedation medications to choose from when sedating for an BAER versus an EEG (Table 12.11.2).

TABLE 12.11.1 EEG sedation regimens

- Oral clonidine
  - <10 kg: 0.05 mg
  - 10–30 kg: 0.1 mg
  - >30 kg: 0.15–0.2 mg
- Dexmedetomidine
  - Oral: 2.9–4.4 mcg/kg
  - Intravenous
    - Load: 1–2 mcg/kg, repeat 1-mcg/kg boluses until asleep
    - Plus continuous infusion: 0.5–1.5 mcg/kg/hour
  - Intramuscular
    - 1.0–4.5 mcg/kg; reduced repeated dose for sedation failure
  - Intranasal
    - 2.5–3 mcg/kg, reduced repeated dose for sedation failure
- Intravenous ketamine
  - 1 mg/kg
- Oral melatonin
  - 2–6 mg; additional dosing as needed

TABLE 12.11.2 BAER sedation regimens

- Intranasal dexmedetomidine
  - 3 – 4 mcg/kg
  - Consider intranasal midazolam adjunct: 0.1–0.2 mg/kg
- Rectal pentobarbital
  - 5 mg/kg
- Intravenous propofol

Medications that may affect brainwave voltage on an EEG will not affect BAER results; however, there are other factors to consider in selecting a sedation agent. If the examination is part of the preoperative evaluation of a patient for cochlear implantation or placement of a hearing amplification device, it will probably be a more time-consuming study than that of an autistic child with speech delay or a child with a recent history of meningitis who requires hearing evaluation. These factors may affect drug selection.

Pediatric sedation providers around the world use a diversity of sedation protocols or regimens to enable the safe and successful completion of these diagnostic procedures. These procedures should be done as part of well-organized system of pediatric sedation care with the appropriate personnel, patient selection, monitoring, and rescue systems in place.

Dexmedetomidine can be an attractive agent for sedating children for either placement of the recording electrodes for EEG or BAER testing or data acquisition. Dexmedetomidine can be administered primarily by the intranasal or intravenous route, or by both routes (see the Appendix). Obviously, the intranasal route is less invasive and painful than with intravenous catheter placement. For BAER sedation, many clinicians use intranasal midazolam as an adjunctive agent, although this is not a good option for EEG sedation.

Many centers use propofol quite successfully in providing sedation to children for BAER examination. This agent does require placement of an intravenous catheter and requires more advanced training and experience in its use and in maintenance of cardiopulmonary function.

Summary

Children who undergo neurodiagnostic testing such as the EEG or the BAER often require sedation so that the study can be done safely with reliable interpretation of the data. The literature describes various sedation regimens that, when administered in the context of an organized sedation system, are safe and efficacious. The intranasal route for sedative administration is very attractive, offers good efficacy, and is less invasive and more comfortable for the patient.

Suggested Reading

Ashrafi MR, Mohammadi M, Tafarroji J, et al. Melatonin versus chloral hydrate for recording sleep EEG. *Eur J Paediatr Neurol.* 2010;14(3):235–238.

Baier NM, Mendez SS, Kimm D, et al. Intranasal dexmedetomidine: an effective sedative agent for electroencephalogram and auditory brain response testing. *Paediatr Anaesth.* 2016;26(3):280–285.

Burkholder DB, Britton JW, Rajasekaran V, et al. Routine vs extended outpatient EEG for the detection of interictal epileptiform discharges. *Neurology.* 2016;86: 1524–1530.

Francois M, Teissier N, Barthod G, Nasra Y. Sedation for children 2 to 5 years of age undergoing auditory brainstem response and auditory steady state responses recordings. *Int J Audiol.* 2012;51(4):282–286.

Mason KP, Lubisch N, Robinson F, et al. Intramuscular dexmedetomidine: An effective route of sedation preserves background activity for pediatric electroencephalograms. *J Pediatr.* 2012;161(5):927–932.

Mehta UC, Patel I, Castello FV. EEG sedation for children with autism. *J Dev Behav Pediatr.* 2004;25(2):102–104.

12.12

Cutaneous

Laceration Repair, Incision and Drainage, Burn Debridement

JUDSON BARBER AND JACINTA COOPER

Cutaneous procedures are some of the most common reasons for using analgesia and sedation in outpatient pediatrics (Table 12.12.1). An individualized approach to each patient and the proposed procedure results in better outcomes and higher patient and family satisfaction. Familiarity with the available analgesia and sedation options allows sedationists to make the best choices for their patients.

Children presenting to outpatient settings, urgent care centers, and emergency departments (EDs) undergo procedures that may be painful or anxiety-producing, such as laceration repair, incision and drainage (I&D) of an abscess, and debridement of burns. The goal is to adequately treat pain and address anxiety while producing the fewest side effects (e.g., allergic reaction, hypotension, inadequate anesthesia, fear of future procedures). Procedural anesthesia aims to address pain and anxiety by using oral, inhalation, or intravenous medications (see Chapter 15 and the Appendix).

The AMPLE mnemonic (allergies, medications, past medical history, last meal, events leading to the need for sedation), the ASA-PS classification system, and the Mallampati scoring system can help the clinician to answer three questions before proceeding with procedural sedation:

TABLE 12.12.1 Sedative and analgesic approaches for cutaneous procedures

	Child Life	*Local Anesthetic*	*Narcotic (PO, IN, IV)*	*Nitrous Oxide*	*Anxiolytic (PO, IN, IV)*	*Deep Sedation*
Simple laceration	++	++++	–	++	++	–
Complex laceration	++	++++	+	++	+++	consider
Abscess I&D	++	++	++++	+++	++	consider
Burn debridement	++	–	++++	++	++	consider

PO, oral; IN, intransal; IV, intravenous.

1. Is the patient a good candidate?
2. What are the risks for a difficult airway?
3. Is all of the equipment readily available to provide a safe environment for procedural sedation?

Once it has been determined that a patient is a good candidate for procedural sedation, the SOAP ME mnemonic (suction, oxygen, airway equipment, pharmaceuticals for the procedure and reversal agents, monitoring equipment, and emergency cart) can be used to gather the necessary supplies for an airway emergency.

Laceration Repair

Analgesia and/or sedation strategies for laceration repair will depend on a number of factors, such as the patient's age (chronologic or developmental); the body area affected; the depth, length, and complexity of the laceration; expected time to complete the procedure; and clinical space. Most laceration repairs will take place in outpatient areas (office, clinic, urgent care center, or ED), so this section will focus on techniques in this setting.

Most lacerations in older children and adolescents can be repaired with only local anesthesia. This can be achieved for small to medium lacerations by using a topical anesthetic gel such as LET (lidocaine, epinephrine, and tetracaine). LET and other topical anesthetics work best in areas of the body that are more vascular (e.g., face and scalp). For larger lacerations or areas not amenable to topical anesthetic, local injection of 1% lidocaine with epinephrine may be used. Regional (including digital) blocks are also an option where appropriate.

Younger children and those with developmental delay or neurobehavioral disorders may require sedation in addition to analgesia. In some cases all that is needed is an anxiolytic such as midazolam (oral or intranasal). Other nonparenteral options include dexmedetomidine (intransal, oral, buccal) and inhaled nitrous oxide. Repairs that require the patient to remain very still (e.g., complex facial lacerations) may require deeper levels of sedation. Deep sedation requires a dedicated sedation provider who is not performing the repair. Use of distraction techniques by child life specialists can often lessen the need for sedation.

Incision and Drainage

As with laceration repair, the need for sedation in addition to analgesia to tolerate abscess I&D depends on the patient's age, the location and depth of the abscess, and the setting of the procedure. In most cases I&D is performed in the outpatient setting (clinic, ED). Large, complex, or anatomically challenging abscesses often require surgical management in the operating room.

Topical anesthetics do not provide adequate analgesia for abscess I&D because the medication does not penetrate the depth of the abscess and the acidic nature of the abscess alters the ability of lidocaine to work. Local injection around the abscess, field blocks, and topical sprays and gels may help with the incision portion of the procedure, but most patients still feel discomfort with manual expression of pus, breaking up loculations, and wound irrigation or packing. It is worth noting that topical anesthetic creams (LMX 4%) will often cause smaller abscesses to spontaneously rupture and drain. Abscess I&D in younger children or those with neurobehavioral disorders may necessitate the use of sedation in addition to analgesia.

Nitrous oxide with or without a narcotic analgesic is useful in settings where it is available (see Chapter 15). Intranasal fentanyl paired with inhaled nitrous oxide provides excellent analgesia and anxiolysis for I&D without the need to start an IV. Child life specialists are very helpful in this situation by not only distracting the patient from the procedure but also aiding with mask acceptance to administer the nitrous oxide.

Deep sedation with ketamine, propofol, or the combination ("ketofol") may be the best option to humanely and safely drain some abscesses. Deep sedation should be considered in large and/or deep abscesses or abscesses that are expected to take a relatively long time to drain.

Burns

Burns are treated in a variety of outpatient and inpatient settings, including specialized burn centers. Superficial and partial-thickness burns may be exquisitely painful. Debridement and dressing of burns are additional painful stimuli. Topical anesthetics and cooling sprays may be used for minor burns. Because the outer layer of skin is damaged, topical anesthetics are easily absorbed, increasing the risk of systemic toxicity. Oral nonsteroidal anti-inflammatory drugs (NSAIDs) and narcotics usually provide adequate analgesia for minor burns.

Patients with 2nd- and 3rd-degree burns often require debridement and therefore require a more detailed approach. At a minimum, a narcotic analgesic should be given (intravenous morphine or fentanyl, intranasal fentanyl, oral hydrocodone). Young children often benefit from an anxiolytic, as do patients of all ages who require serial debridement. Consideration of factors specific to the burn injury (anatomy, depth, complexity of debridement/dressing process) and to the patient (age, pain profile, developmental stage) is vital to the development and provision of a safe, successful procedural sedation for burn management. Patients who have extensive burns and/or major trauma are beyond the scope of this text.

Suggested Reading

Hsu DC, Cravero JP. Selection of medications for pediatric procedural sedation outside the operating room. UpToDate. Waltham, MA, 2016.

Zier JL, Tarrago R, Liu M. Level of sedation with nitrous oxide for pediatric medical procedures. *Analges Anesth.* 2010;110:1399–1405.

12.13

Botox Injections for Spasticity and Sialorrhea

CHRISTINA MANNIX

Botulinum toxin injections have become one of many treatment modalities available for children with cerebral palsy. The procedure consists of intramuscular injections of the botulinum toxin type A (Botox®, Dysport®, Xeomin®) into targeted muscle groups. Botox produces chemical denervation by preventing the release of acetylcholine from the presynaptic terminal of the motor end plate. If the desired degree of decreased spasticity is achieved, repeat treatment every 3–6 months is required for maintenance. The goals of spasticity management are to decrease pain, improve ambulation, facilitate activities of daily life and ease of care, prevent or lessen muscle contractures, increase joint range of motion, and delay the need for surgery.

Procedure

The muscle to be injected is localized by palpation, electromyography, or ultrasound. The injections are given into the muscle belly through the fascia. The total volume of medication injected is typically divided into separate injection sites within each muscle group. The volume of each injection may be 5 mL or more, adding to the painful nature of the procedure.

Sedation Approaches

The level of sedation that is used for this procedure varies among institutions and from patient to patient, ranging from no sedation at all to general anesthesia. Patients often require treatment of multiple muscle groups and thus require multiple injections per visit, and the injections often involve sensitive areas of the body such as the thenar eminence.

Minimal to moderate sedation with nitrous oxide is an effective method of sedation for this painful but quick outpatient procedure. Nitrous oxide has both amnestic and analgesic properties (see Chapter 15). It can be administered easily without the need for placement of an intravenous line. The procedure can usually be started within 2–3 minutes of administering the gas and the patient usually has returned to baseline within 2–5 minutes of stopping the gas, making the recovery time very brief.

In the author's experience, a concentration of >50% nitrous oxide (commonly 60–65%) administered via face mask is most effective for patient comfort. Maintaining minimal stimulation in the procedure room and using calming distraction techniques provided by child life specialists are integral to the success of this type of sedation. If face mask application is stressful and frightening, a useful adjunct can be midazolam administered enterally or intranasally prior to applying the mask.

As with any sedation, one should always be prepared for complications. Emesis is not an uncommon adverse effect of nitrous oxide, especially when used at higher concentrations. Children with cerebral palsy may be more susceptible to aspiration, so one must be prepared to suction quickly if vomiting occurs (see Chapter 11.3).

Some patients have a history of nonresponse to the nitrous oxide, have a contraindication to nitrous oxide use, or have a history of adverse reactions such as hyperstimulation or dysphoria that have caused patient distress in the past. In these cases, other approaches to achieving minimal and moderate states of sedation could include topical analgesia such as EMLA, analgesia with a narcotic such as fentanyl along with an anxiolytic, or intravenous sedation with ketamine or propofol. Obviously enteral or intranasal midazolam will provide no analgesia and will require much longer recovery times compared to the procedure time. Ketamine and propofol have appropriately short half-lives, but the struggle to obtain intravenous access may seem to outweigh the benefit of moderate to deep sedation during particularly a single muscle group injection.

Although not specific to patients with cerebral palsy, the use of Botox injection in the parotid and/or submandibular glands for sialorrhea is increasing in the pediatric population. Performed generally under ultrasound guidance, injection of specific doses of Botox may produce decreased salivation for 2–4 months. Complications include inconsistent effectiveness, injection, and transient muscle weakness that may produce dysphagia. The target glands are small and the risk for iatrogenic injury of adjacent anatomic structures is higher, making ultrasound localization useful. Generally, deeper levels of sedation are required for this indication compared with spasticity to allow localization of the gland and precise delivery of the treatment. Patients with sialorrhea or with pharyngeal dysfunction are at higher risk for airway-related complications during sedation and anesthesia.

Suggested Reading

Brochard S, Blajan V, Lempereur M, et al. Determining the technical and clinical factors associated with pain for children undergoing botulinum toxin injections under nitrous oxide and anesthetic cream. *Eur J Paediatric Neurol.* 2011; 15(4):310–315.

Lungre MP, Halula S, Coyne S, et al. Ultrasound-guided botulinum toxin type A salivary gland injection in children for refractory sialorrhea: 10-year experience at a large tertiary children's hospital. *Pediatr Neurol.* 2016;54:70–75.

Strobel W, Theologis T, Brunner R, et al. Best clinical practice in botulinum toxin treatment for children with cerebral palsy. *Toxins (Basel).* 2015;7(5):1629–1648.

Zier JL, Rivard PF, Krach LE, Wendorf HR. Effectiveness of sedation using nitrous oxide compared with enteral midazolam for botulinum toxin A injections in children. *Dev Med Child Neurol.* 2008;50:854–858.

13

Sedation in the Pediatric Dental Practice

JOHN H. UNKEL

Anxiety and the Dental Environment

A child's oral conditions and parents' concerns regarding oral health are commonly addressed in the dental office. The pediatric dental office serves, more often than most pediatric medical primary care offices, both as a facility for primary oral healthcare assessment and as a location for treatment involving invasive procedures. Preprocedure anxiety in the dental setting is heightened by (1) the parents' anxiety specific to the dental environment that is transferred to the child and (2) the child's temperament and developmental age.

Consequently, guardians become accustomed to accompanying their child for both an evaluation and treatment; these conversations involve a triad interaction, (Figure 13.1). Parental anxiety, specifically dental anxiety, can be easily transferred to the child,[1-4] which may be in addition to the child's own fears. Baier et al found that 20% of children who have dental fear tend to be younger and have been exposed to local anesthesia leading to negative behavior in the dental office.[5] Child temperament[6-8] in toddlers and preschoolers with an immature level of cognitive development[9] further affect the dental encounter.

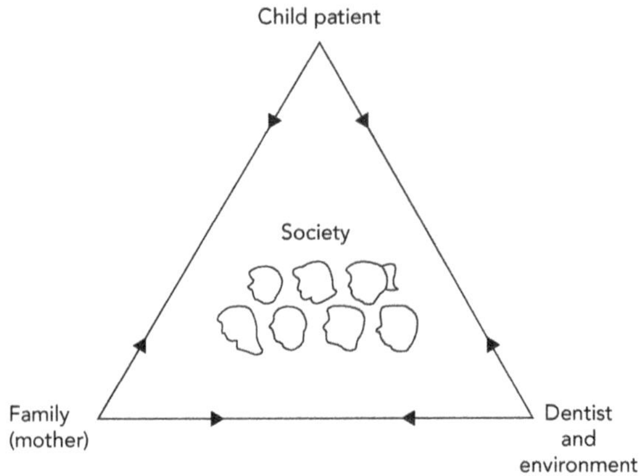

FIGURE 13.1

The pediatric dental triangle illustrates basic relationships in pediatric dentistry

Dental treatment of children frequently involves invasive procedures, such as restoration of carious lesions to return the dentition to form and function or extraction of teeth. Procedural anxiety and fear lead to uncooperative behavior, diminishing the likelihood of successful procedure completion. Specific aspects of dental procedures leading to the need for sedation care include the following:

- Unpleasant tastes and odors of topical anesthetics or equipment in the mouth
- Painful injections of local anesthetics
- Pharyngeal anesthesia, leading to a feeling of impaired ability to control secretions or gag reflex
- The oral-pharyngeal protective barrier used during the procedure to prevent aspiration of dental materials, which may lead to a feeling of impaired breathing
- High-pitched noise and vibrations from the drill and suction devices
- Mandatory positioning in the supine position with mouth held open
- Need to protect proceduralists from human bites.

Preparation for Sedation in the Dental Office

Thorough preparation of the patient, the staff, and the procedural area for sedation is essential in order to deliver effective treatment and safe care. The dental office lies outside of the traditional healthcare theater where invasive care with anesthesia or sedation is more often delivered (e.g., ambulatory surgical centers and hospitals). Those locations are staffed with multiple types of providers who can respond to complications in a patient who is undergoing or recovering from general anesthesia or sedation. The pediatric dental office is frequently operated by a sole provider or a partnership arrangement. Practitioners of pediatric dentistry may serve as the proceduralist and sedationist simultaneously when moderate sedation is employed. The ability to respond to sedation emergencies is often limited to one or two licensed professionals.

Sedation-related adverse events that occur outside the hospital setting are associated with more serious outcomes, which can be lessened with emergency response planning and sedationist recognition and recovery expertise.[1,2] In recognition of the potential for serious complications, the American Academy of Pediatrics and the American Academy of Pediatric Dentistry recommend sedation preparation guidelines to minimize risks that include pre-operatory consent, fasting regimen, history and physical evaluation with emphasis on the airway and other medical risk factors, monitoring during the intraoperative period, and discharge criteria.[3,4]

The appropriate presedation assessment is discussed in Chapter 6. Presedation planning involving medical clearance for sedation requires a close relationship between the medical provider and the dental care provider. The medical care provider may be unaware of the conditions and depth of sedation needed to accomplish the procedure, while the dental provider may not be as aware of medical risk factors in a particular child. The dentist routinely obtains a history using forms completed by the guardian when the child becomes a patient of the office. Unfortunately, parents may omit important information unintentionally, such as birth and infant history, developmental issues, hospitalizations, anesthesia reactions, and so forth on these forms. To minimize sedation risk, the objective is to identify generally healthy patients or patients with controlled mild illness for sedation in the dental office.

Dental surgery is unique in that the procedures are all in the oral airway. Conditions specific to dental procedures of which the sedationist must be aware include the following:

- Teeth requiring extraction or exfoliating as well as materials used for restoration, such as stainless steel crowns, may be inadvertently displaced in the mouth.
- Appropriately placed oropharyngeal barriers, such as the rubber dam or 4×4 gauze (2×2 gauze and cotton rolls are best avoided), will minimize aspiration of secretions and fluids used in the procedure but may become dislodged themselves.
- Dental assistants, while providing retraction, may displace the tongue posteriorly, occluding the oral airway.
- Variation in noise and vibration levels, jaw pressure, and tongue retraction may require adjustment of the level of sedation throughout the procedure.
- Excessive salivation will adversely affect dental restoration quality. Sedatives such as ketamine may not be a good choice for dental procedures without use of antisialagogues.
- Bleeding may occur, particularly from inflamed mucosal surfaces.

Monitoring

Monitoring is covered in detail in Chapter 7 and should be no different in the dental office than in any other procedural site. Delivery of pediatric dental sedation by a procedural sedationist in the dental office is at the minimal to moderate level. Pulse oximetry, heart rate, blood pressure, and respiratory monitors are standard. An electrocardiogram is not usually used for mild and moderate dental sedation of patients with an American Society of Anesthesiologists (ASA) classification of I or II. The use of capnography is encouraged for the delivery of moderate sedation.

Local Anesthesia and Dental Sedation

The oral cavity is extremely sensitive to pain and pressure. Local anesthetics are often required to render invasive dental therapy. Local anesthetics act as analgesics during a painful procedure and provide pain relief for a short time after a procedure (e.g., tooth extraction). Local anesthetics are commonly delivered in two steps to provide pain relief in children. A topical medication is applied initially to anesthetize the oral mucosa from the unpleasant injection of the hypodermic needle that will deliver either an ester or amide. The injected anesthetic then infiltrates through the alveolar bone to the nerves of the dentition or is deposited in proximity to a peripheral nerve (e.g., mandibular inferior alveolar nerve), providing analgesia. Esters are metabolized by plasma cholinesterases and amides are metabolized in the liver, although articaine has both an amide and a thiophene ring ester component. Amides are more commonly used in pediatric dentistry. Some advocate the use of articaine because it may offer the additional advantages of metabolism, quicker onset of action, and more effectiveness for infiltration than lidocaine.[5]

Local anesthetics are not without toxicity in high doses and can produce clinical complications. Elevated concentrations may result in central nervous system (CNS) and cardiac toxicity. CNS toxicity usually occurs at half the plasma concentration of cardiac toxicity with lidocaine (8–10 vs. 20 mg/mL). Pediatric dentistry guidelines state the recommended doses in mg/kg to avoid adverse events.[6] Morbidity and mortality due to dental administration in local anesthetic overdose with and without sedation has been documented. Tissue injuries are common with and without sedation and may occur during the sedation recovery and postoperative periods. Mandibular block (e.g., inferior alveolar or mental) anesthetics may result in maceration of the lip or tongue, whereas maxillary infiltrations usually result in maceration of the lip and buccal cheek abrasions when children curious about the "numb" sensation bite the tissues.

Pain during the procedure is an infrequent consideration once the local anesthetic has been administered. However, delivering the local analgesia to a young child's oral cavity may require sedation. Successful inhalational use of nitrous oxide is very common.

Sedatives

Considerations of commonly used sedatives specific to dental procedures are discussed. One-time enteral delivery of sedatives in addition to nitrous oxide or nitrous oxide as a first-line choice for short procedures is commonly used. Intravenous titratable medications intended to produce minimal to moderate levels of sedation may be considered.

Nitrous Oxide

Nitrous oxide is readily employed by most dental offices for treating anxious children due to its rapid onset and recovery. Desirable properties include anxiolysis, mild sedation, amnesia, and analgesia. A more in-depth description of nitrous oxide sedation is found in Chapter 15. The delivery of nitrous oxide through a nasal hood is unique to dentistry as procedures are performed in the oral cavity. The nasal hood delivery is ideal for children with a fear of suffocation due to the face mask covering the nose and the mouth. When treating children who are fearful, a rapid induction technique may be considered. These children often take large breaths prior to crying and when beginning to cry. The nitrous oxide can be initiated at 60–70%, allowing the child to inhale through the nose or by placing the hood over the nose and mouth area if the child will not accept the nasal hood. The hood can then be placed over the nose when the child becomes calm.

Benzodiazepines

Benzodiazepines are frequently used for dental sedation. They offer multiple desirable effects such as anxiolysis, sedation, hypnosis, amnesia, and muscle relaxation. Triazolam and midazolam are two oral sedative medications used as sole agents for dental sedation. Triazolam does not have active metabolites, whereas midazolam has a minor metabolite, alpha$_1$-hydroxymidazolam, with some activity. Triazolam is the longer-acting of the two. It shortens the preparation time to begin the procedure and may lengthen the working time, unfortunately, as it is supplied only in pill form, and the lack of effectiveness data involving young children would make it best for sedating older children and adolescents.

Midazolam is used as a sole agent or in combination with additional medications for sedating children during invasive dental procedures. Midazolam can be administered safely via the oral, buccal transmucosal, or intranasal route with good effectiveness. Young children given midazolam have been known to display a paradoxical reaction after any route of administration. A delayed paradoxical reaction may last up to several hours, but it seems to be reversible by flumazenil.

Antihistamines

Hydroxyzine may be used as an adjunct during sedation. This H1 histamine blocker offers several benefits, including anticholinergic drying effects, mild sedation, and antiemetic effects. The anticholinergic effects are advantageous when handling dental materials in a wet environment, such as the mouth. Onset is approximately the same as that of oral midazolam (15–30 minutes), which synergistically prolongs the sedation.

Other Agents

Many agents can be titrated by skilled sedationists to produce the moderate levels of sedation appropriate for dental procedures. Ketamine in particular produces a state of moderate to even deep sedation and analgesia that might be ideal for certain dental cases. However, it is associated with increased salivation, which is a deterrent to routine use in the dental office without the additional use of an antisialagogue (e.g., glycopyrrolate or hydroxyzine). There is increasing interest in dexmedetomidine but little literature yet demonstrating advantages or disadvantages in the dental office setting. Propofol, despite its titratability, cannot be recommended for use in the office setting without at a minimum the presence of two separate licensed, credentialed providers functioning separately as the proceduralist and sedationist. Sedation with opioids e.g. meperidine is declining in the dental office setting.

Safety Considerations

Minimizing adverse sedation events in the dental office is critical. Some orally administered medications may last for a significant period of time after completion of the procedure, and time for recovery with trained staffing must be anticipated. Not all children can be safely and adequately sedated for dental procedures by the most common routes and medications in the dental office. Those who fail to respond or are not candidates for moderate sedation approaches will require deeper sedation or general anesthesia, which involves bringing anesthesiologists to the dental office or treating the child at a hospital or ambulatory surgical center. A preoperative history and evaluation are key in avoiding sedation adverse events and possible sedation failure in the dental office. Excellent preparation and planned rescue procedures are crucial when providing minimal or moderate sedation in the dental office.

Suggested Reading

Cravero JP, Tobias JD, eds. *Procedural Sedation for Infants, Children and Adolescents*. Elk Grove Village, IL: American Academy of Pediatrics, 2016.

Malamed SF. *Sedation: A Guide to Patient Management*. 5th ed. St. Louis, MO: Mosby, 2010.

Wilson S, ed. *Oral Sedation for Dental Procedures in Children*. Berlin/Heidelberg/New York/Dordrecht/London: Springer, 2015.

References

1. Coté CJ, Notterman DA, Karl HW, et al. Adverse sedation events in pediatrics: a critical incident analysis of contributing factors. *Pediatrics*. 2000 Apr;105(4 Pt 1):805–814.
2. Coté CJ, Notterman DA, Karl HW, et al. Adverse sedation events in pediatrics: analysis of medication used for sedation. *Pediatrics*. 2000 Oct;106(4):633–644.
3. Coté CJ. American Academy of Pediatrics sedation guidelines: are we there yet? *Arch Pediatr Adolesc Med*. 2012;166 (11):1067–1069.
4. Coté CJ, Wilson S, American Academy of Pediatrics, American Academy of Pediatric Dentistry. Guidelines for monitoring and management of pediatric patients before, during, and after sedation for diagnostic and therapeutic procedures: update 2016. *Pediatrics*. 2016;138(1):20161212.
5. Arrow P. A comparison of articaine 4% and lignocaine 2% in block and infiltration analgesia in children. *Aust Dent J*. 2012;57(3):325–333.
6. Guideline on use of local anesthesia for pediatric dental patients. *Pediatr Dent*. 2015;37(5):71–77.

14

International Approaches to Pediatric Sedation

14.1

The NICE Guidelines and Pediatric Sedation in the United Kingdom

MICHAEL SURY AND SARAH GREENAWAY

Advances in pediatric medicine over the last 20 years have led to an increase in the number of procedures and imaging techniques requiring sedation. Sedation is commonly used in children, but it occasionally may not be sufficiently effective for the intended procedure and, if used in excessive doses, can cause respiratory failure, hypoxia, and death. Sedation failure is distressing for the child and, if the procedure is abandoned, it represents an inefficient use of resources. In the United Kingdom, the National Institute for Health and Clinical Excellence (NICE) is a government organization whose purpose is to provide guidelines to help ensure that patients receive effective, good-value healthcare across the whole of the National Health Service. In 2010 NICE published guidelines "Sedation in under 19s: using sedation for diagnostic and therapeutic procedures (CG112)."[1] This chapter summarizes its key recommendations and describes how pediatric sedation has developed subsequently in the UK.

What the Guidelines Said

The overarching aims were to review the safety and efficacy of sedation for common procedures and to form a consensus view on the necessary resources to do this safely. Of the 10 key recommendations, arguably the most important concerned training, patient assessment, and safe facilities (Table 14.1.1). Other recommendations focused on the choice of sedation technique according to the procedure, competency in theoretical and practical delivery of safe sedation and pediatric life support training, and appropriate use of minimum clinical monitoring.

The NICE guidelines were widely reported and generally accepted, although there was criticism that it did not adequately define the sedation qualifications and training, or the facilities in which potent sedation

TABLE 14.1.1 NICE key recommendations

Establish suitability for sedation by assessing:	Current medical condition and any surgical problems Weight (growth assessment) Past medical problems (including any associated with previous sedation or anaesthesia) Current and previous medication (including any allergies) Physical status (including the airway) Psychological and developmental status
Seek advice from a specialist before delivering sedation:	If there is concern about a potential airway or breathing problem If the child or young person is assessed as ASA 3 or greater For infants, including neonates.
Ensure that the following will be available during sedation:	A healthcare professional and assistant trained in delivering and monitoring sedation in pediatrics Immediate access to resuscitation and monitoring equipment

Source: NICE. Sedation in under 19s: using sedation for diagnostic and therapeutic procedures. Available at nice.org.uk/guidance/cg112.

drugs should be used. The Academy of Medical Royal Colleges, led by the Royal College of Anaesthetists, sought to clarify these issues by organizing another committee to produce improved guidance.

Meanwhile, another report—the Francis Report (2013)—followed a public inquiry into serious failings at a hospital in England. This report defined standards of care and stimulated the Academy of Medical Royal Colleges to publish standards of safety for sedation ("Safe sedation practice for healthcare procedures: standards and guidance")[2] to prevent common problems encountered with sedation of adults (Table 14.1.2). Even though the Academy of Medical Royal Colleges guidance was aimed for adult sedation, we consider that its principles are valid and apply to children as well: they reinforce safe practices in pediatric sedation and support the principles of the NICE guidelines.

The NICE guidelines provided guidance for 4 common sedation settings: painless imaging, painful procedures, endoscopy, and

TABLE 14.1.2 Common problems encountered with sedation

Inadequate presedation assessment
Inadequate monitoring of patients
Excessive doses at extremes of age
Failure to titrate drugs to effect
Lack of appreciation of the risks implicit in the use of drug combinations (e.g., synergism)
Association of the use of flumazenil, a benzodiazepine antagonist, with the use of excessive doses of benzodiazepine and the lack of, or poor, recovery facilities
Minimal training of those administering sedation and the lack of supervision of inexperienced trainees

Source: Academy of Medical Royal Colleges. Safe Sedation Practice for Healthcare Procedures: Standards and Guidance. October 2013. Available at http://www.rcoa.ac.uk/document-store/safe-sedation-practice-healthcare-procedures-standards-and-guidance.

dentistry. One of the themes for debate was the definition of depth of sedation. In the UK the terms describing the levels of sedation (i.e., minimal, moderate, and deep) are the same as for other countries, except that the term *conscious sedation* is preferred by UK dentists. Conscious sedation is a sleepy state from which the patient can be roused easily by the spoken word (rather than any other physical stimulus). Moreover, some UK dentists were promoting the use of potent anesthetic drugs, used in low doses, to enable short-acting conscious sedation. This was a controversial topic and many practitioners believed that such techniques were not safe enough for use outside the hospital setting or by non-anesthetists. Several committees attempted to provide guidance or regulation to prevent accidental deep sedation. The Intercollegiate Advisory Committee for Sedation in Dentistry (ICACSD)[3] published Standards for Conscious Sedation in the Provision of Dental Care in 2015, and the key recommendations in relation to pediatric sedation are presented in Table 14.1.3. In essence

TABLE 14.1.3 Key dental recommendations for pediatric sedation

Pediatric population is defined as ages 0–12 years.
Inhaled Entonox® (nitrous oxide/oxygen) should be the first line for conscious sedation.
Monopharmacy only unless a skilled sedationist is present alongside the dental surgeon.
Monitoring for sedation may be clinical only for Entonox® (nitrous oxide/oxygen), but must include NIBP and pulse oximetry for any technique utilizing benzodiazepines. For any opioid use, end-tidal capnography must also be used.
All dental practices must be regularly inspected by the Care Quality Commission (CQC) with regard to their sedation practice.

Source: Intercollegiate Advisory Committee for Sedation in Dentistry. Standards for Conscious Sedation in the Provision of Dental Care. 2015. Available at https://www.rcseng.ac.uk/dental-faculties/fds/publications-guidelines/standards-for-conscious-sedation-in-the-provision-of-dental-care/.

this set of guidelines limits sedation drugs to simple techniques for which dentists have had training. In particular, it caused all dental practices to be inspected, and if standards were not met the practices were closed (Care Quality Commission: http://www.cqc.org.uk/content/dentists). This was a major step forward and ensured that dental practices' standards matched those of hospital practice.

What Now?

The guidelines and reports discussed have in common the importance of differentiating between anesthetists (all anesthetists are physicians in the UK) and non-anesthetist sedation providers. A national survey of workload by UK anesthetists[4] in 2013 found that few anesthetists provided sedation to children; thus, it is difficult to give practical training in pediatric sedation to anesthetists.

The UK guidelines in all disciplines have reduced the variation in practice outside of the hospital environment. It is our impression that dental surgeons are following the guidance of the ICACSD and that dental offices are being inspected; in fact, some inspections have caused suspension of sedation practice. In endoscopy, anesthesia by anesthetists is dominant. In radiology, sedation by non-anesthetists is still an important service provision. For painful procedures—particularly in the emergency department—ketamine seems to be a reliable and common method and is being used by non-anesthetists.

With respect to ED pediatric sedation, a recent review article[5] drew attention to improvements in UK practices and found that standards were catching up with other developed nations (United States, Canada, New Zealand, and Australia). The main issues were the use of effective agents (such as ketamine) and the training and accreditation of sedation practitioners in ED.

Finally, in the last 5 years, dexmedetomidine has become available in the UK, and this has the potential to offer another very important technique to manage children undergoing painless imaging. This drug may lead to new national guidelines.

Summary

The NICE guidelines led to an increased awareness in healthcare professionals about pediatric sedation and sparked the creation of specialty-specific guidelines. Dental sedation outside the hospital is now limited to simple techniques that are reliable in selected patients and procedures, and this has increased the number of hospital-based dental procedures. Ketamine is being used increasingly in UK EDs; training and credentialing remain the most important issues. Novel sedation agents such as dexmedetomidine are likely to generate further guidelines.

References

1. NICE. Sedation in under 19s: using sedation for diagnostic and therapeutic procedures. Available at nice.org.uk/guidance/cg112.
2. Academy of Medical Royal Colleges. Safe Sedation Practice for Healthcare Procedures: Standards and Guidance. October 2013. Available at http://www.rcoa.ac.uk/document-store/safe-sedation-practice-healthcare-procedures-standards-and-guidance.
3. Intercollegiate Advisory Committee for Sedation in Dentistry. Standards for Conscious Sedation in the Provision of Dental Care. 2015. Available at https://www.rcseng.ac.uk/dental-faculties/fds/publications-guidelines/standards-for-conscious-sedation-in-the-provision-of-dental-care/.
4. Sury MR, Palmer JH, Cook TM, Pandit JJ. The state of UK anaesthesia: a survey of National Health Service activity in 2013. *Br J Anaesth.* 2014;113:575–584.
5. Green SM, Mason KP, Krauss BS. Ketamine and propofol sedation by emergency medicine specialists: mainstream or menace? *Br J Anaesth.* 2016;116:449–451.

15

Non-Intravenous Sedation

15.1

Nitrous Oxide

JUDITH L. ZIER AND MARYKAY FARRELL

History

Nitrous oxide (N_2O) has been used in dentistry since the 1840s and has a lengthy record of safety and efficacy. Due to its low potency, its role in the operating room has been limited to use in combination with more potent general anesthetics. Recently, N_2O has been used to provide maternal labor analgesia and to provide sedation/analgesia for a variety of pediatric and adult medical procedures.

Pharmacokinetics

N_2O is a colorless gas, heavier than air, with a faint sweet smell. Because it is relatively insoluble in blood, alveolar uptake is rapid and equilibrium is reached quickly in vascular-rich tissues such as the brain. Sedative effect may be apparent within the first 30 seconds after initiation of inhalation, with full effect within 5–10 minutes. N_2O is neither metabolized nor stored in tissue; it is eliminated rapidly via expiration. When inhalation is discontinued, the sedative effects of N_2O abate within minutes, with return to baseline psychomotor function in 15–30 minutes.

Mechanism of Action and Clinical Effects

N_2O provides anxiolysis and analgesia in addition to sedation. Its mechanism of action is complex, with sedation involving noncompetitive inhibition of the *N*-methyl-D-aspartate (NMDA) subtype of glutamate receptors, anxiolysis mediated by activation of gamma-aminobutyric acid (GABA) receptors, and analgesia involving activation of opioid receptors as well as descending noradrenergic pathways. N_2O also provides amnesia when used in concentrations suitable for procedural sedation.

Level of Sedation

N_2O has low potency compared to general anesthetic gases. Its minimum alveolar concentration (MAC), the concentration necessary to prevent movement in 50% of subjects responding to a surgical stimulus, is 104%, a level that cannot be achieved outside of a hyperbaric chamber. N_2O administration at a concentration of $\leq$50% without other sedating agents is classified as minimal sedation by the American Academy of Pediatrics. Administration at >50% may produce moderate sedation, though many patients will remain awake and interactive when receiving the maximum deliverable concentration of 70%. N_2O used in combination with other sedating medications (e.g., benzodiazepines or opioids) is more likely to produce moderate to deep sedation. Unlike many inhaled anesthetics, N_2O is safe for patients with malignant hyperthermia.

Equipment for Nitrous Oxide Administration

All N_2O delivery equipment must be equipped with a scavenging system to minimize the risk of occupational exposure. Scavenging removes exhaled N_2O with all system types and removes excess flow with a continuous-flow device. The gas removed by scavenging should be vented into a system appropriate for disposal of waste anesthetic gases. Equipment should be checked before each use to ensure that N_2O flow will cease if the oxygen supply fails (to prevent inadvertent administration of 100% N_2O) and to look for signs of wear that could result in N_2O leakage.

Continuous-Flow, Titratable System

The flowmeter (N_2O/oxygen blender) for this system allows the delivery of a variable percentage of N_2O (0–70%), with oxygen as the remaining gas. Gas flow is continuous while the flowmeter is in use. Titration allows the percentage of N_2O to be matched to individual patient need. However, continuous flow makes the system prone to environmental contamination if a complete patient/mask seal is not maintained. The N_2O concentration and gas flow rates are both adjustable, which may take some practice to master. This is the system used by most dentists in the United States.

Fixed 50% N_2O/50% Oxygen Concentration

The flowmeter for this system mixes N_2O and oxygen in this fixed concentration. The system typically incorporates a demand valve that provides gas flow only when the patient inhales. This is a simple system to use, and the demand valve may decrease the risk of environmental contamination, but young children may have difficulty overcoming the demand valve to initiate gas flow. The N_2O concentration cannot be altered if the patient is over- or under-sedated. This is the most common device used for labor and delivery analgesia in the United States.

Tanks of Premixed 50% N_2O/50% Oxygen

This is a simple system to use, but the concentration cannot be altered if the patient is over- or under-sedated. It is not currently available in the United States.

Procedure Indications

N_2O as a single agent may be adequate for procedures that are distressing but not particularly painful or for minor painful procedures (Table 15.1.1). Although N_2O has analgesic properties, it is most effective when combined with topical or local anesthetics if pain is anticipated. N_2O as a single agent may be inadequate for more

TABLE 15.1.1 Procedural considerations for nitrous oxide sedation/analgesia

Consider nitrous oxide + topical/local anesthetic for:
Urinary catheterization Venipuncture Lumbar puncture Nasogastric tube insertion Gastrostomy or gastrojejunostomy tube replacement Intramuscular injection (e.g., botulinum toxin) Foreign-body removal Peripherally inserted central catheter (PICC) Radiologic imaging (CT, nuclear medicine imaging) Otolaryngology procedures (e.g., cerumen removal, speech endoscopy) Placement of subcutaneous hormonal implant Gynecologic exam, intrauterine device placement
Consider nitrous oxide combined with opioid or benzodiazepine + topical/local anesthetic for:
Fracture reduction Burn wound debridement/dressing changes Bone marrow biopsy Laceration repair Abscess incision and drainage Intra-articular injection/joint aspiration Dermatologic procedures (e.g., nevus excision) Organ biopsy (e.g., thyroid, liver)

intensely painful procedures. Success for more painful procedures may be achieved when N_2O administration is combined with opioids or benzodiazepines given orally, nasally, or intravenously.

Administration Techniques

Because of its rapid onset, N_2O administration may be targeted to a few minutes before a procedure. If a continuous-flow, titratable system is used, a baseline level of anxiolysis may be achieved with a modest concentration of N_2O (e.g., 40–50%) during preparation for the procedure, with a brief increase in concentration to coincide with the most painful part of the procedure (e.g., needle insertion for lumbar puncture). Although it may be tempting to administer the maximum concentration (70%) throughout all procedures, some patients find the maximum concentration uncomfortable and may become agitated. Administration of a high concentration (>50%) for prolonged periods also increases the risk of vomiting.

Administration of 100% oxygen for 3–5 minutes after N_2O is discontinued with the scavenging system in place disposes of residual exhaled N_2O, decreasing the risk of environmental contamination. This also eliminates the risk of "diffusion hypoxia"—the theoretical risk of alveolar oxygen dilution as N_2O leaves the blood.

N_2O sedation/analgesia is most effective when combined with calm distraction (e.g., digital tablet games, movies, storytelling). However, too many distractors or unorganized commotion may overstimulate a child and trigger agitation. The child's temperament also plays a role in the success of N_2O sedation. All involved with the procedure (patient, parents, and procedural provider) must be aware of the expected level of sedation as well as the possibility of failure.

Nursing staff specifically trained in N_2O sedation, including contraindications and side effects, have safely administered N_2O to children for procedural sedation.

Side Effects

Side effects of N_2O are listed in Table 15.1.2. Some deserve additional discussion.

Nausea and vomiting are the most common side effects, with an incidence of ~5%. The incidence of vomiting increases when N_2O is administered at concentration of >50% for >15 minutes, or when N_2O is combined with an opioid.

Expansion of trapped gas occurs due to the rapid diffusion of N_2O into the gas-filled space. Administered at high concentration, N_2O can double the size of a pneumothorax in 10 minutes and triple it in 30 minutes. Gas trapped in a rigid structure will develop increased pressure, and this may cause pain in some circumstances (e.g., blocked sinus).

Inactivation of vitamin B_{12} may lead to bone marrow or neurologic dysfunction in patients with low levels of vitamin B_{12}. Vitamin B_{12}

TABLE 15.1.2 Nitrous oxide side effects

Nausea and vomiting
Euphoria
Dizziness
Tingling of extremities
Headache
Hallucinations
Expansion of trapped gas
Increased pressure of gas trapped in a rigid structure
Vasodilatation in some vascular beds, including the cerebral circulation
Inactivation of vitamin B_{12}
Potential increased pulmonary vascular resistance in patients with pulmonary hypertension
Mildly decreased myocardial contractility
Increased venous tone
Decreased hypoxemic drive
Aspiration, airway obstruction, and/or oxygen desaturation (see text)

deficiency is rare in children but can occur due to inadequate intake (e.g., exclusively breastfed infants of mothers with a strict vegan diet) or malabsorption (e.g., with gastric bypass, short bowel syndrome, ileal resection, or congenital pernicious anemia).

Other serious side effects such as aspiration, airway obstruction, and oxygen desaturation are rare but have been reported. Risk is increased when N_2O is combined with an opioid or benzodiazepine.

Most studies have shown no association between fasting state and risk of adverse events.

The side effects of N_2O lead to a list of contraindications for administration (Table 15.1.3).

Occupational Exposure

Chronic exposure to N_2O has been has been linked to reproductive issues, neurologic deficits, and hematologic disorders. In the United

TABLE 15.1.3 Contraindications to nitrous oxide use

Pneumothorax
Bowel obstruction
Intracranial air[1]
Recent tympanoplasty
Diving within previous 24 hours
Previous intraocular surgery if gas was injected into the vitreous[2]
Severe bullous emphysema
Impaired level of consciousness
Pregnancy[3]
Vitamin B_{12} deficiency
Chronic obstructive pulmonary disease

[1] Intracranial air may remain up to 3 weeks following craniotomy.

[2] Length of risk varies based on the gas injected, but gas may be retained up to 3 months.

[3] Although used as a labor analgesic, nitrous oxide should be avoided in the first 2 trimesters.

States, regulatory bodies have recommended exposure limits of 25 ppm (National Institute for Occupational Safety and Health) or 50 ppm (American Conference of Governmental Industrial Hygienists). Exposure limits vary by country; some European countries allow exposure up to 100 ppm. The risk of environmental exposure is minimized with the use of a scavenging system, adequate room ventilation and air exchanges, routine equipment checks to eliminate leaks, and proper administration technique, including maintenance of a good mask/patient seal and scavenging exhaled N_2O during postprocedure oxygen administration.

Other Issues

N_2O is a known drug of abuse, so N_2O administration equipment and gas cylinders must be securely stored. N_2O is also an environmental greenhouse gas, although the contribution from medical gas use is insignificant compared to naturally occurring and industrial sources.

Suggested Reading

Sanders RD, Weimann J, Maze M. Biologic effects of nitrous oxide: a mechanistic and toxicologic review. *Anesthesiology*. 2008;109(4):707–722.

Tobias JD. Applications of nitrous oxide for procedural sedation in the pediatric population. *Pediatr Emerg Care*. 2013;29(2):245–265.

Tsze DS, Mallory MD, Cravero JP. Practice patterns and adverse events of nitrous oxide sedation and analgesia: a report from the Pediatric Sedation Research Consortium. *J Pediatr*. 2016;169:260–265.

15.2

Intranasal Medications

DANIEL S. TSZE AND JASON REYNOLDS

The intranasal (IN) route is an effective means of administering sedatives and analgesics. It is a needle-free alternative to intravenous (IV) or intramuscular (IM) routes, it is not subject to first-pass metabolism, and its efficacy approaches that of IV administration without requiring IV access. There is absorption through the highly vascular nasal mucosa, as well as utilization of the nose–brain pathway that bypasses systemic circulation and the blood–brain barrier and transports medications directly to the brain. The use of IN medications has been well described for providing procedural sedation for both painful and non-painful procedures in children.

Agents Used

The most common agents administered by the IN route are midazolam, fentanyl, dexmedetomidine, and ketamine.

Midazolam

Midazolam is a benzodiazepine that provides anxiolysis, amnesia, and sedation but not analgesia. IN midazolam as a single agent is typically used to achieve anxiolysis or minimal sedation but has no analgesic effects. It is commonly used for preoperative anxiolysis to promote separation, to facilitate catheter placement for voiding cystourethrography (VCUG) exams, to obtain intravascular access, and to provide anxiolysis for minor procedures such as laceration repairs. There are reports of its use in combination with fentanyl, dexmedetomidine, and nitrous oxide in order to achieve moderate or deep levels of sedation.

Fentanyl

Fentanyl is a potent opioid analgesic. IN fentanyl as a single agent is typically used to provide analgesia and has minimal sedative effects. Its use has been extensively described for the treatment of acute pediatric pain and a wide range of painful pediatric procedures. There are reports of its use in combination with midazolam, dexmedetomidine, and nitrous oxide to achieve moderate or deep levels of sedation.

Dexmedetomidine

Dexmedetomidine is a potent alpha-2 agonist that provides sedation and mild analgesia. IN dexmedetomidine as a single agent in low doses can be used to provide minimal sedation and has been shown to be comparable to midazolam to promote separation in the perioperative setting. In higher doses, IN dexmedetomidine may be used to provide moderate to deep sedation for non-painful procedures. Its utility for auditory brainstem response (ABR) tests, echocardiography, and CT scans has been well established. A recent study from the Pediatric Sedation Research Consortium demonstrated that IN dexmedetomidine in combination with IN midazolam was effective for MRI exams.

Ketamine

Ketamine is a dissociative *N*-methyl-D-aspartate (NMDA) receptor antagonist with analgesic, sedative, and amnestic properties. IN ketamine has been described for providing procedural sedation to facilitate painful or distressing procedures (e.g., laceration repair or dental procedures) and non-painful procedures such as CT scans, both as a sole agent and in combination with other IN medications, such as midazolam. IN ketamine has also been used as an analgesic to treat severe pain in the emergency department setting when administered in sub-dissociative doses.

Reversal Medications

It is important to mention that reversal medications (e.g., naloxone and flumazenil) can also be administered by the IN route to reverse effects due to opioids or benzodiazepines, respectively.

Discussion

There are four keys to successful IN administration:

1. ***Proper positioning of the device during administration.*** If an atomizer is being used, it should be aimed toward the most superior–posterior aspect of the vertex, away from the roof of the nasal vestibule, where there is no absorption. Aiming the device toward the ipsilateral eye maximizes dispersal over the highly vascular nasal turbinates and may optimize absorption into the systemic circulation. We have proposed aiming straight up, without lateral deviation. This may facilitate dispersal over the olfactory region located in the roof of the nasal cavity and a short way down the septum and lateral wall, which may optimize absorption through the nose–brain pathway, in addition to dispersal over the turbinates. We have demonstrated good clinical outcomes using this technique in a prior study and our clinical practice.
2. ***Atomization.*** Atomization of the solution optimizes absorption by decreasing the molecule size and facilitating broader distribution. If an atomizer is not available, the solution can

still be administered as drops using a syringe, and facilitated using the plastic cannula of an IV cannula. However, atomization has been shown to be superior to drops and is therefore preferable.

3. ***Volume of administration.*** Excessive volumes can lead to runoff. It is ideal to use the highest concentration possible so that the smallest possible total volume is required. Up to 1 mL can be administered with comparable clinical effects to lower volumes of administration (e.g., 0.2 mL, 0.5 mL), but we recommend a maximum volume of administration of 0.5 mL. If the total volume to be given exceeds the desired volume of administration, alternate between nares using the desired volume of administration each time until the total volume is achieved.
4. ***Optimizing surface area.*** The total volume should be divided into at least two aliquots and the medication administered to both nares when possible. Doing so effectively doubles the amount of surface area available for absorption.

IN sedatives can be used for a diverse range of procedures. For longer procedures, such as non-contrast MRIs, patients may be successfully sedated with a combination of IN dexmedetomidine (3–4 mcg/kg) and IN midazolam (0.1–0.2 mg/kg), avoiding the need for IV placement. For less stimulating exams like ABRs, echocardiograms, and CT, IN dexmedetomidine may be successful when given in doses of 2.5–4 mcg/kg as a single agent.

When using IN dexmedetomidine, time to achieve adequate sedation varies but is generally 20–30 minutes. Likewise, sedation duration and recovery time vary widely but are closer to those achieved with IV administration techniques without the prolonged clearance sometimes seen with enteral administration. IN dexmedetomidine can be used to achieve adequate sedation for 30–60 minutes depending on the degree of stimulation of the exam. Finally, recovery times are not well documented in the literature, but it has been our experience that most children meet discharge criteria within 60 minutes of arrival in recovery.

IN midazolam has been used to facilitate catheter placement for VCUG. Published doses range from 0.2 to 0.5 mg/kg. Despite providing anxiolysis and the potential for anterograde amnesia, the procedure should always be completed with topical lidocaine jelly unless otherwise contraindicated. IN midazolam does not appear to impact urodynamic variables.

The use of IN medications to facilitate more painful procedures such as fracture reductions or abscess incision and drainage is most successful when local anesthesia is optimized, and/or a sedative and analgesic are combined to achieve deeper levels of sedation. For example, the use of IN fentanyl (1.5–2 mcg/kg) with nitrous oxide (50–70%) has been well described for facilitating closed fracture reductions, with children achieving moderate to deep sedation. IN fentanyl may also be combined with IN midazolam if deeper levels of sedation are desired. When targeting deeper levels of sedation providers must remember to adhere to the same policies and procedures required when these medications are administered IV.

IN midazolam is well described as a safe and effective sedative for facilitating laceration repair in children, with the best chance of success when using doses of 0.4–0.5 mg/kg. However, IN midazolam must always be used in conjunction with topical anesthetics (e.g., lidocaine-epinephrine-tetracaine gel) and integrative strategies (e.g., child life, distraction) to minimize the patient's experience of pain and distress. IN dexmedetomidine (2 mcg/kg) may also be considered for laceration repair, but the time to onset of adequate sedation is significantly longer than IN midazolam (20–30 minutes vs. 5–10 minutes, respectively).

Table 15.2.1 provides IN dosage information and special considerations for the agents discussed in this chapter.

TABLE 15.2.1 IN sedatives and analgesics

Medication	*Dosing*	*Special Considerations*
Midazolam	Anxiolysis: 0.4–0.5 mg/kg Max. total dose 10 mg	Nasal burning with administration. May consider pre- or co-administration of IN midazolam with IN 4% lidocaine (10 mg/0.25 mL per nostril).
Dexmedetomidine	Anxiolysis: 0.5–2 mcg/kg Sedation: 2.5–4 mcg/kg	No clear max. dose; recommend max. dose of 200 mcg, based on volume when using 100-mcg/mL concentration
Fentanyl	1.5–2 mcg/kg Max. total dose 100 mcg	May use up to 200 mcg in opioid-tolerant patients
Ketamine	Analgesia: 1 mg/kg Sedation: 9 mg/kg	Use highest concentration available. No clear max. dose; recommend max. dose of 300 mg, based on volume when using 100-mg/mL concentration.
Naloxone	0.2–0.3 mg/kg Max. total dose 2 mg	Opioid reversal
Flumazenil	40 mcg/kg Max. total dose 200 mcg	Benzodiazepine reversal

Summary

IN administration of sedative and analgesic medications has been shown to be safe and effective for children in a variety of settings. The avoidance of first-pass metabolism and the reliability of delivery (compared to oral medications) make them especially attractive for children. IN administration also provides an opportunity to avoid IV line placement in many situations, which may reduce the pain and anxiety associated with many diagnostic and therapeutic procedures in children. More studies are needed to compare important sedation outcomes between IN and IV sedation regimens in order to guide best practice.

Suggested Reading

Pires A, Fortuna A, Alves G, Falcão A. Intranasal drug delivery: how, why and what for? *J Pharm Pharm Sci.* 2009;12:288–311.

Wolfe TR, Braude DA. Intranasal medication delivery for children: a brief review and update. *Pediatrics.* 2010;126:532–537.

15.3

Oral Medications

REBECCA K. BURGER AND SHOBHIT JAIN

Oral (PO) sedatives are usually well accepted by children when issues of flavor and texture are addressed. They are easily administered in all ages and obviate the pain involved in intravenous (IV) or intramuscular injection. The most commonly administered PO sedative is midazolam, which has a specific enteral formulation with predictable pharmacokinetics and dynamics. Other sedatives (e.g., ketamine, dexmedetomidine) have been administered enterally without necessarily having a specific enteral formulation. These medications may be useful as preprocedure anxiolytics or as sedatives and analgesics when IV access is unavailable but may not be well accepted from a taste standpoint. Medications with specific PO formulations such as melatonin and clonidine have not been used extensively for procedural sedation, but potential benefits will be discussed here. Other agents available for administration by the PO route, such as ketamine, dexmedetomidine, melatonin, the combination of meperidine and hydroxyzine, and clonidine, will also be discussed.

Midazolam

Beneficial Effects

PO midazolam is approved by the U.S. Food and Drug Administration (FDA) for premedication prior to anesthesia. PO midazolam is an ideal premedication in children due to its anxiolytic properties, easing parental separation and reducing sensory input. It also acts as a sedative–hypnotic and muscle relaxant and causes anterograde amnesia. PO midazolam may cause mild to moderate sedation in children but has no analgesic properties.

Pharmacokinetics

- Time to onset: median time of 15 minutes (range 5–55 minutes) in a study of children in the emergency department (ED) who received 0.5 mg/kg for procedural sedation[1]
- Duration of action: 30 minutes in pediatric patients given 0.5 mg/kg as premedication[2]
- Time to recovery (discharge readiness): 60 minutes (range 30–100 minutes)[1]

Uses

PO midazolam should not be used as a sole agent for procedural sedation for invasive or painful procedures. PO midazolam may be useful for simple short procedures, with local anesthetic when necessary, or for brief noninvasive tests. A Cochrane review found "no high-quality evidence to determine if midazolam, when administered as the sole sedative agent prior to a procedure, produces more or less effective sedation than placebo or other medications."[3]

For preprocedural anxiolysis, PO midazolam as a premedication helps reduce separation anxiety from parent and reduces behavioral changes in the first week after the procedure.[4] Minimal to moderate sedation can be achieved with PO midazolam, resulting in amnesia for brief painful procedures such as IV catheter placement, injection of local anesthesia, and nerve blocks. PO midazolam has synergistic effects when used in conjunction with other sedatives, analgesics. or hypnotics, often reducing the total dose of medications used.

Indications for the use of PO midazolam are brief minimally invasive procedures (laceration repair [less successful on facial wounds],[1,5] wound care,[1] foreign-body removal,[1] splint application,[1] nerve blocks,[6] dental cleanings/extractions,[7,8] and upper gastrointestinal endoscopy[9]) and noninvasive imaging/procedures (electroencephalography [EEG][10]).

Unwanted Effects/Adverse Reactions

~1% of children will have a paradoxical reaction (hyperactivity, agitation, and restlessness) from midazolam unrelated to the route of administration.[11] There are no known factors that predict who will experience a paradoxical reaction. Treatment options for a paradoxical reaction are (1) wait for the midazolam to wear off, since it has a short duration and (2) for severe cases, give flumazenil (requires IV or intranasal).

Differing levels of hypoxia have been reported in the literature.

Postprocedural hallucinations and nightmares have been reported in the subsequent week. In a study comparing premedication using PO ketamine versus PO midazolam, there was no difference in visual or auditory hallucinations during recovery nor in the incidence of nightmares in the following week in children 2–10 years old.[12]

Ketamine

Beneficial Effects

Although less frequently used than the IV route, PO administration of ketamine can be a useful approach in certain cases. The FDA-approved uses include procedural sedation and as an adjunct for general anesthesia. Ketamine has been used as a premedication for anesthesia, but its use as a sedative–analgesic is most described in patients with difficult IV access and for dental rehabilitation.

Pharmacokinetics

- Peak effect: 20-45 minutes (slower-acting than IV administration)
- Bioavailability (16%): significantly less than IM or IV route (>90%)[13]
- Wide range of enteral dosing has been described (5–10 mg/kg).

Uses

Ketamine has both sedative and analgesic properties, making it useful in both painful and non-painful procedures. In wound care and laceration repair, PO ketamine was demonstrated to be superior not only to placebo but to PO midazolam as well.[14,15] It can be used for burn management in combination with PO midazolam[16] and can also be used as premedication for elective surgery.

Unwanted Effects/Adverse Reactions

Compared with PO midazolam, ketamine may have higher rates of sedation failure.[14,17] Its bioavailability enterally makes ketamine much less predictable. Postprocedural agitation and hallucinations (emergence phenomenon) may occur, along with nightmares in the subsequent week; this is unrelated to the route of administration. Vomiting is more common with higher doses (6 mg/kg vs. 3 mg/kg); this too is unrelated to the route of administration.

Dexmedetomidine

Beneficial Effects

Dexmedetomidine is a relatively selective alpha-2 adrenergic agonist with sedative characteristics. It may have weak analgesic effects.

Uses

Dexmedetomidine has largely been used as an IV premedication prior to anesthesia and for sedation for mechanically ventilated patients in the intensive care unit. The oral route is much less commonly described. Zub et al.[18] described use in a small number of patients as a premedication for anesthesia induction and procedural sedation and concluded that it was effective even in patients with neurobehavioral disorders. Jannu et al.[19] compared PO dexmedetomidine (4 mcg/kg) with PO midazolam (0.75 mg/kg) as a premedication in patients 1–7 years old and found no difference in the level of preoperative sedation achieved; quicker onset of sedation occurred with midazolam but there was less agitation with dexmedetomidine.

Melatonin

Beneficial Effects

Melatonin induces sleep, is both a sedative and hypnotic, and has anxiolytic properties. There is conflicting evidence regarding its effectiveness as an analgesic.

Uses

- ABR tests[21]
- Noninvasive imaging and EEG[10,22]
- Premedication: Decreased preoperative anxiety in children 5–15 years old without impairing cognitive and psychomotor functions; 0.75 mg/kg of melatonin was more effective than 0.5 mg/kg.
- There are case or case series reports of the use of melatonin as a sedative–hypnotic in ABR testing, imaging studies, EEG, and venipuncture[23]
- Blood draws[24]

Meperidine and Hydroxyzine

The combination of PO meperidine and hydroxyzine has been studied for use in pediatric dental procedures. These drugs in combination were 81% effective or very effective for sedation in pediatric dental patients and <5% of cases were aborted due to behavior; however, this study is limited due to its retrospective methodology.[25] Johnson et al. reported 80% successful sedations using this combination in pediatric dental patients.[22]

Clonidine

Clonidine has analgesic, anxiolytic, and sedative effects. At 4 mcg/kg, PO clonidine given as a premedication produced reliable sedation and intraoperative hemodynamic stability while decreasing the need for postoperative analgesia.[25–28] Clonidine can take up to 45 minutes to produce adequate sedation.

Conclusion

Several PO medications are available for sedation in children. They vary in reliability and timely effectiveness. Midazolam, the best-studied in children, can be used in a variety of settings. Oral ketamine, dexmedetomidine, melatonin, meperidine plus hydroxyzine, and clonidine are other options less commonly used for sedation in children. In general, the enteral route is useful for preprocedure anxiolysis but results in less predictable onset and recovery time.

References

1. Davies FC, Waters M. Oral midazolam for conscious sedation of children during minor procedures. *J Accid Emerg Med.* 1998;15:244–248.

2. Jaffe RA, Schmiesing CA, Golianu B. *Anesthesiologist's Manual of Surgical Procedures*. 2015.
3. Conway A, Rolley J, Sutherland JR. Midazolam for sedation before procedures. *Cochrane Database Syst Rev*. 2016;(5):CD009491.
4. Kain ZN, Mayes LC, Wang SM, Hofstadter MB. Postoperative behavioral outcomes in children: effects of sedative premedication. *Anesthesiology*. 1999;90(3):758–765.
5. Hennes HM, Wagner V, Bonadio WA, et al. The effect of oral midazolam on anxiety of preschool children during laceration repair. *Ann Emerg Med*. 1990;19(9):1006–1009.
6. Mittiga MR, Ruddy RM. Procedures. In: Shaw KN, Bachur RG, eds. *Fleisher & Ludwig's Textbook of Pediatric Emergency Medicine*. 7th ed. Philadelphia: Lippincott Williams & Wilkins, 2016.
7. Uldum B, Hallonsten AL, Poulsen S. Midazolam conscious sedation in a large Danish municipal dental service for children and adolescents. *Int J Paediatr Dent*. 2008;18(4):256–261.
8. Lourenço-Matharu L, Ashley PF, Furness S. Sedation of children undergoing dental treatment. *Cochrane Database Syst Rev*. 2012;3(3):CD003877.
9. Rafeey M, Ghojazadeh M, Feizo Allah Zadeh H, Majidi H. Use of oral midazolam in pediatric upper gastrointestinal endoscopy. *Pediatr Int*. 2010;52(2):191–195.
10. Fallah R, Yadegari Y, Behdad S, Karbasi SA. Melatonin and intravenous midazolam administered orally in drug induced sleep electroencephalography of children: randomized clinical trial of efficacy. *Arch Iran Med*. 2014;17(11):741–745.
11. Del Pizzo J, Fein JA, Selbst SM. Procedural sedation. In: Shaw KN, Bachur RG, eds. *Fleisher & Ludwig's Textbook of Pediatric Emergency Medicine*. 7th ed. Philadelphia: Lippincott Williams & Wilkins, 2016.
12. Funk W, Jakob W, Riedl T, Taeger K. Oral preanaesthetic medication for children: double-blind randomized study of a combination of midazolam and ketamine vs midazolam or ketamine alone. *Br J Anaesth*. 2000;84(3):335–340.
13. Grant IS, Nimmo WS, Clements J. Pharmacokinetics and analgesic effects of IM and oral ketamine. *Br J Anaesth*. 1981;53:805–810.
14. Qureshi FA, Mellis PT, McFadden MA. Efficacy of oral ketamine for providing sedation and analgesia to children requiring laceration repair. *Pediatr Emerg Care*. 1995;11(2):93–97.
15. Younge P, Kendall JM. Sedation for children requiring wound repair: a randomised controlled double blind comparison of oral midazolam and oral ketamine. *Emerg Med J*. 2001;18(1):30–33.

16. Norambuena C, Yañez J, Flores V, et al. Oral ketamine and midazolam for pediatric burn patients: a prospective, randomized, double-blind study. *J Pediatr Surg.* 2013;48(3):629–634.
17. Rubinstein O, Barkan S, Breitbart R, et al. Efficacy of oral ketamine compared to midazolam for sedation of children undergoing laceration repair: a double-blind, randomized, controlled trial. *Medicine (Baltimore).* 2016;95(26):e3984.
18. Zub D, Berkenbosch JW, Tobias JD. Preliminary experience with oral dexmedetomidine for procedural and anesthetic premedication. *Paediatr Anaesth.* 2005;15(11):932–938.
19. Jannu V, Mane RS, Dhorigol MG, Sanikop CS. A comparison of oral midazolam and oral dexmedetomidine as a premedication in pediatric anesthesia. *Saudi J Anaesth.* 2016;10(4):390–394.
20. Godwin SA, Caro DA, Wolf SJ, et al. Clinical policy: Procedural sedation and analgesia in the emergency department. *Ann Emerg Med.* 2005;45(2):177–196.
21. Schmidt CM, Knief A, Deuster D, et al. Melatonin is a useful alternative to sedation in children undergoing brainstem audiometry with an age-dependent success rate—a field report of 250 investigations. *Neuropediatrics.* 2007;38(1):2–4.
22. Johnson K, Page A, Williams H, et al. The use of melatonin as an alternative to sedation in uncooperative children undergoing an MRI examination. *Clin Radiol.* 2002;57(6):502–506.
23. Kurdi MS, Patel T. The role of melatonin in anaesthesia and critical care. *Indian J Anaesth.* 2013;57(2):137–144.
24. Marseglia L, D'Angelo G, Manti S, et al. Analgesic, anxiolytic and anaesthetic effects of melatonin: new potential uses in pediatrics. *Int J Mol Sci.* 2015;16(1):1209–1220.
25. Lenahan M, Wells M, Scarbecz M. A retrospective study of 248 pediatric oral sedations utilizing the combination of meperidine and hydroxyzine for dental treatment. *J Clin Pediatr Dent.* 2015;39(5):481–487.
26. Nishina K, Mikawa K, Maekawa N, Obara H. The efficacy of clonidine for reducing perioperative haemodynamic changes and volatile anaesthetic requirements in children. *Acta Anaesthesiol Scand.* 1996;40(6):746–751.
27. Nishina K, Mikawa K, Shiga M, Obara H. Clonidine in paediatric anaesthesia. *Paediatr Anaesth.* 1999;9(3):187–202.
28. Mikawa K, Nishina K, Maekawa N, Obara H. Oral clonidine premedication reduces postoperative pain in children. *Anesth Analg.* 1996;82(2):225–230.

15.4

Topical and Local Anesthetics

AMY E. VINSON AND CONSTANCE S. HOUCK

Procedural sedation can significantly reduce the pain and anxiety children experience with medical procedures. Despite this, the moment that the patient and family often remember most clearly is the placement of the intravenous catheter (IV) and any associated discomfort. Attempts have long been made to minimize this pain, with easier and faster methods becoming more common as topical anesthetic delivery methods have evolved:

- 1980s—topical anesthesia for laceration repair using a solution of tetracaine, adrenaline (epinephrine), and cocaine (TAC).[1] As the use of cocaine was eliminated this was replaced by a topical solution of lidocaine, epinephrine, and tetracaine (LET).
- Prior to 1990—anesthesia for intact skin achieved by injecting local anesthetic (LA) subcutaneously with small (30-gauge) needles
- Early 1990s—development of topical LA creams (eutectic mixtures of local anesthetics [EMLA]), usually requiring long application times (>60 minutes) to provide local anesthesia
- Late 1990s to the present—newer and faster-acting creams/devices, such as the Synera® topical patch, liposomal lidocaine (LMX4®), and jet propulsion injectors (J-Tip™) providing topical anesthesia in <30 minutes.

While anesthetizing the skin is helpful for IV placement, these same strategies can also be used at procedural sites (e.g., lumbar puncture or PICC line site) to decrease the sharp sensation associated with the needle penetration at the initiation of the procedure, thereby decreasing the depth of sedation required. LAs can also aid in anesthetizing the pharynx for endoscope placement, although this approach does carry some risk.

Topical Local Anesthetics

Traditional aqueous LAs cannot penetrate the skin's stratum corneum to render the tissue insensate, but topical LAs have been modified to be more lipophilic and therefore able to penetrate the epidermal lipid bilayers.

Creams and Gels

- **EMLA® cream** (eutectic mixture of local anesthetics; Astra Zeneca, Wilmington, DE, USA)
  - Mixture of lidocaine and prilocaine
  - First commercially available for use on intact skin
  - Reduces pain of venipuncture/cannulation in 85% of the population[2]
  - Long onset time (at least 60 minutes) and shallow penetration
  - Causes vasoconstriction, potentially making cannulation more difficult[3]
- **LMX4®** (previously marketed as ELA-Max 4%®, Ferndale Laboratories, Ferndale, MI, USA)
  - Liposomal encapsulation of lidocaine designed to penetrate the epidermis and resist degradation
  - Faster onset than EMLA, with improved efficacy[4–6]
  - An occlusive dressing is not required, as with EMLA.

- **Synera® topical patch** (Endo Pharmaceuticals, Chadds Ford, PA, USA)
  - Utilizes CHADD™ (controlled heat-assisted drug delivery) to speed the onset of cutaneous absorption and anesthesia to 20 minutes
  - Contains a eutectic mixture of lidocaine and tetracaine as well as a heating element and bio-occlusive dressing.
  - Has been shown effective for venipuncture in children[7,8]
  - May cause vasodilation at the site, a benefit for vascular access
- **AMETOP Gel 4%™** (Smith & Nephew Healthcare Ltd., Hull, UK)
  - Topical aqueous gel preparation of 4% tetracaine
  - Available in Europe and Canada, but not the United States
  - Faster onset than EMLA, with added vasodilation[9]

Jet-Propulsion Injector

- **J-Tip™ injector** (National Medical Products, Inc. Irvine, CA, USA)
  - Needleless, handheld, single-use device that uses a compressed gas source to propel a local anesthetic through the epidermis and into the dermal layer
  - Depth of effect: 3–8 mm
  - Designed to be "loaded" with up to 0.25 mL of lidocaine (can be buffered to reduce irritation)
  - In a pediatric trial, demonstrated greater analgesia after 1–3 minutes than EMLA after 60 minutes[10]

Vapocoolant Spray

- **Pain Ease®** (Gebauer Company, Cleveland, OH, USA)
  - Nonflammable ethyl chloride preparation
  - Can be used on both intact skin and minor open wounds
  - Rapid onset but ultrashort-acting

- Has demonstrated similar efficacy to EMLA for immunization pain[11,12]

Local Anesthetic Use to Alleviate Pain Associated with Propofol Injection

The pain associated with the injection of propofol has been demonstrated in 70% of patients and results from the activation of capsaicin receptors, hence the "burning" feeling reported. The C-fibers responsible for pain transmission are not particularly responsive to opioids but do respond to LAs.[13] In a systemic review, the only reliable technique that reduced the pain associated with propofol was a modified Bier block (injection of lidocaine while a tourniquet is inflated) prior to propofol administration.[14] The pain is also lessened when the propofol is injected into larger veins, such as those in the antecubital fossa.

Aerosolized Benzocaine Sprays

Benzocaine sprays can be efficacious for anesthetizing the mucous membranes of the pharynx for procedures such as upper endoscopy but must be used with caution (see "Risks of Local Anesthetics"):

- **HurriCaine® Spray** (Beutlich LP Pharmaceuticals, Bunnell, FL, USA): benzocaine 20%
- **Cetacaine® Spray** (Cetylite Industries, Inc., Pennsauken Township, NJ, USA)
  - Benzocaine 14.0%, butamben 2.0%, tetracaine hydrochloride 2.0%
  - Mixture available in spray, gel, and liquid form.

- **Lidocaine 4% solution (Hikma Pharmaceuticals, London, UK)** Disposable mucosal atomization devices (e.g., MADgic®, MAD Nasal™ Atomization Device; Teleflex Inc., Wayne, PA, USA) are available that allow the local anesthetic solution to be sprayed in the nose and onto respiratory tissues.

Risks of Local Anesthetics

While the topical use of LA is generally safe, careful titration of dosage based on the patient's age and weight and the drug's side-effect profile is important to prevent toxicity. Specific information regarding the onset, duration, benefits, and risks of each LA can be found in Table 15.4.1.[15]

Methemoglobinemia

Acquired methemoglobinemia can occur following the use of certain LAs, including prilocaine and benzocaine, when absorbed in sufficient quantities. This may manifest as persistent cyanosis and tissue hypoxia due to the left shift of the hemoglobin dissociation curve. Prompt treatment with methylene blue is indicated. EMLA® cream (containing prilocaine) and HurriCaine® and Cetacaine® sprays (both containing benzocaine) have been implicated.[16]

Local Anesthetic Systemic Toxicity

Several commonly used LAs carry the risk of local anesthetic systemic toxicity (LAST), severe, life-threatening cardiovascular collapse precipitated by the intravascular injection or absorption of LAs. In addition, procedural sedation may be required to facilitate procedures where larger doses of LA may be used (e.g., peripheral nerve blocks, dental procedures). LAST generally begins with central

TABLE 15.4.1 Pharmacology of topical local anesthetics

Name	*Composition*	*Onset*	*Duration*	*Benefits*	*Limitations*
EMLA® cream	Lidocaine and prilocaine	60–120 minutes	60–120 minutes (after removal)	Vasoconstriction at site may be desirable (e.g., lumbar puncture, intramuscular injections).	Long onset time, shallow penetration. Vasoconstriction can make IV placement difficult. Potential methemoglobinemia with overdose from prilocaine.
LMX4®	Lidocaine (liposomal encapsulation)	30 minutes	60 minutes (after removal)	Ease of application, no occlusive dressing needed, faster onset than EMLA	May cause itching, redness, or swelling at application site
Synera® topical patch	Lidocaine and tetracaine Uses CHADD™ (controlled heat-assisted drug delivery)	20–30 minutes	120 minutes (after patch removal)	Ease of application; vasodilation may facilitate venipuncture	May cause redness, swelling, and/or irritation
AMETOP Gel 4%™	Tetracaine 4%	30–40 minutes	3–4 hours (after removal)	Faster onset than EMLA; vasodilation (may facilitate venipuncture)	Not available in the United States Vasodilation at site may be undesirable (e.g., lumbar puncture)

J-Tip™ injector	Delivery system, typically loaded with lidocaine with or without sodium bicarbonate	1–2 minutes	15–20 minutes	Rapid onset Depth 3–8 mm	May cause venous puncture if administered directly over a vein, especially with tourniquet engaged
Pain Ease®	Pentafluoropropane tetrafluoroethane vapocoolant (nonflammable)	<5 seconds	10–60 seconds	Can be used on minor open wounds Rapid onset	Short duration Overapplication can cause frostbite.
HurriCaine® Spray	Benzocaine 20%	30 seconds	10–15 minutes	Ease of administration Rapid onset	Potential methemoglobinemia with benzocaine overdose
Cetacaine® Spray	Benzocaine 14.0%, butamben 2.0%, tetracaine HCl 2.0%	30 seconds	30–60 minutes	Ease of administration Longer duration	Potential methemoglobinemia with benzocaine overdose
Lidocaine Solution	Lidocaine 4%	2–5 minutes	15–60 minutes	No concern for methemoglobinemia Less expensive than benzocaine sprays	Longer onset time

TABLE 15.4.2 Checklist for treatment of local anesthetic systemic toxicity

• Get help
• Initial focus o Airway management: ventilate with 100% oxygen o Confirm or establish adequate IV access o Seizure suppression: benzodiazepines are preferred; be prepared to treat resultant hypoventilation
• Management of cardiac arrhythmias o Confirm and monitor continuous electrocardiography, blood pressure, and SaO_2 o Pediatric Advanced Life Support (PALS) may require adjustment of medications and perhaps prolonged effort o Avoid vasopressin, calcium channel blockers, beta blockers, or local anesthetic. o Treat hypotension with small doses of epinephrine (≤1 mcg/kg).
• Lipid emulsion (20%) therapy o Bolus 1.5 mL/kg (lean body mass) IV over 1 minute o Start continuous infusion of 0.25 mL/kg/min o Repeat bolus every 3–5 minutes (up to 4.5 mL/kg total dose) until circulation is restored. o Increase the rate to 0.5 mL/kg/min if blood pressure remains low or declines. o Continue infusion for 10 minutes after hemodynamic stability is restored. o Max. total Intralipid 20% dose: 10 mL/kg over first 30 minutes
• Monitor and correct acidosis, hypercarbia, and hyperkalemia.
• Consider alerting nearest cardiopulmonary bypass/extracorporeal membrane oxygenation (ECMO) center and intensive care unit if no return of spontaneous circulation after 6 minutes.

Adapted from reference 18 and SPA Critical Events Checklist (http://www.pedsanesthesia.org/wp-content/uploads/2017/06/SPACriticalEventsChecklists.pdf).

nervous system excitation (irritability, restlessness, seizures) and then can lead to rapid cardiovascular deterioration (dysrhythmias, myocardial depression, reduced systemic vascular resistance, and cardiac arrest). Treatment depends on prompt administration of Intralipid while providing high-quality cardiopulmonary resuscitation.[17] A checklist describing current recommendations for the treatment of LAST can be found in Table 15.4.2.

Conclusion

Often one of the only experiences remembered by a patient receiving procedural sedation is the placement of the IV catheter. Local anesthetics are a useful tool to improve the overall experience, decrease stress, reduce pain, lower analgesic requirements, and prevent fear of subsequent medical encounters.

References

1. Pryor G, Kilpatrick W, Opp D. Local anesthesia in minor lacerations: topical TAC vs. lidocaine infiltration. *Ann Emerg Med.* 1980; 9:568–571.
2. Fetzer SJ. Reducing venipuncture and intravenous insertion pain with eutectic mixture of local anesthetic: a meta-analysis. *Nurs Res.* 2002;51(2):119–124.
3. Wahlgren CF, Quiding H. Depth of cutaneous analgesia after application of a eutectic mixture of the local anesthetics lidocaine and prilocaine (EMLA cream). *J Am Acad Dermatol.* 2000;42(4):584–588.
4. Eichenfield LF, Funk A, Fallon-Friedlander S, Cunningham BB. A clinical study to evaluate the efficacy of ELA-Max (4% liposomal lidocaine) as compared with eutectic mixture of local anesthetics cream for pain reduction of venipuncture in children. *Pediatrics.* 2002;109(6):1093–1099.
5. Taddio A, Soin HK, Schuh S, et al. Liposomal lidocaine to improve procedural success rates and reduce procedural pain among children: a randomized controlled trial. *CMAJ.* 2005;172(13):1691–1695.

6. Koh JL, Harrison D, Myers R, et al. A randomized, double-blind comparison study of EMLA and ELA-Max for topical anesthesia in children undergoing intravenous insertion. *Paediatr Anaesth.* 2004;14(12):977–982.
7. Shoemaker TS, Zhang J, Love G, et al. Evaluating skin anesthesia after administration of a local anesthetic system consisting of an S-Caine patch and a controlled heat-aided drug delivery (CHADD) patch in volunteers. *Clin J Pain.* 2000;16(3):200–204.
8. Sethna NF, Verghese ST, Hannallah RS, et al. A randomized controlled trial to evaluate S-Caine patch for reducing pain associated with vascular access in children. *Anesthesiology.* 2005;102(2):403–408.
9. O'Brien L, Taddio A, Lyszkiewicz DA, Koren G. A critical review of the topical local anesthetic amethocaine (Ametop) for pediatric pain. *Paediatr Drugs.* 2005;7(1):41–54.
10. Jimenez N, Bradford H, Seidel KD, et al. A comparison of a needle-free injection system for local anesthesia versus EMLA® for intravenous catheter insertion in the pediatric patient. *Anesth Analg.* 2006;102(2):411–414.
11. Cohen Reis E, Holubkov R. Vapocoolant spray is equally effective as EMLA cream in reducing immunization pain in school-aged children. *Pediatrics.* 2997;100(6):E5.
12. Berberich FR, Landman Z. Reducing immunization discomfort in 4- to 6-year old children: a randomized trial. *Pediatrics.* 2009;124(2):e203–e209.
13. Fischer MJ, Leffler A, Niedermirtl F, et al. The general anesthetic propofol excites nociceptors by activating TRPV1 and TRPA1 rather than GABAA receptors. *J Biol Chem.* 2010;285:34781–34792.
14. Picard P. Tramer MR. Prevention of pain on injection with propofol: a quantitative systematic review. *Anesth Analg.* 2000;90:963–969.
15. http://www.fda.gov/Drugs/DrugSafety/PostmarketDrugSafetyInformationfor PatientsandProviders/ucm124350.htm. Accessed February 16, 2016.
16. Taleb M, Ashraf Z, Valavoor S, Tinkel J. Evaluation and management of acquired methemoglobinemia associated with topical benzocaine use. *Am J Cardiovasc Drugs.* 2013;13(5):325–330.
17. El-Boghdadly K, Chin KJ. Local anesthetic systemic toxicity: continuing professional development. *Can J Anaesth.* 2016;63(3):330–349.
18. Neal JM, Mulroy MF, Weinberg GL. American Society of Regional Anesthesia and Pain Medicine checklist for managing local anesthesia systemic toxicity: 2012 version. *Reg Anesth Pain Med.* 2012;37:16–18.

PART 3

BEYOND SEDATION

16

Multiprofessional Team

16.1

Physician Training and Perspective

ANDREA R. CARBERRY AND

GREGORY A. HOLLMAN

Institutions vary in the requirements used to define whether a provider is competent to perform moderate and deep procedural sedation. Regardless of institutional variation, attaining sedation competency requires a multitiered approach that (1) incorporates the individual practitioner's specialty and previous training and experience; (2) encompasses a variety of teaching methods; and (3) uses different methods of assessment.

Within an institution, requirements for moderate versus deep sedation privileges may vary based on subspecialty background and prior experience and training. Regardless of the institutional variation in requirements, competency in procedural sedation requires the incorporation of a provider's cognitive, psychomotor, and affective skills to achieve the desired outcome (Figure 16.1.1). The following section will focus on different types of training, education, and expertise for practitioners, with a brief discussion of assessment.

Subspecialty Background and Formal Training and Education

Several specialties outside of anesthesiology routinely provide pediatric procedural sedation services. These specialties often perform

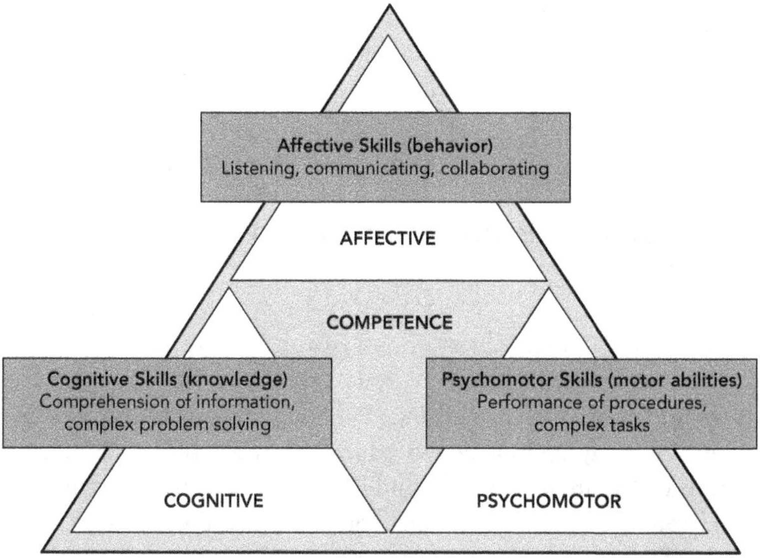

FIGURE 16.1.1.

Integration of a practitioner's cognitive, psychomotor, and affective skills to achieve a desired outcome. Cognitive skills in procedural sedation can be taught through didactic written materials and lectures, while psychomotor skills and affective skills can be addressed through interactive small-group sessions, medical simulation, and clinical experience/mentoring.

pediatric sedation as an integral part of their clinical practice and frequently receive formal training during their fellowship. The most common pediatric specialties other than anesthesiology that provide sedation services include pediatric critical care medicine (PCCM), pediatric emergency medicine (PEM), and pediatric hospital medicine (PHM).

Pediatric procedural sedation is a fundamental part of PCCM and PEM fellowship training. Consequently, completing a fellowship in PCCM or PEM often satisfies an institution's "core" privileging requirements for moderate sedation and in some centers deep sedation. PHM physicians, however, often do not receive formal procedural sedation education and experience during training. Thus, providers in PHM often need additional training and experience to fulfill competency requirements for becoming privileged in moderate and deep sedation.

Additional Training, Education, and Expertise

Additional training, education, and expertise are required when a physician's training and previous experience do not meet the threshold criteria for privileging at an individual institution. While there are many approaches to education and training, in general methods that are multimodal and interactive in nature are superior to any one individual educational format. The following list outlines some of the most common approaches, with a description and discussion of advantages and disadvantages:

- Didactic written materials
  - Deliver factual information in printed form and include manuals, policies, articles, etc.
  - Provide a large amount of information at a pace the individual practitioner can dictate. For example, most published written instruction in sedation discusses the presedation risk assessment, fasting guidelines, definitions of sedation levels, pharmacology of sedative drugs, sedation monitoring, sedation-related complications and their management, and postsedation recovery and discharge criteria.
  - Convey only cognitive information (factual knowledge).
- Didactic lectures
  - Provide factual information in a variety of formats including live talks, online lectures, and videos
  - Deliver a large amount of information while emphasizing certain points

- Summarize written materials, typically covering what the instructor feels is most relevant to the audience
- Allow some interaction (e.g., question and answers) between student and instructor during live lectures
- Provide only cognitive information, similar to written material.

- Interactive small-group sessions
  - Provide instruction in the form of hands-on small-group case- and problem-based discussions and scenarios
  - Facilitate higher-order cognitive skills, including comprehension, reasoning, and evaluation
  - Can provide hands-on teaching for motor skills such as airway positioning or bag-mask ventilation
  - Encourage formative assessments and feedback from instructors that can promote reflection
  - Require prior review of written didactic materials on an individual basis to be most efficacious.
- Medical simulation
  - Creates an environment that realistically attempts to present a medical situation to the learner. Examples include partial task simulation that teaches specific skills (e.g., intubation heads); standardized patients for objective structured clinical examinations; and high-fidelity human simulations that use life-sized manikins with physiologic capabilities.
  - Teaches healthcare professionals communication and psychomotor skills and other important attributes for procedural sedation
  - Promotes higher cognitive functioning skills such as clinical decision-making, technical abilities, and teamwork
  - Provides the best educational experience outside the clinical setting for mimicking "real-life" events
  - Can create and standardize reproduction of uncommon clinical scenarios for students

  - Requires a baseline foundation of factual knowledge to be most beneficial.
- Clinical experience and mentoring
  - Provides experience in a real-life setting working directly with patients and staff in an actual sedation environment
  - Offers the best overall educational environment to learn sedation when coupled with a supervising mentor
  - Affords hands-on experience that incorporates higher educational cognitive, psychomotor, and behavioral skills needed for sedation competencies
  - Encourages instructor feedback and assessment of skills individualized to the practitioner
  - Fosters patient safety, as instructor can intervene if needed
  - Can be challenged by time constraints, mentor commitment, and individual practice styles.

Assessing Sedation Competencies

Assessment is an important component of privileging and should be summative in nature to evaluate a practitioner's competency at specific procedures and clinical activities. As clinical practice is complex and multifaceted, more than one assessment method is often needed to assess for medical competence. Assessment methods should all be reproducible, reliable, and valid for the intended skill or competency. The competence pyramid introduced by Miller describes competence based at four levels: *knows, knows how, shows how,* and *does.* Figure 16.1.2 describes Miller's hierarchal framework for clinical assessment as it relates to procedural sedation. The following list outlines assessment methods, with a description and brief discussion of advantages and disadvantages:

- Written examinations
  - Assess factual knowledge (*knows*) and clinical reasoning and decision-making (*knows how*), most commonly through multiple-choice questions

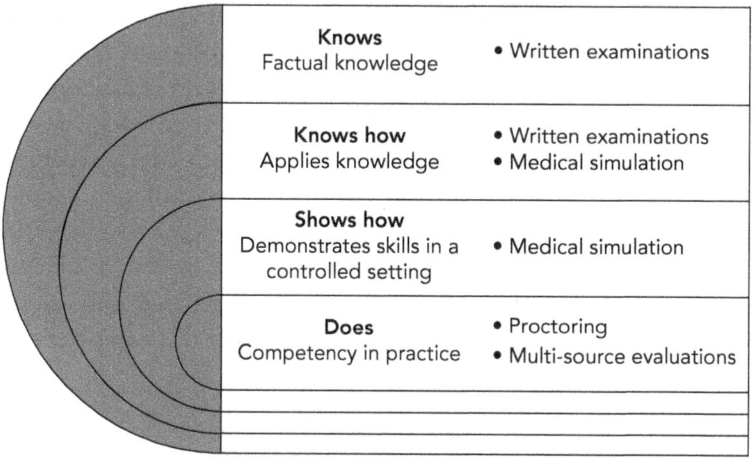

FIGURE 16.1.2.

Miller's hierarchy of clinical competence as it can be applied to assess competency for procedural sedation.

    - Assess cognitive skills with a minimum score for passing
    - Promote efficiency, ease of performing, and reliability
    - Exclude assessment of psychomotor skills, communication, and teamwork (*shows how*).
- Medical simulation
    - Promotes a reproducible and realistic environment that can assess specific educational objectives
    - Assesses higher-level functioning such as problem-solving and decision-making as well as procedural skills through case- and problem-based medical stimulation (*shows how*)
    - Evaluates communication and teamwork skills.
- Direct assessment of clinical practice (proctoring and multisource evaluations)
    - Evaluates a practitioner's performance under real-life circumstances (*does*) and usually involves a preset number of cases

- Provides information about interpersonal skills, ability to work as a team member, and professionalism by other staff members through multisource (360-degree) evaluations.

Institutions vary in their requirements for determining competency and subsequent privileging in pediatric procedural sedation. Pediatric subspecialties that are not anesthesiology-based are assuming a greater role in providing procedural sedation services in children. Based on the individual practitioner's prior training and experience, a multimodal approach to education, training, and assessment is most effective to encompass the multifaceted competencies required for procedural sedation.

Suggested Reading

Hollman G. Pediatric sedation credentialing and privileging. In: Tobias J, ed. *Procedural Sedation for Infants, Children, and Adolescents.* Elk Grove Village, IL: American Academy of Pediatrics, 2016:236–247.

Kamat R, Hollman G, Harold K, et al. Current state of institutional privileging profiles for pediatric procedural sedation providers. *Hosp Pediatr.* 2015;5(9):487–494.

Miller GE. The assessment of clinical skills/competence/performance. *Acad Med.* 1990;65(9 Suppl):S63–S67.

16.2

Nursing Perspective

MICHELLE M. RHOADS, EILEEN BRIENING,
NANCY CREGO, KIMBERLY PAULA-SANTOS,
AND LAUREN HUSTER

The Nursing Process

Nursing practice is guided by the nursing process, a framework that consists of (1) assessment, (2) nursing diagnosis, (3) planning, (4) intervention, and (5) evaluation.[1] This framework may be applied to the numerous roles nurses have in ensuring the safe and effective delivery of pediatric sedation care by multidisciplinary teams. Nurses contribute to the direct care of sedated patients by developing competency and expanding knowledge and expertise within their specialty, described later in this chapter. While the provision of care to patients and families is of paramount importance, ensuring an environment conducive to the delivery of safe, quality care by the healthcare team is another fundamental aspect of nursing.

Organizations such as the Agency for Healthcare Research and Quality (AHRQ; https://www.ahrq.gov/) provide numerous educational resources, tools, and data that can be referenced and used by nurses across settings.[2] The AHRQ highlights four areas in which nurses contribute to providing high-quality care to patients: patient-centered care, work environment, quality improvement, and safety.[2]

This section will focus on the application of the nursing process to the work environment, quality improvement, and safety aspects of the nurse's role within the multidisciplinary sedation team.[3] Table 16.2.1 includes examples of how the nursing process can be used to address each of the AHRQ components.

Assessment

Nurses begin the nursing process by collecting objective and subjective data. Information may include process data routinely collected such as the frequency of sedation cancellations, late starts, and adverse events or may come from patients, other departments, other members of the sedation team, advisory committees, unit meetings, or patient surveys. The purpose of the assessment is to develop an understanding of the sedation process and to provide relevant information to share with the multidisciplinary team.

Nursing Diagnosis

In this part of the process, data from the assessment and collaboration with the team are analyzed and used to identify an actual or potential problem. Once the problem is identified, the role of the nurse is to identify those aspects of the problem that fall within the nursing professional, regulatory, and practice role within the sedation team.

Planning

Nurses collaborate with teams to develop a plan to solve the identified problem and to set goals and objectives. Plan development may involve obtaining more data on evidence-based nursing practices, nursing regulations, nursing standards of care, or support from the organization, such as the education department.

TABLE 16.2.1 Examples of nursing contributions to multidisciplinary sedation teams

Nursing Process	*Clinical Care*	*Patient Safety*	*Patient Satisfaction*
Assessment	• Staffing/care needs	• Equipment and training	• Policies and unit practices
Nursing Diagnosis	• Identifies when additional human resources/expertise are necessary	• Identifies changes in equipment needs/ technologies necessary to meet patient needs	• Identifies policies/unit practices that are not optimal in meeting patient needs
Planning	• Consults with team members to define and prioritize needed resources	•Consults with team members to define training/equipment needs and possible resources to address these	• Consults with team members to develop specific policies or practices necessary to meet patient needs
Intervention	• Work flow redesign • Explores internal/external sources of expertise and how these can be integrated • Collects data that support needed change in clinical care	• Obtains needed equipment, develops training and method to track data on outcomes • Develops content and training method (online, certification, simulation) • Tracks data on changes in performance	• Uses current sedation guidelines, networks with other similar institutions or uses internal resources (e.g., child life, parent advisory boards) to address policies/ practices that meet patient needs
Evaluation	• Evaluates data on staffing, sedation adverse events	• Evaluates data on equipment utilization, procedure length, adverse events, staff satisfaction with training	• Evaluates patient satisfaction scores, on-time procedure times, recovery times, and follow-up calls

Implementation

Once a plan is developed, nurses work with the team to implement the plan. This may require changes in unit policies or practices that require approval outside of the unit-based team, staff meetings, in-services, emails, or collaboration with other departments. Furthermore, consideration of how evaluation data (frequency, method, and reporting) will be collected is part of the implementation phase.

Evaluation

Nurses are involved in several aspects of evaluation, including documenting care so that data can be collected and reviewed by other team members and orienting new staff to newly implemented practices/policies. Evaluation data are shared with all team members to determine effectiveness, unforeseen consequences, or the need to revise changes to processes.

Team Concept

Much progress has been made in the field of pediatric sedation with the introduction of a multidisciplinary approach. Demonstration of professional respect for all team members is fundamental to the overall success of a multidisciplinary pediatric sedation service. To provide optimal sedation, analgesia, and anxiolysis to our patients, the clinical knowledge of various disciplines must be combined. That being said, it is important to recognize and appreciate the diversity of each team member while acknowledging the unique contributions each brings to the sedation team.

The universal goals among the various disciplines include the following:

- To minimize patient and caregiver distress
- To enhance patient comfort

- To ensure quality procedural and diagnostic outcomes
- To return the patient to baseline status

A multidisciplinary approach that incorporates a safe, efficient environment, addresses underlying issues surrounding patient and family distress, and manages sedation and analgesia using a standardized approach will optimize patient comfort and improve outcomes.[4] This approach allows for professional collaboration and utilization of the varied skill sets of all the disciplines.

Specialty Certification

The development of a sedation nurse specialty certification has been viewed as essential. Specialty certification is noted to be positively linked to nurses' job satisfaction, sense of empowerment, and sense of collaboration with other healthcare team members.[5] The benefits of specialty certification have far-reaching implications, not only for nurses but for patients, families, and the institution. It has been demonstrated that certified nurses are more likely to provide care based on evidence-based guidelines, have greater confidence in their decision-making, increase patient safety, and produce higher patient satisfaction.[6] Certification is the formal recognition of specialized knowledge, skills, and experience demonstrated by achievement of standards identified by a nursing specialty to promote optimal health outcomes.[7] It is an indicator of quality that attracts patients and families.

The development of the scope and standards of specialty nursing certification is a long and arduous task. However, the benefits associated with specialty certification extend beyond the individual nurse to impact patients, families, and employers.

Specialty Credentialing

Credentialing is a process that allows a healthcare provider to provide patient care in an institution. Despite the growth of sedation services, there is limited information about the credentialing models and practices of the sedation providers involved with the various pediatric sedation programs in the United States.[8] Opportunity exists for benchmarked credentialing for providers of moderate and deep procedural sedation.

For nurse practitioners, the hospital credentialing process involves a review of their education, certifications, training skills, and licensure. Advanced practice nurses who are credentialed as moderate sedation providers are uniquely qualified to use their skills, experience, and competency to deliver safe moderate sedation to children. In order to help advanced practice nurses meet the Joint Commission's requirements for credentialing, some states have developed specific credentialing forms. In addition to hospital credentialing, nurse practitioners should be credentialed by health insurance companies as well as Medicare and Medicaid plans.

Registered nurses are also credentialed to administer or monitor sedation. These nurses must be accountable for their own practice within the guidelines of the institution, regulatory agencies, state nursing board requirements, professional standards of practice, and guidelines for sedation. The credentialed pediatric sedation nurse ensures safe and appropriate levels of sedation as well as pain management.

The nurse's role in pediatric sedation continues to evolve as the specialty grows. As members of a pediatric sedation team, nurse practitioners and registered nurses have the opportunity to be involved in a multidisciplinary specialty that values their experience, knowledge, and compassion while providing safe and effective care to children.

Nursing Competencies

Nurses play an integral role in the multiprofessional sedation team, but their skills and knowledge base can vary greatly, given the myriad of experiences within the nursing profession. It is therefore imperative to establish competency in order for sedation nurses to provide high-quality and safe care to sedation patients. Sedation nurses must possess a strong understanding of the sedation process, proficient assessment and monitoring skills, and expertise in emergency preparedness. They must have previous experience in a critical care setting, such as an intensive care unit, emergency department, or postanesthesia care unit. Sedation nurses must be under the supervision of a pediatric intensive care specialist or qualified sedation provider.[9] The entire team will benefit from participating in simulation or mock codes on a regular basis, ensuring that their roles are defined. It is paramount to have a standardized competency for all roles, particularly nursing, in order for procedural sedation to be safe and effective.

Each institution should carefully consider and develop its own sedation nursing competency tool. Such a qualifying instrument should include, but not be limited to, demonstration of a thorough knowledge and assessment skill base to care for sedation patients. The competent sedation nurse is proficient in carrying out the following:

- Perform a presedation assessment of the patient: Review past medical history, any active conditions, allergies, NPO status, weight, and current vital signs.
- Educate the patient and family: Engage them in discussion of the sedation process, expectations, and outcomes. Thorough and timely preparation of the sedation patient serves to enhance the patient and family experience.
- Perform an active timeout prior to the start of all sedation procedures to ensure that the following are correct: patient, procedure, site (if applicable), procedural staff, and necessary equipment. The nurse must confirm that the appropriate method for obtaining informed consent was used.[10]
- Monitor vital signs: The nurse must recognize deviation from the patient's baseline status in accordance with published guidelines for sedation that include protocols for minimal,

moderate, and deep sedation.[11] The nurse must be aware of the imperative of early recognition of vital sign deterioration in the sedated patient.

- Manage airways: Assist, when needed, with bag-valve-mask ventilation. Familiarity with inserting oral/nasopharyngeal airways should also be considered.
- Place and maintain intravenous access when applicable.
- Participate in mock codes and emergency simulation.
- Understand the pharmacology of the sedative, analgesic, and reversal agents that may be administered during procedural sedation. Understanding of appropriate preparation and administration of common medications should also be demonstrated.
- Properly recover the patient and continue to monitor vital signs, respiratory rate and effort, and level of consciousness until the patient has reached his or her appropriate Modified Aldrete score of 8 or greater.
- Provide the patient and family with postsedation care instructions, including restrictions, guidelines, and recommendations for care at home. Careful consideration of the procedure as well as the sedation medications used should be included in the discussion with those involved in caring for the patient following discharge.
- Perform a follow-up telephone call 24 hours after the procedure to ensure there were no reactions or untoward side effects noted subsequent to discharge; answer questions related to sedation, procedure, and further follow-up care.

Prior to participating in procedural sedation, a completed competency checklist is required. Competent sedation nurses foster a safe context for procedural success for the patient, and this facilitates trust by the family. Qualified sedation nurses are fundamental to the multiprofessional team and are committed to competency with the skills, knowledge, and highest quality of care.

Suggested Reading

Finnell DS, Thomas EL, Mehring WM, et al. Best practices for developing specialty nursing scope and standards of practice. *OJIN: Online Journal of Issues in Nursing*. 2015;20(2): manuscript 1.

Murphy JS. Credentialing process for nurse providers of moderate sedation. *J Radiol Nurs*. 2013;32(1):10–18.

References

1. Ackley BJ, Ladwig GB. *Nursing Diagnosis Handbook: An Evidence-Based Guide to Planning Care*. 10th ed. St. Louis, MO: Mosby Elsevier, 2011:26–34.
2. Agency for Healthcare Research and Quality. QI Guide on Improved Nursing Care. U.S. Department of Health and Human Services website. https://www.ahrq.gov/professionals/systems/monahrq/myqi/nursing.html—resources. Reviewed September 2017. Accessed February 12, 2018.
3. American Nurses Association. The Nursing Process. American Nurses Association website. http://www.nursingworld.org/TheNursingProcess. Accessed February 11, 2018.
4. Sessler CN, Grap MJ, Brophy GM. Multidisciplinary management of sedation and analgesia in critical care. *Semin Respir Crit Care Med*. 2001;22(2):211–226.
5. Wade CH. Perceived effects of specialty nurse certification: a review of the literature. *AORN J*. 2009;1:183–192.
6. Kaplow R. The value of certification. *AACN Adv Crit Care*. 2011;22(1):25–32.
7. Promoting excellence in nursing certification: A position statement on the value of specialty nursing certification. ABNS. Approved May 5, 2005. https//www.aaacn.org/sites/default/files/images/ABNS-cert-stat.pdf. Accessed April 19, 2017.
8. Kamat PP, Hollman GA, Simon HK, et al. Current state of institutional privileging profiles for pediatric procedural sedation providers. *Hosp Pediatr*. 2015;5(9):487–494.
9. Lavoie L, Vezina C, Paul-Savoie E, et al. Procedural pediatric sedation by nurses: available, competent, and safe. *Int J Pediatr*. 2012;2012:820209.

10. Connors JM, Cravero J, Lowrie L, et al. *Core Competencies for Pediatric Providers Who Deliver Deep Sedation*. Society for Pediatric Sedation, 2016.
11. Langhan M, Mallory M, Hertzog J, et al. Physiologic monitoring practices during pediatric procedural sedation. *Arch Pediatr Adolesc Med.* 2012;166(11):990–998.

16.3

Child Life Specialists and Nonpharmacologic Interventions

LAURA MITCHELL AND CHRISTINE TATEM

Role of the Child Life Specialist

Child life specialists (CLSs) "provide evidence-based, developmentally appropriate interventions including therapeutic play, preparation and education that reduce fear, anxiety, and pain for infants, children, and youth. Their education and training involves the developmental impact of illness and injury."[1] Historically, CLSs have provided care for inpatients and their families; however, with the shift toward ambulatory care, opportunities have arisen to incorporate the role of the CLS into the sedation team. The specialists working in this area can help reduce the emotional trauma that can be associated with medical procedures. CLSs are an integral component of the multidisciplinary sedation team. Their assessments can help the team develop a plan of care, and they offer insight into how to provide developmentally appropriate education as well as psychosocial and emotional support to pediatric patients and their families.

The core of child life practice is for patients and families to perceive the CLS as inherently nonthreatening. To be effective, the relationship needs to be both supportive and therapeutic. This unique balance allows the CLS to be nurturing while also providing expertise. This bond can be tenuous and care must be taken to avoid crossing professional boundaries. The relationship between the CLS and child should not undermine the established attachments to family or interfere with the building of a relationship with the medical team. The CLS acts as both advocate and facilitator, helping patients, families, and healthcare professionals understand and appreciate each other's point of view.[2]

Assessing the Patient

In determining how to effectively interact with patients, CLSs use screening tools to determine the patient's risk for experiencing increased distress during an encounter. The Psychosocial Risk Assessment in Pediatrics (PRAP) is used to evaluate a child's potential response to a healthcare experience based on these factors:

- Developmental considerations
- Ability to communicate
- Anxiety level
- Parental stress level
- Special needs
- Temperament
- Invasiveness of procedures
- Previous medical experiences
- Parental support.

In addition to providing insight into developing a plan of care, the PRAP also includes a database that can be used for benchmarking capabilities among participating facilities. Use of this tool is limited to the initial assessment of risk because it is not reliable once sedation medications have been administered. Consequently, further evaluation relies on more informal needs assessment tools.

Developing a Plan

Based upon an initial assessment, the CLS uses a family-centered care strategy and incorporates information from the treatment team to develop an individualized education and coping plan designed to reduce anxiety, increase cooperation, and promote mastery (Figure 16.3.1). On a sedation unit, the CLS may not be able to remain with one patient during the entire visit. Thus, if the specialist is developing a plan based solely on personal observation, CLS information and assessment may be incomplete or inaccurate. But by educating the healthcare team about the tenets of child life work, nurses and physicians can help with this process.[3] This multidisciplinary approach is applicable to sedation planning.

Depending on the need, a preprocedural education/play session can provide the patient opportunities to touch and manipulate medical supplies, look at images of the treatment area, or watch videos of other children having a similar experience. These sessions are designed

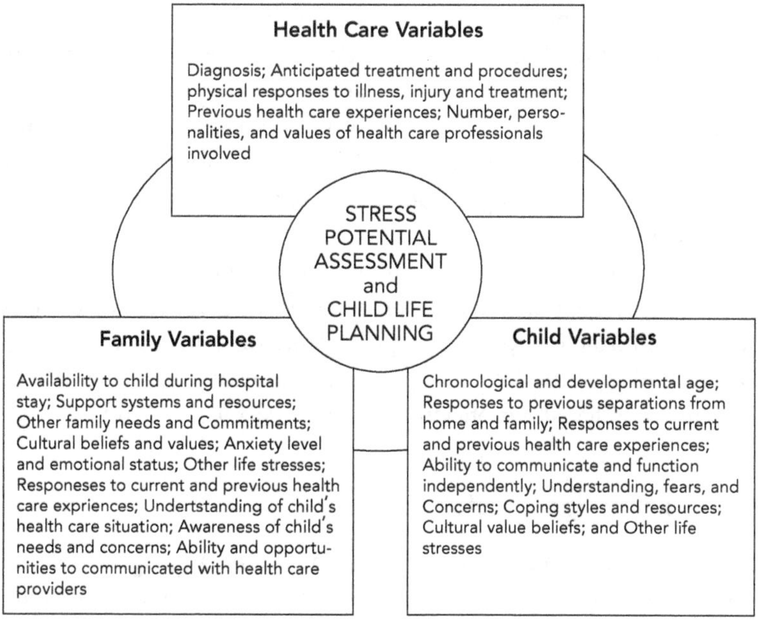

FIGURE 16.3.1.

Stress potential assessment process

Reprinted with permission of the Child life council.

to prepare patients, and by extension their families, for what they could experience during a healthcare encounter. The goal is to reduce the fear and anxiety associated with these experiences and promote positive coping both in the short and long term. These interventions exist on a continuum, with child-directed medical play experiences on one end and specialist-directed procedural preparation on the other.[2]

A child-directed medical play session provides both recreation and education; allowing the child to retain a sense of autonomy. A procedural preparation session, by contrast, is completely directed by the CLS and does not include a dramatic play component. Depending on the need, the CLS can incorporate sensory information about the procedure into the session, including what the child may see, hear, smell, feel, and even taste. During a preparation session, the CLS provides information through multiple modalities (e.g., images, verbal communication, videos) and gives the child an opportunity to manipulate medical equipment that may be used during the procedure. A goal is to impart information in order to clarify misconceptions. This is also an opportunity to develop a coping plan for the procedure. When appropriate, the patient can be given choices about various elements of the procedure, such as positioning and parental involvement. CLSs work with patients to help them develop a strategy for managing their pain and anxiety by applying nonpharmacologic techniques. There may also be an opportunity for role-rehearsal so that the child can feel more comfortable implementing the plan. For example, a CLS may review and practice different approaches to breathing so the patient becomes familiar and proficient with this relaxation method.[2,4]

Using Language Carefully

When communicating with patients, the use of language should be considered. Information presented should be honest and concrete, without being overwhelming. Whenever possible, nonthreatening language should be used. For example, when starting intravenous fluids, tubing should be "connected" or "attached" as opposed to "hooked up." Medical terminology and hospital jargon may confuse both children and their parents. Instead, descriptive phrasing can be used to simplify complex processes; "fluoroscopy" becomes "a moving X-ray picture." When discussing sedation, it's important to distinguish medication-induced "sleep" from the normal napping and sleeping patterns that children experience. Avoid euphemisms like "put to sleep," as a child may relate this to a time when a beloved pet was euthanized. Other common fears related to sedation are often centered on a loss of control and fear of either waking up in the middle of a procedure or not waking up at all.[2,5]

In addition to providing information that is concise and developmentally appropriate, it is important for the sedation team to use consistent language with patients and their families, a technique that demonstrates close communication among team members, reduces confusion, and promotes continuity of care. This collaboration becomes especially important in larger hospitals or health networks. The CLS can work with sedation colleagues to develop scripting options that meet the developmental and cultural needs of their patients and families.[2]

Parental education is also a component of child life practice on a sedation unit. CLSs provide parents with information about developmental norms and how to better understand how their child is coping. CLSs can prepare parents and caregivers for what they may see during the medical procedure and model supportive language and techniques. Parents can also receive guidance about educating and supporting siblings at home.[2]

After the Procedure

For a variety of reasons, preprocedural interventions are not always possible or even recommended. Scheduling challenges or parental preferences may prevent the CLS from providing preprocedural education. The CLS may also assess that due to the patient's heightened level of anxiety, this intervention would not be beneficial and, in fact, may cause more distress. In these situations, postprocedural play/education sessions can be just as valuable. Preschool and school-age children can benefit from a postprocedural medical play session to help them emotionally process their experiences. Postprocedural play opportunities can help a patient develop mastery over the experience, which will help him/her to cope during future medical experiences. This can be especially important for a patient with a chronic condition who will need to return to the hospital or clinic for continued monitoring or treatment. After discharge, children may even continue to process their experiences on their own by engaging in dramatic play with a pronounced medical theme.[2,4,5]

After the procedure, older school-age children and adolescents may be interested in learning more about the details of a procedure to help them develop their own narrative about their healthcare experiences. Another value to postprocedural interventions is that they help children to process the experiences that occurred while they were receiving sedation and/or anesthesia. A multitude of factors will determine how a child's memory will be affected by the sedation experience. For some children, the amnestic effect of sedation can be stressful and they may ask the CLS what occurred while they were "asleep." Other patients may need support from the CLS to reframe their experiences. This is especially true for patients who report having dreams during their sedation experience. These dreams can vary in mood from playful to menacing, and sometimes children need reassurance that these vivid images were not real. Other patients may experience incomplete recall and require the help of the CLS to fill in the gaps for them. This is an opportunity to provide positive reinforcement so that the child feels a sense of accomplishment and mastery moving forward.[2]

Patients Transitioning to Adult Care

Another critical concern is the best way to support chronic patients who are making transition from pediatric to adult care, where procedural sedation may not be available. The sedation practitioner and CLS can educate adolescent patients and families about the differences in treatment models and even advocate, if appropriate, for tapering off of sedation medications during their routine procedures. By initiating these changes while still in the pediatric realm, patients can benefit from child life interventions to further develop their own coping style and will have the chance to practice in a supportive environment.

Nonpharmacologic Interventions

For many children, undergoing potentially painful or invasive procedures can create fear and anxiety. This often results in avoidance or uncooperative behaviors and can lead to an increased need for sedation in order to complete the procedure successfully. There are a number of nonpharmacologic techniques that can be used with children to decrease their anxiety and perhaps even their experience of pain, leading to increased cooperation and potentially reducing the need for sedation. These techniques include providing a child-friendly environment, parental presence, positioning for comfort, distraction, and more advanced techniques such as guided imagery and hypnosis.

Environment

Procedure rooms can be overwhelming to children because of the amount of stimulation present both in terms of equipment and people. Creating a child-friendly environment involves minimizing the sensory information in order to help the child remain calm and feel in control.

- Set up the room as much as possible before the child enters, including covering medical equipment or keeping it out of sight until needed. Remove anything that is not necessary.
- Consider using local lighting to minimize the need for bright overhead lights.

- Minimize the number of adults in the room. If there are people who need to be present but are not directly involved in the procedure, have them stand back and away from the child.
- Minimize the amount of noise in the room. Keep voices low and side conversations to a minimum. Discussion about the procedure should happen outside the room.
- Designate one person to be the "voice" for the child. When many people are talking to either give directions or provide reassurance, it is confusing for the child to know which voice to listen to; this increases his or her anxiety.
- Be aware of the language you use and the effect it may have. Suggestions of language to use and language to avoid are included in Table 16.3.1.[6]

Parental Presence

Parental presence can also be effective in reducing the child's anxiety. Parents can engage their child in distraction and provide comfort through touch or their voice. They may also be able to assist by supporting their child in a comfortable position. It is important to assess the parent's own anxiety before engaging him/her; an anxious parent may find it difficult to support the child. In all situations, parents should be prepared for what to expect and coached in their role.

Positioning for Comfort

Placing children in a supine position often creates distress and should be avoided whenever possible. Positioning for comfort allows the child to be held by the parent in a way that is supportive for the child and appropriate for the procedure being performed while giving the child a sense of control. Comfort positions can include:

- Chest to chest with child straddling parent and arm extended

TABLE 16.3.1 Suggested language for parents or healthcare providers

Language to Avoid	*Language to Use*
You will be okay; there is nothing to worry about (reassurance) This is going to hurt/this won't hurt (vague; negative focus) The nurse is going to draw your blood (vague information)	What did you do in school today? (distraction) It might feel like a pinch (sensory information) First, the nurse will clean your arm, you will feel the cold alcohol pad, and next . . . (sensory and procedural information)
You are acting like a baby (criticism) It will feel like a bee sting (negative focus) The procedure will last as long as . . . (negative focus)	Let's get your mind off of it; tell me about that movie (distraction) Tell me how it feels (information) The procedure will be shorter than . . . (television program or other familiar time for child) (procedural information, positive focus)
The medicine will burn (negative focus) Tell me when you are ready (too much control)	Some children say they feel a warm feeling (sensory information; positive focus) When I count to 3, blow the feeling away from your body (coaching to cope; distraction; limited control)
I am sorry (apologizing) Don't cry (negative focus) It is over (negative focus)	You are being very brave (praise; encouragement) That was hard; I am proud of you (praise) You did a great job doing the deep breathing, holding still . . . (labeled praise)

Words or phrases that are helpful to one child may be threatening to another, so parents and healthcare providers should select their language carefully.

- Side sitting on parent's lap with parent holding child's head against the chest
- Parent sitting on stretcher with child leaning against the chest and parent's legs extended or placed gently over child's legs to prevent kicking

Many child life programs have developed posters illustrating these positions. They are often available on the hospital's website and displayed in treatment or procedure rooms.

Distraction

Distraction is a widely used nonpharmacologic approach to reduce pain and anxiety in children undergoing procedures. Techniques shown to be effective include bubble blowing and deep breathing, playing interactive games, reading books, listening to music, viewing videos, guided imagery, and hypnosis.[6–8]

Distraction focuses the child's attention away from the procedure while allowing him or her to engage in a more pleasant activity. The method of distraction used should be suitable to the child's age, developmental level, and interests (Table 16.3.2). Providing children the opportunity to choose their preferred distraction method allows them to feel involved and gives them a sense of control.

During the procedure, a child's attention may shift from the chosen distraction method. It is important that a parent, CLS, or other care provider is available to redirect the child's focus and keep him/her engaged in the activity.

While hypnosis can be effective in reducing children's pain and anxiety,[9] it requires advanced training and should only be provided by those qualified to do so.

Infants

Special consideration should be given to infants <12 months of age. For young infants, breastfeeding and administering a sweet-tasting

TABLE 16.3.2 Age-appropriate distraction techniques

Age	*Distraction and Nonpharmacologic Techniques*
Infant	Swaddling, sucking, parental presence, skin-to-skin contact, music, rocking
Toddler	Parental presence, preparation, comfort positioning, interactive books (lift the flaps, hidden pictures), bubbles, music, singing, light & sound toys
Preschool	Parental presence, preparation, comfort positioning, bubbles, pinwheels, counting, interactive books (hidden pictures), singing, storytelling
School age	Parental presence, preparation, comfort positioning, blowing, deep breathing, interactive games (tablet, phone), storytelling, guided imagery
Adolescent	Preparation, talking about interests, music with headphones, guided imagery

liquid are evidence-based strategies to reduce pain. While this may not be possible for those receiving sedation, it should be considered as an option for less invasive procedures such as heelsticks and intravenous line placement. Nonnutritive sucking (i.e., using a pacifier) may be an alternative to provide comfort when breastfeeding is not an option. Swaddling and skin-to-skin contact can also provide security for infants and reduce distress.

Summary

A variety of nonpharmacologic techniques can be used with children to reduce pain and anxiety. These techniques are often most effective when used in combination.[10,11] Preparation and coaching for both the parent and child further enhances the success of these methods.

TABLE 16.3.3 ONE VOICE©

ONE VOICE
One voice should be heard during procedure
Need for parental involvement
Educate patient before the procedure about what is going to happen
Validate child with your words
Offer the most comfortable, nonthreatening position
Individualize your game plan
Choose appropriate distraction to be used
Eliminate unnecessary staff not actively involved with the procedure

For more information, visit www.onevoice4kids.com

Providing a calming environment that includes parental presence and soft language sets the stage for making a child feel safe and comfortable. Using comfort positions and distraction gives the child a sense of control and participation, which can lead to increased cooperation. ONE VOICE© (Table 16.3.3)[12] provides a framework to guide practice when working with pediatric patients. It incorporates the concepts discussed in this chapter and is easily incorporated into daily use. Following this model ensures that the provider is using a child-friendly approach to deliver care to the pediatric patient.

Suggested Readings

Krauss BS, Calligaris L, Green S, Barbi E. Current concepts in management of pain in children in the emergency department. *Lancet* 2016;387:83–92.

Kuttner L. *A Child in Pain: What Health Care Professionals Can Do to Help.* Carmarthen, Wales, and Bethel, CT: Crown House Publishing, 2010.

References

1. Association for Child Life Professionals. http://www.childlife.org/. Published 2017. Accessed April 16, 2017.
2. Thompson RH, ed. *The Handbook of Child Life: A Guide for Pediatric Psychosocial Care.* Springfield, IL: Charles C. Thomas Publisher, Ltd. 2009.
3. Martin SR, Chorney JML, Tan ET, et al. Changing health care providers' behavior during pediatric inductions with an empirically based intervention. *Surv Anesthesiol.* 2012;56(1):27–28.
4. Veselis RA. Effects on Memory and Amnesia. In: Mason KP, ed. *Pediatric Sedation Outside of the Operating Room: A Multispecialty International Collaboration.* New York: Springer New York, 2015.
5. KazakAE, PenatiB, BrophyP, HimelsteinB. Pharmacologicandpsychologic Interventions for procedural pain. *Pediatrics.* 1998;102(1):59–66.
6. Cohen LL. Behavioral approaches to anxiety and pain management for pediatric venous access. *Pediatrics.* 2008;122(Suppl. 3):S134–S139.
7. Mutlu B, Balci S. Effects of balloon inflation and cough trick methods on easing pain in children during the drawing of venous blood samples: a randomized controlled trial. *J Spec Pediatr Nurs.* 2015;20:178–186.
8. Nillson S, Hallqvist C, Sidenvall B, Enskar K. Children's experiences of procedural pain management in conjunction with trauma wound dressings. *J Adv Nurs.* 67;7:1449–1457.
9. Butler LD, Symons BK, Henderson SL, et al. Hypnosis reduces stress and duration of an invasive medical procedure for children. *Pediatrics.* 2005;115:e77–e85.
10. Alexander M. Managing patient stress in pediatric radiology. *Radiol Technol.* 2012;83(6):549–560.
11. Powers SW. Empirically supported treatments in pediatric psychology: procedure-related pain. *J Pediatr Psychol.* 1999;24:131–145.
12. ONE VOICE: Creating a Less Threatening Environment for Children Undergoing Medical Procedures. http://www.onevoice4kids.com/index.html Published 1996. Updated 2017.

17

Guidelines, Regulatory Issues, and Reimbursement

17.1

Society Guidelines

URMILA TIRODKER

In the past several decades the practice of procedural sedation and analgesia has evolved into a distinct skill set and a service that has rapidly grown in terms of indications, need, practitioner types, and practice settings. Subsequently, several subspecialty societies and regulatory institutions have published and revised guidelines and standards to enhance patient safety by standardizing various aspects related to the monitoring and management of procedural sedation and analgesia and its recovery.

The American Academy of Pediatrics (AAP), American Society of Anesthesiologists (ASA), and American College of Emergency Physicians (ACEP) have published the most widely disseminated, comprehensive guidelines. These will be discussed here. All of the guidelines share the following characteristics:

1. Recommendations for best practices for safe sedation delivery systematically developed by current evidence analysis, expert opinion, open forum commentary, and clinical feasibility data
2. Based on the understanding that sedation is a continuum and practitioners should be able to monitor and rescue patients from a level of sedation deeper than intended
3. Not intended as "standards" or absolute requirements
4. Designed to be applicable to sedated procedures in varied settings performed by non- anesthesiologists

5. Mostly applicable to patients receiving moderate or deep sedation
6. Exclude patients who are not undergoing a diagnostic or therapeutic procedure and patients who are mechanically ventilated in critical care units.

AAP Guidelines for Procedural Sedation and Analgesia

In the 1970s and 1980s there was an increase in medical technology and procedures requiring sedation in children. In 1985, in response to several sedation-related deaths, the AAP (Committee on Drugs, Charles J. Coté, MD, and Theodore Striker, MD) first established sedation guidelines. The AAP defined three depths of sedation (conscious sedation, deep sedation, and general anesthesia) and outlined a systematic approach to delivering safe sedation care based on well-established anesthesia concepts.[1]

In 1992 the AAP revised the 1985 guidelines. The revised guidelines emphasized the sedation continuum and its rescue and discouraged the administration of sedation medications at home.[2]

In 2002, the AAP replaced the term "conscious sedation" with "moderate sedation." The American Academy of Pediatric Dentistry (AAPD), the ASA, and the Joint Commission endorsed the new definitions of sedation.[3]

The 2006 AAP and AAPD revision emphasized sophistication of monitoring and rescue skills and pharmacologic expertise of the practitioner. Capnography use was "encouraged."[4]

In the most recent AAP and AAPD revision (2016), capnography use was "required" for deep sedations, and management algorithms for complications were suggested.[5] A summary of the guidelines for moderate and deep sedation in this most recent update follows.

- Patient selection
  - Patients in ASA classes I and II are often considered appropriate candidates. Patients in ASA class III and children

with special needs, anatomic airway abnormalities, or obstructive sleep apnea may need anesthesia consultation.
  - Patient must be accompanied by a parent/legal guardian and preferably two adults for infants in a car seat.
- Must have immediately available facilities, personnel, on-site equipment, rescue drugs, and established protocols for rescue systems. The availability of emergency medical personnel does not replace the practitioner's responsibility to provide initial rescue from adverse events.
- Preprocedure fasting before elective sedation (Table 17.1.1)
- Presedation documentation: informed consent, specific instructions to parents; focused history, airway evaluation, and systemic examination

TABLE 17.1.1 Preprocedure fasting guidelines for elective sedation

Ingested Material	*Minimum Fasting Period (hours)*
Clear liquids (water, clear tea, black coffee, carbonated drinks)	2
Breast milk	4
Infant formula	6
Non-human milk	6
Light meal (toast and clear liquids) *Fried and fatty meals, meat may require longer gastric emptying times.*	6

For emergent sedation, balance the depth of sedation versus the risk of possible aspiration.

Adapted from reference 8. Available at https://www.asahq.org/For-Members/Practice-Management/Practice-Parameters.aspx.

- Documentation after treatment: time of discharge, condition at discharge, recommended usage of validated recovery scales prior to discharge
- Encourage the use of high-fidelity patient simulator training for sedation providers to manage adverse events.
- Continuous quality improvement and tracking of significant adverse events and interventions.

Table 17.1.2 provides more information on the 2016 AAP guidelines for moderate and deep sedation.

ASA Guidelines for Sedation and Analgesia by Non-Anesthesiologists

In 1996 the first practice guidelines were put forth in a report from the ASA's Task Force on Sedation and Analgesia by Non-Anesthesiologists.[6] These guidelines were updated in 2002 (Table 17.1.3).[7]

In 1999 the ASA issued practice guidelines for preoperative fasting in healthy patients undergoing elective procedures to reduce the risk of pulmonary aspiration.[8] In 2004 the group differentiated monitored anesthesia care from moderate sedation/analgesia (conscious sedation).[9] In 2010 an advisory was issued on granting privileges for deep sedation to non-anesthesiologist sedation practitioners; it was approved by the ASA House of Delegates in October 2010.[10] The ASA Committee on Standards and Practice Parameters in 2014 recommended that new practice guidelines focusing on moderate procedural sedation and analgesia should be generated.

A summary of the active guidelines for both levels of sedation follows.

A. Preprocedure evaluation and patient counseling.
B. Preprocedure fasting (see Table 17.1.1)

TABLE 17.1.2 2016 AAP guidelines: comparison of moderate and deep sedation

AAP/AAPD	*Moderate Sedation*	*Deep Sedation*
Personnel	An observer trained in Pediatric Advanced Life Support (PALS) who monitors the patient but also may assist in interruptible tasks	A PALS-trained independent observer who cannot assist in other tasks
Responsible provider	PALS trained and able to rescue the patient from known sedation complications, including bag-valve-mask (BVM) and continuous positive airway pressure (CPAP)	PALS trained and able to manage sedation complications, including BVM, CPAP, tracheal intubation, and cardiopulmonary resuscitation
Monitoring and documentation	Pulse oximetry, heart rate (HR), blood pressure (BP), respiratory rate (RR) required Electrocardiography (ECG) and capnography recommended Parameters recorded every 10 minutes	Pulse oximetry, HR, BP, RR required ECG and capnography required Parameters recorded every 5 minutes
Emergency checklists and appropriately stocked crash carts	Required	Required
Recovery	Dedicated recovery area with rescue equipment and drugs recommended Vital signs monitored every 10 minutes until awake	Dedicated recovery area recommended Vital signs recorded every 5 minutes until awake
Discharge	Safe discharge criteria via use of validated recovery scales required with longer observation times for specific patient populations	Safe discharge criteria via use of validated recovery scales required with longer observation times for specific patient groups

Adapted from reference 5.

TABLE 17.1.3 2002 ASA guidelines: comparison of moderate and deep sedation

	Moderate Sedation	*Deep Sedation*
Monitoring and recording: Data recorded at appropriate intervals before, during, and after procedure, in recovery, and at discharge (5-minute intervals for both levels of sedation)	Level of consciousness (LOC), pulse oximetry, heart rate, blood pressure REQUIRED Capnography should be considered in all patients who are separated from caregiver. Electrocardiogram (ECG) in patients with significant cardiovascular disease	LOC, pulse oximetry, heart rate, blood pressure, capnography, ECG REQUIRED for all patients
Emergency equipment	Suction, oxygen source, bag-valve-mask (BVM), airway equipment and adjuncts, basic resuscitative medication and rescue carts, antagonists, intravenous equipment Defibrillator immediately available for patients with cardiac disease	Suction, oxygen source, BVM, airway equipment and adjuncts, basic resuscitative medications and rescue carts, antagonists, intravenous equipment Defibrillator immediately available for ALL patients
Personnel	Person monitoring patient may assist with short, interruptible tasks provided adequate monitoring is maintained.	Person monitoring sedation has no other responsibilities.
Personnel training requirements	Trained in sedation pharmacology and in recognition and management of complications Ability to rescue from deep sedation Basic life support skills present and advanced life support skills within 5 minutes	Trained in sedation pharmacology and in recognition and management of complications Ability to rescue from general anesthesia Advanced life support skills in the procedure room at all times
Supplemental oxygen	Oxygen administered if hypoxia occurs	Oxygen administered to ALL patients unless contraindicated

Adapted from reference 7.

C. Choice of agents and dose titration: medications titrated to effect, appropriate dose reduction for concurrent use of medications
D. Recovery: monitoring and use of validated discharge criteria to minimize risk

In 2018 new guidelines replace the Practice Guidelines for Sedation and Analgesia by Non-Anesthesiologists: An Updated Report by the American Society of Anesthesiologists.[11] New Guidelines: Practice Guidelines for Moderate Procedural Sedation and Analgesia 2018.[11]

- These guidelines do not focus on mild or deep sedation. It is likely, that at a later date a separate document will focus on deep procedural sedation.
- A multidisciplinary group of physicians with representation from several medical and dental organizations with the purpose of focusing on the issue of moderate procedural sedation for the in-hospital and out-of-hospital settings.

ACEP Clinical Practice Guidelines for Procedural Sedation and Analgesia in the Emergency Department

In 1998 the ACEP first published "Clinical Policy for Procedural Sedation and Analgesia in the Emergency Department." Procedural sedation was defined and recommendations were made for personnel, patient assessment, consent, equipment and supplies, monitoring and documentation, postprocedure and discharge management, and quality assurance.[12] In the 2005 revision, depths of sedation, including dissociative state, were defined, and expanded support, including level of evidence (A, B, C), was provided for the 1998 recommendations, plus preprocedural fasting.[13] A clinical policy revision was issued in 2014 (summarized below).[14]

In 2004 a clinical practice guideline was published for emergency department (ED) ketamine dissociative sedation in children.[15] A 2011 update addressed indications and contraindications, the role of anticholinergics and benzodiazepines, personnel and monitoring requirements, and recovery associated with ketamine sedation.[16]

In 2007 the ACEP issued "Fasting and Emergency Department Procedural Sedation and Analgesia: A Consensus-Based Clinical Practice Advisory." The goal was to create a tool to help choose a sedation depth and timing in light of fasting status, type of meal intake, patient risk factors, and the degree of urgency of the procedure in the emergency department.[17]

A summary of the current guidelines follows.

1. Preprocedural fasting in the ED and risk of emesis or aspiration: Procedural sedation should not be delayed in adults or children in the ED based on fasting times. Preprocedural fasting has not been demonstrated to reduce the risk of either emesis or aspiration in ED patients receiving procedural sedation.
2. In the sedated ED patient, capnography may be used as an adjunct to detect hypoventilation and apnea earlier than pulse oximetry and/or clinical judgment alone.
3. Personnel needed: A nurse or other qualified individual should be present for continuous monitoring of the patient in addition to the provider performing the procedure.
4. Ketamine and propofol and its combinations can be safely administered to children in the ED.

Summary

As the practice of pediatric procedural sedation has evolved, diversified, and grown over the decades, several societies, such as AAP/AAPD, ASA, and ACEP, have created guidelines for delivery of pediatric sedation. These society guidelines form an important resource and framework for best practices in the safe and effective delivery of pediatric sedation. Sedation providers must be familiar and abide by these guidelines, evidence-based practices, and their own institutional policies and regulatory standards.

References

1. American Academy of Pediatrics Committee on Drugs, Section on Anesthesiology. Guidelines for the elective use of conscious sedation, deep sedation, and general anesthesia in pediatric patients. *Pediatrics.* 1985;76(2):317–321.
2. Committee on Drugs, American Academy of Pediatrics. Guidelines for monitoring and management of pediatric patients during and after sedation for diagnostic and therapeutic procedures. *Pediatrics.*1992;89(6 pt 1):1110–1115.
3. Committee on Drugs, American Academy of Pediatrics. Guidelines for monitoring and management of pediatric patients during and after sedation for diagnostic and therapeutic procedures: addendum. *Pediatrics.* 2002;110(4):836–838.
4. Coté CJ, Wilson S, American Academy of Pediatrics, American Academy of Pediatric Dentistry; Work Group on Sedation. Guidelines for monitoring and management of pediatric patients during and after sedation for diagnostic and therapeutic procedures: an update. *Pediatrics.* 2006;118(6):2587–2602.
5. Coté CJ, Wilson S, American Academy of Pediatrics, American Academy of Pediatric Dentistry. Guidelines for monitoring and management of pediatric patients before, during, and after sedation for diagnostic and therapeutic procedures: update 2016. *Pediatrics.* 2016;138(1):e1–31.
6. Practice guidelines for sedation and analgesia by non-anesthesiologists: a report by the American Society of Anesthesiologists Task Force on Sedation and Analgesia by Non-Anesthesiologists. *Anesthesiology.* 1996;84:459–471.
7. Practice guidelines for sedation and analgesia by non-anesthesiologists: an updated report by the American Society of Anesthesiologists Task Force on Sedation and Analgesia by Non-Anesthesiologists. *Anesthesiology.* 2002;96:1004–1017.

8. Practice guidelines for preoperative fasting and the use of pharmacologic agents to reduce the risk of pulmonary aspiration: application to healthy patients undergoing elective procedures. A report by the American Society of Anesthesiologist Task Force on Preoperative Fasting. *Anesthesiology.* 1999;90:896–905.
9. American Society of Anesthesiologists. Distinguishing Monitored Anesthesia Care (MAC) from Moderate Sedation/Analgesia (Conscious Sedation). 2004.
10. American Society of Anesthesiologists. Granting Privileges for Deep Sedation to Non-Anesthesiologist Sedation Practitioners, 2010. Available at: http://www.asahq.org/~/media/sites/asahq/files/public/resources/standards-guidelines/advisory-on-granting-privileges-for-deep-sedation-to-non-anesthesiologist.
11. American Society of Anesthesiologists. Practice guidelines for moderate procedural sedation and analgesia 2018. *Anesthesiology.* 2018;128:437–479.
12. American College of Emergency Physicians. Clinical policy for procedural sedation and analgesia in the emergency department. *Ann Emerg Med.* 1998;31:663–677.
13. Godwin SA, Caro DA, Wolf SJ, et al. American College of Emergency Physicians. ACEP clinical policy: procedural sedation and analgesia in the emergency department. *Ann Emerg Med.* 2005;45:177–196.
14. Godwin SA, Burton JH, Gerardo CJ, et al. American College of Emergency Physicians. Clinical policy: procedural sedation and analgesia in the emergency department. *Ann Emerg Med.* 2014;63(2):247–258.
15. Green SM, Krauss B. Clinical practice guideline for emergency department ketamine dissociative sedation in children. *Ann Emerg Med.* 2004;44:460–471.
16. Green SM, Roback MG, Kennedy RM, et al. Clinical practice guideline for emergency department ketamine dissociative sedation: 2011 update. *Ann Emerg Med.* 2011;57(5):449–461.
17. Green SM, Roback MG, Miner JR, et al. Fasting and emergency department procedural sedation and analgesia: a consensus-based clinical practice advisory. *Ann Emerg Med.* 2007;49:454–461.

17.2

Regulatory Issues

JESSE J. STURM AND JERARD (MICK) CONNORS

In 2009, the Center for Medicare and Medicaid Services (CMS) released interpretive guidelines for the provision of Anesthesia Services and Condition of Participation for Hospitals. This initial guideline was revised in 2011 in response to concerns about clarity regarding the distinctions between administration of sedation and anesthesia and possible restrictions on provision of sedation by non-anesthesiologists. The 2011 revisions clarified that hospitals are responsible for establishing policies and procedures that differentiate anesthesia from analgesia/sedation and specified that hospitals were responsible for determining the qualifications for practitioners who administer sedation based on nationally recognized guidelines. The regulations and corresponding interpretive guidelines issued by CMS require the anesthesia service in CMS-certified hospitals to develop hospital policies and procedures governing the provision of all categories of anesthesia services, including specifying the minimum qualifications for practitioners permitted to provide procedural sedation. State survey agencies, which may include departments of health and accrediting organizations, follow CMS interpretive guidelines to determine a facility's compliance with the Medicare Conditions of Participation. State laws, health department requirements, professional boards, accrediting organization standards, and facility bylaws and policy may exceed the CMS requirements.

In the 2011 Interpretive Guidelines, CMS reaffirmed its longstanding definition of anesthesia to mean general anesthesia, regional anesthesia, or deep sedation/monitored anesthesia care (MAC). The CMS definition of deep sedation or MAC is "a drug-induced depression of consciousness during which the patient cannot be easily aroused but respond purposefully following repeated or painful stimuli. The ability to independently maintain a patent airway and spontaneous ventilation may be inadequate." CMS guidelines further state that "anesthesia exists along a continuum and for some medications there is no bright line that distinguishes . . . the physiologic transition from analgesic [moderate sedation] to anesthesia [deep sedation] effects. Furthermore, each patient may respond differently to different types of medications. " Joint Commission guidelines clarify that "individuals administering moderate sedation be qualified to rescue patients at whatever levels of sedation is achieved, either intentionally or unintentionally" (Table 17.2.1).

CMS clearly defines those individuals permitted to administer "anesthesia" as qualified anesthesiologists, non-anesthesiologist MD/DOs, certified registered nurse anesthetists and anesthesiology assistants, dentists/oral surgeons, and podiatrists who are qualified to administer anesthesia under state law. CMS does not clarify the circumstances under which a non-anesthesiologist MD or DO, a dentist, or an oral surgeon is permitted to administer anesthesia but requires that a hospital's anesthesia/sedation policies must clearly address this issue. In the case of a dentist, oral surgeon, or podiatrist, administration of anesthesia must be permissible under state law and comply with all state requirements concerning qualifications. The guidelines do not specifically prescribe how these policies are to be written but state that "hospitals should conform to generally accepted standards of anesthesia care when establishing policies governing anesthesia administration by these types of practitioners as well as MDs or DOs who are not anesthesiologists."

CMS states that each hospital that provides anesthesia services must establish policies and procedures based on nationally recognized guidelines that address whether specific clinical situations involve

TABLE 17.2.1 Joint Commission sedation provider qualification

Sedation Level	*Sedation Provider Qualifications*
Minimal sedation (anxiolysis)	None
Moderate sedation (formerly "conscious sedation")	Individuals administering moderate sedation are qualified and have credentials to manage and rescue patients at whatever level of sedation or anesthesia is achieved, either intentionally or unintentionally.
Deep sedation	Individuals administering deep sedation are qualified and have credentials to manage and rescue patients at whatever level of sedation or anesthesia is achieved, either intentionally or unintentionally.
Anesthesia	Individuals qualified to administer general anesthesia include anesthesiologists, doctors of medicine or osteopathy other than anesthesiologists, doctors of podiatric medicine, certified registered nurse anesthetists with supervision, and anesthesiologist assistants supervised by an anesthesiologist.

Source: Joint Commission International, *Comprehensive Accreditation Manual for Hospitals*. Oak Brook Terrace, IL: Joint Commission Resources, 2011.

anesthesia versus analgesia/sedation. Furthermore, CMS encourages hospitals to address whether sedation provided outside of the operating room, in procedural locations or the emergency department, involves anesthesia or analgesia/sedation. In "establishing such policies, the hospital is expected to take into account the characteristics of the patients, the skill set of the clinical staff in providing the service, as well as the characteristics of the sedation medications used in the various clinical settings." The hospital-site directors of anesthesia services should define site-specific anesthesia policies and procedures and guidelines on privileging that will be made locally. Finally, CMS notes that it is expected that the anesthesia services policies will undergo "periodic re-evaluation that includes analysis of adverse events, medication errors and other quality or safety indicators related not only to anesthesia, but also to the administration of medications in clinical applications that the hospital has determined involve analgesia/sedation rather than anesthesia." This requirement includes the provision of mild, moderate, and deep/MAC sedation events.

The practical implication of current CMS regulations is that the responsibility for the oversight of administration of deep sedation falls under the purview of the director of anesthesia services at a hospital or outpatient center, whether or not an anesthesiologist administers the sedation. These regulations mean that while qualified personnel who are locally privileged may provide deep sedation, the parameters for privileging practitioners and for quality assurance of deep sedation care are the responsibility of the director of anesthesia services.

Based on CMS guidelines, for deep sedation/MAC, a preanesthesia evaluation must be performed for each patient who receives general, regional, or monitored anesthesia. While current practice dictates that the patient receiving moderate sedation be monitored and evaluated before, during, and after the procedure by trained practitioners, a preanesthesia evaluation performed by someone qualified to administer anesthesia as specified in §482.52(a) is not required because moderate sedation is not considered to be "anesthesia," and thus is not subject to that requirement under this regulation. Minimum components of the preanesthesia evaluation include a review of the medical history, including anesthesia history/medication/allergies, interview of the patient (if possible), and documentation of an examination. If not performed on the day of the procedure, CMS requires that under no circumstances may these elements of the preanesthesia evaluation be performed >30 days prior to a procedure requiring anesthesia services. Review of these elements must be conducted, and updates documented, within 48 hours prior to the scheduled procedure.

For patients receiving MAC, CMS requires an intraprocedure anesthesia record that identifies the following:

- The patent and hospital ID, the proceduralist, the sedation practitioner
- Name, dosage, route, and time of administration of drugs
- Patient position(s), including the insertion/use of any intravascular or airway devices
- Name and amounts of intravenous fluids, including blood or blood products if applicable
- Time-based documentation of vital signs as well as oxygenation and ventilation parameters
- Any complications or adverse reactions, including time and description of symptoms, vital signs, treatments rendered, and patient's response to treatment

CMS regulations §482.52(b)(3) require that a postanesthesia evaluation must be completed and documented no later than 48 hours after surgery or a procedure requiring anesthesia services. The evaluation is required any time general, regional, or monitored anesthesia has been administered to the patient. While current practice dictates that the patient receiving moderate sedation be monitored and evaluated before, during, and after the procedure by trained practitioners, a postanesthesia evaluation for moderate sedation is not required under this regulation §482.52(a). For deep sedation/MAC, the regulations do not permit delegation of the postanesthesia evaluation to practitioners who are not qualified to administer deep sedation. The postanesthesia evaluation should not begin until the patient has recovered sufficiently from the anesthesia to appropriately participate in the assessment.

Moderate Sedation

Moderate sedation is defined by CMS as "a drug-induced depression of consciousness during which patients respond purposefully to verbal commands, either alone or accompanied by light tactile stimulation. No interventions are required to maintain a patent airway and ventilation is adequate with maintenance of cardiovascular function." CMS, consistent with American Society of Anesthesiolists guidelines, does not define minimal or moderate sedation as anesthesia. Therefore, few of the above requirements are placed upon encounters that include only minimal or moderate sedation. Regulations state that while pre-evaluation/documentation, intraprocedure monitoring, and postsedation evaluations are common in moderate-sedation encounters, since moderate sedation does not qualify as deep sedation/anesthesia, these strict requirements do not apply. Nevertheless, the local director of anesthesia services should define the minimum requirements for pre- and post-sedation evaluations in these cases.

By CMS regulations, the hospital anesthesia policy is expected to address the minimum qualifications and supervision requirements for each category of practitioners who are permitted to provide moderate sedation. Specifically, this requires that medical staff bylaws "include criteria for determining the privileges to be granted to individual practitioners." For instances where nursing staff may administer sedation, the CMS guidelines (§482.23) state that the "nursing staff be assigned to provide care based on qualifications and competence, medications be prepared and administered in accordance of federal/state laws, and if intravenous medications are to be administered by personnel other than MD/DO, the personnel have special training for this duty."

Nursing

A consensus recommendation on nursing competencies and nursing qualifications to administer moderate and deep sedation is lacking.

The Joint Commission and CMS guidelines do not state whether or not RNs meet the qualifications to deliver moderate or deep sedation. These agencies refer to medical staff credentialing but do not specify the manner in which RNs may be credentialed to provide sedation, and no uniformly accepted training exists. State boards of nursing determine the scope of practice for RNs within their state. To date, "current RN sedation regulation in the United States remains fragmented and poorly documented."

Suggested Reading

American Society of Anesthesiologists. Granting privileges for deep sedation to non-anesthesiologist sedation practitioners. Approved by the ASA House of Delegates on October 20, 2010. Retrieved from: http://www.asahq.org/publicationsAndServices/sgstoc.htm. Accessed March 6, 2017.

American Society of Anesthesiologists, Task Force on Sedation and Analgesia by Non-Anesthesiologists. Practice guidelines for sedation and analgesia by non-anesthesiologists. *Anesthesiology.* 2002;96:1004–1017.

Centers for Medicare & Medicaid Services. *Conditions for coverage and conditions of participation.* May 11, 2012. Retrieved from www.cms.gov/Regulations-and-Guidance/Legislation/CFCsAndCoPs/index.html. Accessed March 6, 2017.

Crego N. Procedural sedation practice: a review of current nursing standards. *J Nurs Regulation.* 2015;6(1):50–56.

Joint Commission International. Comprehensive Accreditation Manual for Hospitals. Oak Brook Terrace, IL: Joint Commission Resources, 2011.

17.3

Hospital and Professional Reimbursement

DAVID BANKS AND DAVID WERNER

The viability of a sedation service depends on its ability to generate revenue, both for the providers and for the facility/institution. A thorough understanding of the process of coding and billing to achieve maximum reimbursement is essential for planning a new sedation service, as well as maintaining and expanding an existing one.

Deep Sedation Coding and Billing

Coding and billing for deep sedation involves using Current Procedural Terminology (CPT) codes for anesthesia services. Anesthesia CPT codes are based on the 5-digit CPT code for the procedure being performed for which sedation is required and the 4-digit Anesthesia bridge or "Crosswalk" code.

Deep sedation services are billed as a combination of base units plus time units. The base units charge includes all services provided by the sedationist during the presedation assessment phase, the immediate presedation assessment, the initiation of sedation, and the postsedation recovery phase. A specific number of units is assigned for the various categories of procedures. For instance, 3 base units are billed for the sedation for a forearm fracture reduction, 5 for the sedation for a lumbar puncture, and 7 for the sedation for an MRI.

Services that are performed as part of the presedation assessment of the patient include chart review of past history and previous anesthetic or sedation procedures, taking a history, performing a physical exam, making an assessment of risk, and creating a sedation plan. Services provided during the postsedation and recovery phase involve intervening for any sedation events that occur in recovery and managing any postprocedure complications, along with making reassessments to determine discharge readiness. Other services routinely provided by the sedationist that are covered under the base units charge include the following:

- Transporting, positioning, and preparing patients for the initiation of sedation and the procedure
- Applying monitoring devices and then monitoring pulse oximetry, capnography, temperature, and electrocardiogram
- Placing intravenous catheters, urinary catheters, and airway adjuncts
- Interpreting laboratory study results.

Time units for deep sedation are billed in 15-minute increments based on the total time of the sedation. Sedation start time occurs when the sedation team is present with the patient and ready to begin and the sedationist's time is dedicated to the patient. Many sedation services use the "procedure timeout" time as the start time for the sedation. The end time occurs when the procedure is complete, sedation has been discontinued, and the patient has sufficiently emerged from sedation so that he or she can be safely turned over to the recovery team. The total time is determined and then divided by 15 to determine the time units. Billing is based on total units, base units plus time units.

While providing the service of deep sedation the sedationist commonly provides multiple services that have their own CPT code for billing, such as starting a peripheral intravenous line or administering intravenous medications. When provided during the course of

TABLE 17.3.1 Common sedated procedures and CPT codes

Procedure	*CPT Code*	*ASA Bridge CPT Code*	*Base Units*
Auditory brainstem response	92585	0300	5
Bone marrow aspirate, biopsy	38220, 38221	1112	5
Fracture reduction, distal radius, radial shaft	25605, 25505	1820	3
Incision and drainage of abscess, simple, complicated	10060, 10061	0400	3
Lumbar puncture, diagnostic, therapeutic	62270, 62272	0635	4
Magnetic resonance imaging, brain	70551	1922	7

delivering deep sedation, these services are considered part of the sedation process and are not billed separately.

Table 17.3.1 shows the CPT codes and base units for some of the common procedures for which sedation is provided by a typical pediatric sedation service.

Moderate Sedation Coding and Billing

Coding and billing for moderate sedation involves the use of the moderate sedation CPT codes that were updated for 2017; the previous moderate sedation codes (99143–99150) are no longer used.

- CPT code 99151 is used for moderate sedation performed by the physician or other qualified healthcare provider who will also be performing the procedure on a patient who is <5 years of age. The presence of an independent trained observer to assist in monitoring the patient's level of consciousness and physiologic status is required.
- CPT code 99152 is used in the same circumstance for a patient who is >5 years of age also requiring a trained observer to assist in monitoring the patient.
- CPT code 99155 is used for sedation performed by a physician or other qualified healthcare provider other than the proceduralist for a patient who is <5 years of age.
- CPT code 99156 is used in the same circumstance for a patient who is >5 years of age.

The codes for moderate sedation include the services of presedation assessment, the ordering and administration of sedation medications, and the monitoring of the patient during the procedure. The start time of the sedation is the time medication is administered. The end time is considered to be the time when the procedure is complete and the patient is stable and no longer requires the presence of the sedationist. The above-mentioned CPT codes include sedation time up to 15 minutes after medication administration. If the procedure extends beyond the initial 15 minutes, and the presence of the sedationist is still medically necessary, then additional time is billed in 15-minute increments using CPT code 99153 for a sedation performed by the proceduralist and 99157 for a sedation performed by a separate sedationist.

To bill moderate sedation codes, the sedating physician must be present at the time of medication administration and remain present until the end of the procedure. A sedation time of at least 10 minutes must be recorded to bill CPT codes 99151, 99152, 99155, and 99156. To bill for additional segments of time using CPT codes 99153 and 99157, a minimum of an additional 8 minutes of sedation time, beyond the preceding 15 minutes, must be recorded in the record. The ability to bill moderate sedation codes for nonphysician providers to state Medicaid programs may vary from state to state.

Table 17.3.2 lists CPT codes for age and provider.

Consultation—Provider

At times the sedationist may perform a presedation evaluation for a patient who is deemed to not be an appropriate candidate for sedation, or whose procedure is subsequently canceled, and therefore no longer requires sedation services. The sedationist may then submit a claim for reimbursement for the assessment using the CPT codes for consultation or standard evaluation and management (E&M) codes.

Medicare has discontinued paying claims for consultation services (CPT codes 99241–99245 and 99251–99255), and many state Medicaid programs have followed suit. For these payers, physicians should submit claims based on the appropriate E&M codes:

- 99201–99205 (new office/outpatient visit)
- 99211–99215 (established office/outpatient visit)
- 99221–99223 (initial hospital care) (inpatient)
- 99231–99233 (subsequent hospital care)

Anesthesia/Deep or Procedural Sedation Coding—Facility Fees

Coding and billing for hospital services associated with providing deep sedation involves the use of facility revenue codes, specifically code 370. The fee associated with this code is inclusive of the physical space, the necessary supplies and equipment, and the nursing and support staff necessary to provide appropriate care to a patient undergoing a procedure requiring sedation, from presedation assessment to discharge from the area. The various

TABLE 17.3.2 CPT codes for age and provider

CPT1/ HCPCS	*Description*	*Work RVUs*	*Non-Facility PE RVUs*	*Facility PE RVUs*	*Malpractice RVUs*	*Total Non-Facility RVUs*	*Total Facility RVUs*
99151	Moderate sedation, same physician/ qhp <5 years	0.50	1.63	0.12	0.05	2.18	0.67
99152	Moderate sedation, same physician/ qhp 5/> years	0.25	1.18	0.08	0.02	1.45	0.35
99153	Moderate sedation, same physician/ qhp ea	0.00	0.30	n/a	0.01	0.31	n/a
99155	Moderate sedation, other physician/ qhp <5 yrs	1.90	n/a	0.56	0.17	n/a	2.63
99156	Moderate sedation, other physician/ qhp 5/> years	1.65	n/a	0.35	0.15	n/a	2.15

17.4

Credentialing and Recredentialing for Pediatric Sedation

JOSEPH D. TOBIAS AND GREGORY A. HOLLMAN

As procedural sedation guidelines have expanded and undergone several rounds of review and revisions over the years since their introduction, the recommendations have expanded to include not only the sedation event itself but also the presedation phase, the recovery phase, and the personnel responsible for providing sedation and monitoring the patient. The guidelines outline the training and skills required to provide procedural sedation with the recommendation for provision of appropriate level of monitoring. Furthermore, given the potential for adverse effects on hemodynamic, respiratory, and upper airway function, the practitioner must be able to intervene and rescue the patient when needed. The most recent edition of the guidelines, which appeared in the July 2016 issue of *Pediatrics*, provided algorithms for the treatment of the most common respiratory and upper airway events, including apnea, laryngospasm, and upper airway obstruction. As such, it is expected that the practitioner, who is credentialed to provide sedation, has the knowledge and technical skills required to treat and reverse these events. These technical skills include the ability to open and maintain the airway, suction secretions, provide continuous positive airway pressure, and even bag-valve-mask ventilation should apnea occur. While many of these skills are taught in advanced resuscitation courses such as Pediatric Advanced Life Support (PALS), such training uses only manikins with limited live scenarios requiring rapid decision-making. Therefore, additional hands-on training in airway management may be necessary, using simulation scenarios or in real-life situations in the operating room or procedural sedation environment.

Such training and credentialing is needed first and foremost to ensure the safe conduct of the sedation encounter. Additionally, hospital accreditation and credentialing organizations such as the Joint Commission on Accreditation of Healthcare Organizations and the Center for Medicare and Medicaid Services (CMS) recognize the potential for morbidity and mortality during procedural sedation. As such, they mandate that healthcare institutions establish sedation practice models that promote patient safety and welfare. This extends to the credentialing of the practitioner; as the Joint Commission's statement on a provider's qualifications states: "Individuals administering moderate or deep sedation are qualified and have the appropriate credentials to manage and rescue patients at whatever level of sedation or anesthesia is achieved, either intentionally or unintentionally." The Joint Commission further states that the responsibility of defining and implementing the privileging process rests with the individual hospital and must be "an objective, evidence-based process."

The diversity of practitioners providing sedation is clearly shown by the growth of the role of non-anesthesiologist–based practitioners in providing sedation services to children. Non-anesthesiologists now represent >80% of sedation practitioners submitting data to the national Pediatric Sedation Research Consortium. Given the complexity of the knowledge and skills required, compounded by the diversity of sedation practitioners (pediatric intensivist, pediatric emergency medicine, pediatric hospitalist, or advanced practice provider), a formal process for training and credentialing is recommended.

To ensure safe sedation practice, hospitals must have a concise and well-defined process for credentialing and delineating sedation privileges to only those individuals who are qualified. The following section discusses options for the medical staff process of granting privileges to licensed independent practitioners and allied health professionals (i.e., advanced-practice nurses, nurse practitioners, and physician assistants) for performing procedural sedation in children.

Credentialing

Credentialing is the process by which hospitals collect and review a practitioner's qualifications for membership to the medical staff and represents the initial step in granting clinical privileges. Although there are no specific guidelines for this process, regulatory boards mandate that each institution have a process in place for granting privileges in various clinical arenas, including procedural sedation. Therefore, each institution must develop its own rigorous and consistent process that clearly defines the training, education, and experience that practitioners need to ensure they are competent to perform sedation. The credentialing procedure should be clearly defined in the institution's medical staff bylaws. It should clearly define the criteria for clinical privileges based on the practitioner's credentials (e.g., practitioner type, current licensure, education and training credentials, board certification).

In general, institutions may divide privileges into core privileges and special/additional privileges. In many cases, procedural sedation falls into the latter category. Core privileges are granted to an individual practitioner who is deemed qualified to perform these duties based upon successful completion of a residency or fellowship in a particular specialty. Following the successful completion of a fellowship in pediatric critical care medicine, core privileges would include care of any child with a life-threatening illness, initiation and management of mechanical ventilation, and procedures such as placement of central venous catheters. The privilege process may require nothing more than documentation of successful completion of the fellowship with board certification or eligibility. Additional or special privileges may be those that are not necessarily part of the specific residency or fellowship. Specific privileges outside the core privileges are frequently considered more specialized and higher risk and require additional education, training, and/or experience. As noted above, procedural sedation frequently falls into this category. With the expansion of pediatric critical care fellowships and the involvement of this group in procedural sedation, there may be recent graduates of fellowships whose credentialing process for procedural sedation falls under the category of core privileges more than special or additional privileges based on their education and fellowship training.

The credentialing and privileging process may therefore use different criteria based on whether the practitioner recently completed fellowship, obtained sedation experience during fellowship, or is new to the institution or was at the institution previously and is requesting new privileges. A requirement to demonstrate skills in a proctored setting may vary as to whether or not subspecialty training provided the core competencies for, and significant experience in, procedural sedation. Review of a procedural sedation log may suffice for those with robust sedation experience. As such, the following scenarios may occur in which the healthcare provider needs to be credentialed:

1. Recent graduate of a fellowship with experience in procedural sedation. This may vary and may need to be investigated when one is looking at the pathway to privilege acquisition.
2. Physician joining the faculty from another institution with prior procedural sedation experience
3. Physician already at the institution who desires to start providing procedural sedation
4. Physician already at the institution who is pursuing a change in the level of sedation provided or the medication used (e.g., the physician wants to start using propofol or ketamine for more invasive procedures)
5. Physician who is part of a specialty that has the recognized skill set as part of everyday practice (pediatric anesthesiologist). For this group, the core privileges will include not only general anesthesia but also procedural sedation.

Sedation Skills

The skills necessary for procedural sedation may be broken down into three general categories:

1. Cognitive: Cognitive or intellectual abilities include knowledge base, the learning or processing of information, and the ability to recall information. The knowledge base includes basic information about the procedural sedation pathway, including presedation assessment, monitoring during the procedure, and an understanding of the medications used, including their pharmacology and adverse effect profile.
2. Psychomotor abilities encompass the motor skill aspects of procedural sedation, including the ability to rescue and resuscitate, such as advanced airway management skills (e.g., bag-valve-mask ventilation and placement of airway devices [supraglottic airway or endotracheal tube]).
3. The affective component concerns a practitioner's behavior and is considered the most difficult quality to assess. Effectively listening to, communicating with, and collaborating with medical staff, patients, and families are examples of affective skills.

Failure to rescue and failure to monitor are key factors leading to poor outcomes, including death, and are often secondary to insufficient integration of these three skills. These reports mandate that the credentialing process clearly demonstrates that the practitioner can identify upper airway, respiratory, and hemodynamic compromise early and provide appropriate intervention. Specific areas of deficiency that may lead to adverse outcomes include inadequate performance of a presedation risk assessment, lack of knowledge about sedative drug pharmacology and dosing, inadequate airway and resuscitation skills, incomplete understanding and use of sedation monitoring, lack of appropriate response to monitoring information, and insufficient recovery and discharge procedures. As respiratory compromise related to hypoventilation or upper airway obstruction remains the sentinel event in the vast majority of cases, the practitioner must understand a sedative drug's effect on upper airway tone and respiratory drive, be able to interpret information from direct patient observation as well as monitoring equipment (pulse oximetry and capnography), and intervene with advanced airway skills to treat hypoventilation, apnea, upper airway obstruction, or laryngospasm.

Tables 17.4.1 and 17.4.2 summarize some of the key cognitive, psychomotor, and affective skills required for performing sedation. As needed, these may be included in a checklist when reviewing a practitioner's request for procedural sedation privileges.

Core Sedation Competencies

Clinical competency can be defined as the ability of a practitioner to apply his or her cognitive, psychomotor, and behavioral skills to a particular clinical task or activity and achieve the desired outcome. Procedural sedation is a complex, multifaceted clinical activity of varying degrees with different components that require diverse skills and competencies. The skills required to perform a presedation risk assessment, including taking a history and performing a physical examination, are vastly different than those needed to manage the patient with sedation-related upper airway obstruction. A practitioner who is competent to perform procedural sedation applies and integrates the necessary cognitive, psychomotor, and behavioral skills to all aspects of the sedation encounter within the practice context. As such, "sedation competency" requires the practitioner to perform a number of distinct tasks proficiently throughout the entire sedation process. The Joint Commission requires hospitals to define the competencies of its practitioners who provide patient care. Published sedation guidelines from the American Academy of Pediatrics (AAP), American College of Emergency Physicians (ACEP), American Society of Anesthesiologists (ASA), and Joint Commission describe the general competencies required by sedation practitioners to safely and effectively conduct procedural sedation, including:

TABLE 17.4.1 Cognitive skills for sedation competencies

1.	Perform a thorough, systems-oriented presedation assessment including a physical examination with identification of features that suggest a problematic or difficult airway scenario. This should identify risk factors (historical or physical features) that may predispose the patient to sedation-related complications. This includes the identification of physical features that may predispose to difficulties with airway management.
2.	Understand the basic pharmacology of sedative medications and their effects on upper airway tone, respiratory drive, and hemodynamic function.
3.	Assignment of an appropriate American Society of Anesthesiologists (ASA) physical status.
4.	Describe the presedation preparation process to patients and caregivers, including information about the objectives of sedation, anticipated changes in behavior following sedation, and the sedation risks, benefits, and alternatives.
5.	Understand the informed consent and "timeout" process.
6.	List the monitoring equipment required for conducting procedural sedation. Explain the principles, indications, and use of the following monitoring tools: blood pressure, electrocardiograph, pulse oximetry, capnography, and pretracheal/precordial stethoscope.
7.	Interpret information derived from pulse oximetry (oxygen saturation) and capnography (carbon dioxide values and waveforms). Recognize the adequacy of oxygenation and ventilation by direct observation and respiratory monitoring.
8.	List the resuscitation equipment required during procedural sedation.
9.	Demonstrate in-depth knowledge of the pharmacology, clinical indications, dosing, and drug interactions of common sedative/analgesic medications and their antagonists.
10.	State fasting guidelines based on age for liquids and solids.

(*Continued*)

TABLE 17.4.1 Continued

11.	Define the sedation levels as defined by the American Society of Anesthesiologists and the American Academy of Pediatrics. Explain the concept of "rescue" from a deeper-than-planned level of sedation.
12.	List the most common sedation-related adverse events that result in the potential for morbidity and mortality, including oxygen desaturation, upper airway obstruction, apnea, and laryngospasm. Specify and be familiar with the respiratory and airway maneuvers that may be required to treat these problems, including the administration of oxygen, repositioning of the airway, performance of a jaw thrust, bag-mask ventilation, suctioning, placement of an oral, nasopharyngeal, or laryngeal mask airway, and endotracheal tube intubation.
13.	Describe the roles of the personnel involved in the sedation process.
14.	List the equipment required in the postsedation recovery environment.
15.	Know the postsedation recovery phases and monitoring requirements.
16.	Understand the discharge criteria.

1. Performance of a presedation risk assessment, including a history and physical examination
2. Administration of sedative medications and their antagonists
3. Evaluation and monitoring of the patient during the sedation process
4. Recognition and management of sedation-related effects and complications
5. Recovery and discharge of patients following sedation.

TABLE 17.4.2 Psychomotor and affective skills for sedation competencies

Psychomotor (Technical) Skills
1. Set up and use age- and size-appropriate monitoring equipment, including noninvasive blood pressure, pulse oximetry, end-tidal carbon dioxide, pretracheal/precordial stethoscope, and continuous electrocardiography.
2. Troubleshoot monitoring equipment.
3. Administer supplemental oxygen using various devices, including nasal cannula, simple and advanced face-mask systems.
4. Perform oropharyngeal suctioning with airway positioning and the application of continuous positive airway pressure.
5. Perform bag-valve-mask ventilation.
6. Place oropharyngeal, nasopharyngeal, and laryngeal mask airways.
7. Perform direct laryngoscopy with placement of an endotracheal tube.
8. Conduct cardiopulmonary resuscitation according to established guidelines, including Pediatric Advanced Life Support.
Affective (Behavioral) Skills
1. Listen and communicate effectively with patients and the family members.
2. Communicate and collaborate with sedation team members, including closed-loop communication.
3. Work effectively as a team member.
4. Be attentive to changes in the patient's medical condition.

At times, the required core competencies have been guided by the depth of sedation that was intended. However, it has become readily apparent that irrespective of medication, dose, and route of administration, the significant interpatient variability in the response results in an inability to ensure that the intended depth of sedation is achieved and not exceeded.

Table 17.4.3 lists the "core" sedation competencies compiled from the ASA, AAP, ACEP, Joint Commission, and CMS. The training, education, and experience that many institutions use to qualify an individual for procedural sedation privileges are discussed in greater detail in the following section.

Achieving Sedation Skills and Core Sedation Competencies

Sedation competency requires training, education, and experience in the field of pediatric sedation. The requirements for sedation privileges may be included as part of their core privileges, based on successful completion of a pediatric subspecialty in which formal sedation training is part of the educational curriculum, such as pediatric emergency medicine or pediatric critical care medicine. As some institutions will likely continue to distinguish the qualification requirements between moderate and deep sedation, moderate sedation may be part of a practitioner's core privileges whereas additional training and experience may be required for deep sedation privileges. When procedural sedation is not part of an individual's formal training program, additional experience, training, and education will likely be required to receive sedation privileges.

Formal Training and Education

Several pediatric subspecialties outside of anesthesiology have assumed a greater role in providing sedation services. Much of this has resulted from a relative shortage of pediatric anesthesiologists. For pediatric critical care medicine physicians, sedation during mechanical ventilation is an integral part of their clinical practice,

TABLE 17.4.3 Pediatric sedation core competencies

Presedation
1. Perform a focused preprocedural and sedation health history and physical examination that accurately identifies comorbid medical conditions that increase sedation risk.
2. Complete the informed consent process. Counsel and prepare patients and/or legal guardians with appropriate information as to the anticipated effects, risks, and benefits of sedation and alternatives to sedation.
3. Perform an effective and efficient "timeout" prior to the procedure. Engage and prepare the team members for the sedation process, including the sedation plan and the roles of the individual participants.
During Sedation
1. Administer and titrate the sedative medications in an effective manner that achieves the desired clinical effect while avoiding adverse effects.
2. Assess the depth of sedation accurately and maintain a rapid response to changes in sedation depth.
3. Monitor the patient's respiratory and cardiovascular condition such that changes in upper airway patency, oxygenation, ventilation, and cardiovascular status are immediately recognized and responded to rapidly to avoid deleterious physiologic effects.
4. Treat the above conditions so that the event does not progress to a severe sedation-related complication.
5. Rescue patients who progress to a deeper-than-planned level of sedation.
Postsedation
1. Recover patients following sedation systematically in a structured environment that promotes patient and family well-being and safety.
2. Educate and support patients and their families on discharge such that they are well informed and highly satisfied.

providing them with ample experience and knowledge of the same medications that are used for procedural sedation. Furthermore, these physician, along with pediatric emergency medicine physicians, may have many of the advanced airway management and monitoring skills required.

Pediatric critical care medicine physicians, pediatric emergency medicine physicians, and more recently pediatric hospital medicine physicians are the three largest non-anesthesiologist–based pediatric subspecialties performing procedural sedation in children. Following completion of fellowship, both pediatric emergency medicine and pediatric critical care medicine physicians are expected to be proficient in procedural sedation. Pediatric emergency medicine and pediatric critical care medicine fellows receive formal training and experience in cardiorespiratory monitoring, advanced airway management, and cardiopulmonary resuscitation, as well as cognitive and psychomotor skills directly applicable to sedation practice. By virtue of their training and experience, pediatric emergency medicine and pediatric critical care medicine physicians are often well suited for procedural sedation privileges as part of their core privileges.

Pediatric hospital medicine physicians have assumed a greater role in some institutions in providing pediatric sedation due to their role in caring for children within a hospital setting. Deep/propofol sedation privileging for pediatric hospital medicine physicians may consist of anesthesia experience in the operating room and 25 supervised propofol sedations. The recent development of the pediatric hospital medicine core competencies specifically addresses the core knowledge, skills, and behaviors needed for the hospitalist to perform procedural sedation. Many pediatric hospitalist medicine fellows are now completing training with the needed education, training, and experience to receive credentialing for procedural sedation along similar pathways as pediatric emergency medicine and pediatric critical care medicine physicians. Depending on the institution, various other pediatric subspecialties (e.g., pediatric hematologists performing moderate sedation for invasive oncology procedures) may receive privileges in performing sedation (usually moderate) and often for a specific patient population.

Additional Training, Education, and Experience

Additional training, education. and experience are required when an individual's formal training and experience do not meet the threshold criteria for receiving sedation privileges at a hospital. Additionally, it may be that some practitioners who received formal training have not maintained their skills and experience and hence require retraining. While each of the educational and training approaches described below has advantages and disadvantages, interactive teaching approaches (e.g., case discussions, simulation) are superior to "passive" educational techniques (e.g. didactic lectures) in changing physician behavior and performance. Educational methods, including simulation, complement but do not substitute for education and training that occurs during patient care (clinical mentoring).

Written materials and lectures provide the learner with cognitive knowledge (e.g., factual information). Written materials such as articles, manuals, and policy statements present the required factual information in print or online at a pace determined by the learner. These written materials, such as the AAP policy statement on procedural sedation, discuss the presedation risk assessment, fasting guidelines, definitions of sedation levels, pharmacology of sedative drugs, sedation monitoring, sedation-related complications and their management, and postsedation recovery and discharge criteria. The various resources can be included as online modules on the hospital's intranet to provide educational resources for those wishing to obtain credentials in procedural sedation. Alternatively, some of the organizations focusing on sedation offer sedation provider courses. Regardless of the format, these didactic courses are followed by formal testing using standardized multiple-choice tests to demonstrate the acquisition and retention of an acceptable knowledge base. Some hospitals and sedation provider courses are now also using simulation to teach and/or test the materials.

Assessing Sedation Competencies

Assessment remains the key piece in determining if an individual has the qualifications for being granted specific privileges. Performance assessment tools should be reproducible and consistent (reliable) and test the intended skill or competency (validity). They should include a means to assess the various cognitive, psychomotor, and affective skills required for procedural sedation (as mentioned earlier).

Written Exams

Multiple-choice questions that test recall of factual information are efficient, easily graded, and highly reliable. More difficult is designing multiple-choice questions that assess the higher intellectual skills of comprehension, clinical reasoning, and problem-solving. Although multiple-choice tests are frequently used to assess cognitive skills in sedation by establishing a minimum score for passing, concern is frequently expressed that they may seem unnatural and too far removed from clinical practice. However, given their ability to test the recall of factual information, they remain one of the key elements used to evaluate competency for procedural sedation credentialing. However, written exams cannot be used to test the psychomotor skills needed for sedation and have limited applicability in assessing attitudinal attributes such as communication and the ability to work within a team.

Medical Simulation

Given the inability of written tests to effectively evaluate critical thinking, the decision-making process, and psychomotor skills, medical simulation has gained acceptance as a means of testing cognitive, technical, and behavioral skills. Simulation promotes a reproducible and realistic environment that can be tailored to assess specific educational objectives. Simulation testing can be designed to target specific performance measures that occur in real-life procedural sedation scenarios (e.g., airway repositioning maneuvers in response to upper airway obstruction, or identifying hypoxemia and its cause). Case- and problem-based medical simulation is particularly useful in assessing higher-level intellectual functioning (e.g., analysis, problem-solving, and decision-making) as well as procedural skills (e.g., bag-mask-valve ventilation). Medical simulation can also be used to assess affective functions such as communication with patients and families as well as teamwork and collaboration with other healthcare professionals.

Proctoring

Proctoring assesses a practitioner's performance under real-life circumstances. It usually involves a defined period of time or a specific number of cases. This direct observation and evaluation allows an assessment of performance during all phases and aspects of the procedural sedation encounter. Performance measures that cannot be assessed by written testing, such as interactions with patients and families, communication with medical staff, or working as a team member, can be readily assessed during the proctoring process. Proctoring can also be interactive and informative, providing learners with valuable feedback and information to improve performance or serve as part of their on-boarding or orientation process. Procedural sedation performance is particularly amenable to proctoring as it is a finite clinical activity with specific and discrete phases (i.e., presedation, sedation, and postsedation) that can be assessed individually or as a whole. Difficulties with proctoring include the subjective nature of the process, practice variability among proctoring physicians, and the inability to provide specific clinical scenarios that the proctor may want to assess. Indeed, the supervising physician may not witness a practitioner's response to an uncommon sedation-related event (e.g., laryngospasm) due to the infrequency with which such events occur. Despite these drawbacks, institutions may use supervised performance of a set number of procedures (e.g., 25 propofol sedations) as part of their training process.

Multisource (360-Degree) Evaluations

Assessments by members of the clinical team (e.g., sedation nursing staff), colleagues, and patients and families can provide valuable information about a practitioner's interpersonal skills, ability to work as a team member, and overall professional behavior. While not routinely used as an assessment tool in procedural sedation performance, it has great potential to provide the types of information that cannot be readily assessed through other evaluative methods. In particular it gives an indication of how well the practitioner will perform with other healthcare professionals within the environment where he or she will work. It may be particularly valuable as one moves forward from the initial credentialing process to subsequent recredentialing.

Summary

Procedural sedation in children is a complex, high-risk clinical activity. Institutions should have a formal credentialing and privileging process that ensures only individuals who are qualified to administer sedation are allowed to do so. Individual institutions are responsible for defining the qualification requirements for a practitioner to be eligible to receive procedural sedation privileges. Formal training and experience provide the foundation for a provider's qualifications. Depending on the specialty and its core competencies, this alone may be sufficient for credentialing in procedural sedation. If an individual's formal fellowship training is not sufficient to meet the credentialing requirements, there may be alternative pathways to credential the individual or provide additional training, education, and experience to achieve procedural sedation privileges. Demonstration of the necessary cognitive, psychomotor, and behavioral skills for procedural sedation may require demonstration of significant clinical experience in the area by the provision of sedation logs, successful completion of sedation courses, passing of a formal written examination, or demonstration of competence using simulation. The cognitive information can be supplemented as needed by various techniques, including classroom or didactic models (intranet-based modules, formal lectures, or video-recorded instruction). Ideally, some level of training and performance assessment should take place in the actual sedation setting using a formal proctor or mentor who observes the clinician during the sedation process. Additionally, given the need for airway skills, many institutions rely on certification in standard resuscitation courses (PALS) as evidence of such competency. As part of the privileging process, practitioners agree to follow the AAP guidelines for procedural sedation, including fasting guidelines, sedation monitoring, and recovery and discharge guidelines. Most importantly, the proceduralist cannot be the person conducting the sedation. The credentialing process is generally repeated at 2- to 3-year intervals along with renewal of hospital privileges. Recredentialing of privileges may follow a different pathway from the initial process, with more focus on the practitioner's experience and demonstration of competency through the quality improvement process and the Focused Professional Practice Evaluation (FPPE).

Suggested Reading

Coté CJ, Wilson S, American Academy of Pediatrics, American Academy of Pediatric Dentistry. Guidelines for monitoring and management of pediatric patients before, during, and after sedation for diagnostic and therapeutic procedures: update 2016. *Pediatrics.* 2016;138:e20161212.

Couloures KG, Beach M, Cravero JP, et al. Impact of provider specialty on pediatric procedural sedation complication rates. *Pediatrics.* 2011;127:e1154–1160.

Epstein RM. Assessment in medical education. *N Engl J Med.* 2007;356:387–396.

Epstein RM, Hundert EM. Defining and assessing professional competence. *JAMA*. 2002;287:226–235.

Klass D. Reevaluation of clinical competency. *Am J Phys Med Rehabil.* 2000;79:481–486.

Krauss B, Green SM. Training and credentialing in procedural sedation and analgesia in children: lessons from the United States model. *Paediatr Anaesth.* 2008;18:30–35.Turmelle M, Moscoso LM, Hamlin KP, et al. Development of a pediatric hospitalist sedation service: training and implementation. *J Hospital Med.* 2012;7:335–339.

18

Administrative Organization

18.1

A Sedation Unit Approach

JOHN S. KOPEC

Justification, Structure, and Organization

The concept of a pediatric sedation unit (PSU) developed as the need for a sedation service outside of the operating room became legitimized and essential to hospitals with a large pediatric population. Initially, pediatric sedation was often limited to a small number of nurses and physicians with a travel cart or a single room commonly in or adjacent to an intensive care unit, operating suite, or emergency department. As the number of noninvasive (primarily radiologic) and invasive procedures grew, this model has often been replaced by a unit-based model in which patients are transported to a specific area of the hospital where the procedure will take place. A PSU does not fully replace the need for mobile sedation; there will remain highly specialized units where the patients are not able to travel, such as a burn unit, radiation therapy, and interventional radiology. A PSU may be defined in terms of its location, equipment, and structure, but also by its personnel, with nursing staff, technical staff, and physicians trained and committed to pediatric sedation.

A dedicated PSU can offer the following benefits:

- Added efficiency via one-point scheduling, quick room turnover, recovery, and decreased staff travel time
- Enhanced safety in terms of proximity of dedicated staff and resuscitation equipment

- Limited movement of staff, equipment, and patients, potentially in a stage of sedation or recovery
- Limitation of personnel with sedation privileges as sedation is easily accessible
- Less redundancy of supplies, medications, and potentially costly equipment
- Nursing and technician cross-coverage with other areas such as radiology
- Decompression of the operating room and postanesthesia care unit
- Provision of identity and recognition of a sedation service
- Improved family and patient satisfaction due to dedicated staff and space.

Structural Organization: Considerations for Design, Location, and Function

Physical space should enhance organization. A PSU footprint may vary considerably depending on location as well as the number and type of procedures expected. Most PSUs exist within a hospital and provide services to both inpatients and outpatients; ideally they afford easy access to both. Since radiology is usually the most frequent customer of sedation services, proximity to radiology is a common request. Many PSUs are 4–6 beds, but may range from 1 to 15. The number and size of rooms required must take into consideration the number and length of procedures, the complexity of the procedure (needing extra staff and/or equipment), the sedation agents used, recovery times, and number of available staff.

Many support spaces may be shared with other adjacent units. A workroom for staff should be centrally located; if warranted, a separate room may be added for scheduling, screening, intake, and follow-up phone calls, which may be disruptive in the general work area. An electronic whiteboard, also accessible through the hospital intranet, displays patient list, modality, arrival and procedural start time, room, and staff assigned. Consideration can be given to alternative uses for sedation rooms after hours, such as overnight sleep studies and electroencephalograms.

Summary

The pertinent design and administration of a PSU will vary based on the local medical climate and needs of a given region. The PSU is highly integrated into the hospital and, once established, is virtually essential to the provision of safe and efficient care of children. Integration with the hospital, study modalities, and subspecialties can be facilitated by easy access to the PSU for inpatients and outpatients, enhanced communication using the electronic medical record, an organized scheduling and screening process, and attention to improvement and growth. Brief daily meetings of the staff, periodic multidisciplinary meetings, and parental feedback help promote discussion, enhance safety and organization, and improve family experience.

Suggested Reading

Blike GT, Cravero JP. Pride, prejudice, and pediatric sedation: a multispecialty evaluation of the state of the art. Dartmouth Summit on Pediatric Sedation. September 2000.

Lowrie L, Weiss AH, Lacombe C. The pediatric sedation unit: a mechanism for pediatric sedation. *Pediatrics*. 1998; 102(3):E30.

18.2

A Sedation Team Approach

MICHAEL TURMELLE

When considering the administrative organization of a sedation service, the Centers for Medicare and Medicaid Services (CMS) has published regulations for the oversight of such services:

> The anesthesia services must be under the direction of one individual who is a qualified doctor of medicine (MD) or doctor of osteopathic medicine (DO). Consistent with the requirement at 482.12(a)(4) for it to approve medical staff bylaws, rules and regulations, the hospital's governing body approves, after considering the medical staff's recommendations, medical staff rules and regulations establishing criteria for the qualifications for the director of the anesthesia services. Such criteria must be consistent with State laws and acceptable standards of practice.[1]

Another portion of the CMS document is also worth noting:

> The regulation at 42 CFR 482.52(a) establishes the qualifications and, where applicable, supervision requirements for personnel who administer anesthesia. However, hospital anesthesia services policies and procedures are expected to also address the minimum qualifications and supervision requirements for each category of practitioner who is permitted to provide analgesia services, particularly moderate sedation.[1]

With these two statements, CMS makes it clear that although one individual must have oversight of sedation services, institutions have the flexibility to meet their sedation needs in a variety of ways. The sedation unit (see Chapter 18.1) is one organizational approach to providing safe sedation. A sedation team is an alternative strategy for delivering care within a hospital system.

A sedation team allows more flexibility to function outside the four walls of one set unit. The team could function throughout the hospital or potentially at off-campus sites. This flexibility offers potential benefits and detriments, which must be weighed in the context of a respective institution's needs and mission.

The team approach may look fairly similar to the unit approach. A mobile sedation team may involve sedation delivery by a practitioner who requires supervision. The supervisor must be close enough to the location of the sedation to respond to an emergency, the logistical impact and determination of which will vary among facilities.

The providers who deliver the sedation may vary within the team. The specialty of the sedation providers may include those trained in anesthesiology, critical care, emergency medicine, hospital medicine, pediatric nurse practitioners, or registered nurses, depending on state and institutional regulations. The sedationist is generally accompanied by another provider (e.g., nurse, medic, nurse assistant) who is available to assist with sedation delivery, monitoring, and documentation. The sedationist and assistant focus on the sedation care of the patient, enabling the proceduralist to attend to the interventional task at hand.

If available, the presence of a certified child life specialist dedicated exclusively to the team is incredibly valuable. If not a member of the sedation team, a child life specialist assigned to the clinical procedural unit will enhance the team's success by being involved in the sedation process from pre-planning through emergence and recovery.

Although not visible to the patient, two integral team members are the scheduler and coder. The scheduler receives all requests for sedation and has an understanding of what types of procedures can be accomplished outside of the operating room or dedicated sedation unit. The scheduler also communicates the sedation plan for the day to the other team members. Mobile sedation units may be the team that takes responsibility for short-notice, add-on cases. Working add-ons into the schedule can be difficult but can pay great dividends in keeping the throughput of the entire hospital moving. Spending another day in the hospital for a sedated MRI, PICC line insertion, and so forth is frustrating to patients, families, primary treatment teams, and hospital administrators. For a sedation service to remain financially viable, having a dedicated person for billing and coding is ideal.

How this system is organized will be as variable as the sedation team itself. Defining the respective institutional relationship with the hospital or university simplifies the complexity of billing, collections, and compensation, and makes ongoing negotiations with hospital leadership or university administration much easier.

Although there are many ways to structure a sedation team, the key to success is having a flexible yet well-organized approach that works in the given system and meets the needs of the patients who need procedural sedation care.

Suggested Reading

Campbell K, Torres L, Stayer S. Anesthesia and sedation outside the operating room. *Anesth Clinics*. 2014;32:25–43.

Lalwani K, Michel M. Pediatric sedation in North American children's hospitals: a survey of anesthesia providers. *Pediatr Anesth*. 2005;15:209–213.

Reference

1. Centers for Medicare & Medicaid Services (CMS). State Operations Provider Manual, Appendix A—Survey Protocol, Regulations and Interpretive Guidelines for Hospitals, Certification. Revised. Appendix A, Interpretive Guidelines for Hospitals §482.52 Condition of Participation: Anesthesia Services, Interpretive Guidelines §482.52. 2011.

19

Quality Improvement in Pediatric Sedation

ASHWIN KRISHNA AND CHERI LANDERS

Successful pediatric sedation programs must have processes in place to optimize outcomes for all patients undergoing procedural sedation. Achieved by performing continuous, systematic reviews of existing practice followed by actions to improve the experience, efficiency, and safety of pediatric sedation, quality improvement in pediatric sedation practice involves the following:

- Identification of deficits in care
- Implementation of processes to address deficits
- Tracking of data to ensure that the implemented processes have the intended effect.[1]

Along with institution-specific processes and delivery systems, wide variation in pediatric sedation practice exists between institutions with regards to practitioner training and experience, as well as provider-specific practice.[2] Intra-institutional review serves to identify key processes that affect the respective system's sedation delivery, yet sedation services benefit greatly by sharing data and best practices with others in order to improve their own methods. The need for collaboration among different institutions with varying practice experience led to the founding of the Pediatric Sedation Research Consortium (PSRC) in 2003.[3] The PSRC consists of 52 healthcare institutions devoted to improving the quality of care, processes, and outcomes for children undergoing procedural sedation. The largest database of its kind, the PSRC has demonstrated the outcomes that can be achieved by highly motivated, well-organized pediatric procedural sedation centers.[3]

To narrow the gap between current care and the high-quality care healthcare professionals intend to deliver, the Institute of Medicine (IOM) described 6 aims for improvement (STEEEP):

- Safe
- Timely
- Effective
- Efficient
- Equitable
- Patient-centered care.[4]

The "Great Expectations" article in the *Journal for Healthcare Quality*[5] and the Society for Pediatric Sedation (SPS)'s Center of Excellence Consensus Statement[6] are excellent references for sedation quality and use these same 6 aims as a framework to approach quality in pediatric sedation. This framework is how this discussion will be organized as well.

Safe Care

Healthcare systems and healthcare providers ought to provide care that minimizes injuries or adverse effects to patients. This goes beyond the Hippocratic maxim "do no harm." Instead, the goal should be for safety to be an essential component of the entire patient experience.[4]

In centers contributing to the PSRC, there is zero mortality or irreversible injury reported as a result of sedation, and less severe adverse events such as apnea, desaturation, upper airway obstruction, or laryngospasm are uncommon.[7] Quality sedation programs ought to have an incidence of adverse events that compares favorably with the outcomes reported by the PSRC.

System processes and characteristics that contribute to safe sedation outcomes include the following:

- Well-trained, highly skilled multidisciplinary teams
- Strong presedation screening processes, identifying patients and procedures at higher risk[8]
- Identification and tracking of adverse outcomes
- Well-delineated emergency rescue systems
- Didactic and simulation educational programs such as the SPS Sedation Provider course to advance the following:
  - Education covering the entire sedation encounter from presedation assessment through managing adverse events, recovery, and discharge[9]
  - Ongoing assessment of provider competencies
- Emergency response simulations
- Multidisciplinary reviews of unexpected events.

Population subgroups and procedures posing higher risk for adverse events during sedation include the following:[10,11]

- Premature infants
- Obese patients
- Patients with upper respiratory infections
- Patients undergoing esophagogastroduodenoscopy
- Patients undergoing bronchoscopy.

Table 19.1 shows examples of metrics that centers may track to monitor safe sedation.

TABLE 19.1 Suggested pediatric sedation quality metrics in each Institute of Medicine domain

Safety	*Timely/ Efficient*	*Equitable*	*Patient-Centered*	*Effective*
Apnea rate	Average time from sedation request to sedation start	Rate of IV starts offered topical anesthetic	Rate of child life involvement per sedation encounter	Rate of inadequate sedation encounters
Desaturation rate	Average on-time starts	Rate of presedation phone calls made in language of choice	Rate of cases prescreened for behavioral assessment	Rate of IV success on first attempt
Airway obstruction rate	Next available appointment		Rate of topical anesthetic use prior to minor procedures	
Laryngospasm rate	Same day add-on availability		Rate of parental presence during induction/ procedure	
Mortality or cardiac arrest rate	Rate of same-day referral to anesthesia		Family likelihood to recommend service to others	
Airway interventions needed	Schedule utilization (utilized time per provider time)			

TABLE 19.1 Continued

Safety	*Timely/ Efficient*	*Equitable*	*Patient-Centered*	*Effective*
Emergency anesthesia consult	Cancellation rate			
Reversal agent needed	No-show rate			
	Number of prolonged recoveries			

Timely and Efficient Care

Efficiency and timeliness are closely related and difficult to separate from a practical standpoint. Simplistically, timeliness refers to reducing wait times, while efficiency involves reducing overall waste and using resources wisely. For the purposes of measurement, wait times can be evaluated in segments:

- Request to appointment time
- Patient arrival to sedation start
- Procedure time
- Recovery time.

Improving timeliness often improves efficiency. Efforts that may impact a service's timeliness and efficiency include the following:

- Robust prescreening that identifies patients needing alternative sedation providers
- Streamlined scheduling process
- Appropriate staffing model and availability

- Robust communication with parents prior to arrival to the sedation unit/procedure.

The goal is to eliminate waiting that does not confer or provide information. For patients, waiting on the telephone to receive presedation information, waiting at the sedation unit, or waiting for the proceduralist or provider to be available to start a case is not only time-consuming but emotionally taxing and has the potential to result in medical harm.

Metrics that may suit sedation services for monitoring how timely and efficient their program is are also shown in Table 19.1.

Equitable Care

Healthcare disparities for vulnerable populations remain a weakness for healthcare systems. Pediatric sedation services should strive to provide care of equal quality to all individuals regardless of the following:

- Gender, race, age, ethnicity, socioeconomic status, geographic location, or sexual orientation[4]
- Cultural traditions, personal preferences and values, family dynamics and lifestyles
- Whether they enter the system via the emergency department, the sedation suite, or the inpatient unit.

System characteristics that support equitable care include the following:

- On-site interpreters for common languages spoken in the service area
- Telephone interpreter services for less common languages

- Sensitivity training for staff to understand the concerns regarding vulnerable populations.

Challenges exist, however, with regard to metrics that are easily monitored in this area, and administrators at each center should choose what works best for them. Possible metrics are shown in Table 19.1.

Patient-Centered Care

Sedation services must center their efforts on providing the best, most comfortable experience for the patient as well as the parent/guardian. Sedation can be an uncomfortable experience for a child as it may involve placement of an intravenous line, medications that alter consciousness, and separation from parents in an unfamiliar environment. The most comprehensive patient-centered experience involves the following:

- Providing age-appropriate information in preparation for sedation
- Active participation in the care plan by the patient and guardians
- Measures to alleviate the discomfort associated with the experience, including:
  - Child life services as a part of the sedation team
  - Presedation surveys regarding the child's tolerance of discomfort and separation
- Adoption of universally recognized comfort measures, including:
  - Positioning at the comfort of the patient
  - Distraction techniques
  - Topical anesthetics before intravenous line placement and on the procedure site[12]

  - Parental presence for difficult tasks, including intravenous line placement and induction
- Follow-up after discharge.[4]

Such measures not only improve the patient sedation experience, but can also help with future encounters, especially avoiding needle phobia.[13] Part of patient-centered care includes more innovative, nontraditional ways of communicating with providers and access to protected health information such as through secure websites, text messaging, and social media for appointment reminders and email updates regarding test results. All of these innovations allow for a more streamlined but meaningful patient experience.

Patient-centered care metrics can come from follow-up survey questions and can also include the list shown in Table 19.1.

Effective Care

Most importantly, the care provided by a pediatric sedation service must be effective. This involves more than just getting the procedure done; it also includes the following:

- Completing the procedure
- The appropriate amount of anxiolysis, analgesia, and amnesia
- No discomfort to the child
- Avoidance of physical restraint
- Avoidance of sedation if not warranted.[4]

Ideally, no procedure should fail due to an inability to achieve effective sedation.[10] The unmeasured cost of inadequate sedation or analgesia may not be quantifiable in dollars, but results in increased patient fear, hyperalgesia, and anxiety with future procedures.[14] While assessment of discomfort can be very subjective, attempts to objectify the assessment of sedation efficacy, such as the Pediatric Sedation State Scale, have been made.[15]

Metrics to track in the area of effectiveness are listed in Table 19.1.

Conclusion

Quality improvement is an integral part of any high-functioning pediatric sedation program. Tracking appropriate metrics and making changes to pediatric sedation practice and process in order to maintain benchmarks and improve current practice can help institutions improve the quality of the sedation experience for patients, families, and providers. Tools that help collect information about sedation events can be developed to match each institution's needs. One such example is illustrated in Figure 19.1. Trending outcomes over time can be presented in the form of a scorecard that tracks institutional quality metrics alongside PSRC established benchmarks or institutional targets for each metric. Such a scorecard or dashboard, as shown in Figure 19.2, can help an institution identify areas of strength and where improvement is needed. Pediatric sedation programs, regardless of resources, provider type, or institutional constraints, will benefit from using data to create processes that correctly identify and address obstacles to high-quality sedation care.

SEDATION PERFORMANCE IMPROVEMENT

Date:	◯ NO EVENT	◯ EVENT	
Sedation Practitioner:		Resident/Fellow:	
Procedure:		Surgeon/Medical Specialist:	
Location:		Elective/Urgent/Emergency:	
◯ Minimal	◯ Moderate	◯ Deep	◯ $ETCO_2$
Medications Given:	◯ Midazolam	◯ Fentanyl	◯ Ketamine
◯ Dexmedetomidine	◯ Nitrous Oxide	◯ Propofol	◯ Other:

X	EVENT DESCRIPTION
	ADMISSIONS
	Unexpected hospital admission
	Unexpected ICU admission
	AIRWAY/RESPIRATORY
	Upper Airway Obstruction/Stridor
	Placement of Oral Airway or N/P Airway
	Apnea (>20 seconds)
	Aspiration
	Bronchospasm
	Severe coughing (requiring intervention/interrupts scan)
	Delayed return to normal respiratory pattern
	Unplanned intubation
	Placement of LMA
	Failed LMA placement
	Hypercapnia
	Hypoxemia 90-95%
	Hypoxemia 80-89%
	Hypoxemia <80%
	Intubation: DIFFICULT
	Intubation: Esophageal
	Laryngospasm: MEDICATION REQUIRED
	Laryngospasm: RE-INTUBATION
	Laryngospasm:RELIEVED W/POSITIVE PRESSURE
	Non-Cardio (Negative Pressure) Pulmonary Edema
	Respiratory Arrest
	Vomiting
	Unexpected post-op ventilator assistance
	BEHAVIOR
	Emergence agitation
	"Rage"
	Medication for emergence agitation
	Reversal agent for emergence agitation
	CANCELLATIONS
	Case cancelled after sedation
	Case cancelled because of NPO guidelines
	Case cancelled for further medical work-up
	Case cancelled due to acute illness
	Case cancelled for late arrival
	CARDIOVASCULAR
	Bradycardia 20% change from baseline
	Bradycardia 30% change from baseline
	Cardiac Arrest
	Cardiogenic Pulmonary Edema/CHF
	Dysrhythmia
	Hypertension 10% change from baseline
	Hypertension 20% change from baseline
	Hypotension 20% change from baseline
	Hypotension 30% change from baseline
	Myocardial Ischemia by ECG changes
	Tachycardia
	DEATH
	Patient death

X	EVENT DESCRIPTION
	EQUIPMENT
	Sedation equip malfunction/failure - cancellation/delay
	Sedation equip malfunction/failure - prolonged sedation
	Sedation equipment not available
	Procedure equip malfunction/failure - cancellation/delay
	Procedure equip malfunction/failure - prolonged sedation
	Procedure equipment not available
	IMAGING STUDY
	Interrupted - pt movement
	Interrupted - airway
	LABORATORY
	Erroneous lab result
	Hypoglycemia
	LEVEL OF SEDATION
	Unintended deeper level of sedation ____ (# events)
	Inadequate level of sedation
	Use of restraints
	Failed sedation (procedure not completed)
	LINES/IV
	In-situ failed line/complication (Floor ____)
	Failed line placement
	Unplanned catheter removal
	MEDICATIONS
	Adverse drug reaction
	Adverse contrast reaction
	Allergic reaction
	Anaphylaxis
	Failed Reversal: MEDICATION
	Mislabeled/Wrong medication or dose given
	Overdose
	Pre-Medication-Administered at inappropriate time
	Pre-Medication-Excessive sedation
	Reversal agent used
	Vomiting-MEDICATION
	NEUROLOGIC
	Delayed emergence (30 minutes)
	Headache
	Seizure
	PATIENT INJURIES
	Eye injury
	Lip injury
	Nose injury
	Skin injury
	Tongue injury
	Tooth injury
	Other injury:________________
	THERMOREGULATION
	Hypothermia (<35.5 C/ 95.9 F)
	Hyperthermia (>38.5 C/ 101.3 F)
	TIMEOUT FOR PROCEDURE
	Not performed
	OTHER (ex. Social Issues,etc.)

EVENT DESCRIPTION:

PATIENT LABEL

FIGURE 19.1.

Example of data collection tool used by Texas Children's Hospital Sedation Services for quality assurance.

	Pediatric Sedation Service Dashboard	Jan	Feb	Mar	Targets: Threshold (red)	Targets: Minimum (yellow)	Targets: Goal (green)
Quality/Safety	# Mortality	0	0	0	any	NA	0%
	# Cardiac Arrest	0	0	0	any	NA	0%
	% Need for BVM ventilation, not just CPAP	7.7	4	10.1	>8%	>5-8%	0-5%
	% Need for LMA	1.1	4	1	>2%	>1-2%	0-1%
	% Need for ETT	0	0	0	>1%	>0-1%	0%
	# Need for Increased Level of Care	0	0	0	>5%	>2-5%	0-2%
	% Cancellation Due to Issue related to Sedation	0	0	1	>5%	>2-5%	0-2%
	% Use of Reversal Agents	0	0	0	>2%	>1-2%	0-1%
	% Emergent anesthesia consult	0	0	0	>2%	>1-2%	0-1%
	% Pre-Sedation Checklist Complete	97%	91%	83%	<95%	95-<98%	98-100%
Efficiency	# First Cases >30 min late start	3	3	7	>3	2-3	0-1
	3rd next available (days) MRI+Sed	10.7	13.2	12.8	>19	11-19	<11
	3rd next available(days) Sed Service only	4.2	5.7	5	>19	11-19	<11
	% No show within 24 hour	7%	16%	10%	>14%	8-14%	0-8%
	Rescheduled to GA for complexity	0	0	0	>5	4-5	0-3
	% Scheduling + Add-On Utilization	79%	70%	89%	<70%	70-80%	80-100%
	% Scheduling utilization	74%	68%	78%	<65%	65-75%	75-100%
	% Performed Sedation Utilization	56%	46%	54%	<60%	60-70%	70-100%
Efficacy	% Unable to achieve sedation needed to complete the procedure	0%	0%	0%	>1-2%	>0-1%	0%
	% Immobilizer success rate	0%	100%	none	<60%	60-80%	80- 100%
Service	% cases IV on first attempt	95%	74%	78%	<70%	70-80%	>80%
	>3 IV attempts %	0%	0%	0%	>4%	>2-4%	0-2%
	% received topical anesthetic prior to IV start	95%	91%	100%	<80%	80-94%	≥95%
	% Would refer our service to others	100%	100%	100%	<80%	80-90%	90- 100%
	% Answered "no" to anything we could improve upon?	100%	100%	100%	<80%	80-90%	90- 100%

FIGURE 19.2.

Example of sedation service dashboard. Monthly metrics can be shaded in stoplight colors to represent target level.

Used with permission from Kentucky Children's Hospital Sedation Service, Lexington, KY.

References

1. U.S. Department of Health and Human Services Health Resources and Services Administration. Quality Improvement, https://www.hrsa.gov/quality/toolbox/508pdfs/qualityimprovement.pdf. Accessed February 2017.
2. Langhan ML, Mallory M, Hertzog J, et al. Physiologic monitoring practices during pediatric procedural sedation: a report from the Pediatric Sedation Research Consortium. *Arch Pediatr Adolesc Med.* 2012;166(11):990–998.
3. Society for Pediatric Sedation. Pediatric Sedation Research Consortium. http://www.pedsedation.org/resources/research/. Published 2016. Accessed February 2017.
4. Institute of Medicine. *Crossing the Quality Chasm: A New Health System for the 21st Century*. Washington, DC: National Academy Press, 2001.
5. Connors JM, Cravero JP, Kost S, et al. Great expectations—defining quality in pediatric sedation: outcomes of a multidisciplinary consensus conference. *J Health Qual.* 2015;37(2):139–154.
6. Society for Pediatric Sedation. Center of Excellence. http://www.pedsedation.org/resources/quality-safety/center-of-excellence/consensus-statement/. Published 2016. Accessed February 2017.
7. Cravero JP, Blike GT, Beach M, et al. Incidence and nature of adverse events during pediatric sedation/anesthesia for procedures outside the operating room: report from the Pediatric Sedation Research Consortium. *Pediatrics*. 2006;118(3):1087–1096.
8. Grunwell JR, Marupudi NK, Gupta RV, et al. Outcomes following implementation of a pediatric procedural sedation guide for referral to general anesthesia for magnetic resonance imaging studies. *Paediatr Anaesth.* 2016;26(6):628–636.
9. Hollman GA, Banks DM, Berkenbosch JW, et al. Development, implementation, and initial participant feedback of a pediatric sedation provider course. *Teach Learn Med.* 2013;25(3):249–257.
10. Cravero JP, Beach ML, Bilke GT, et al. The incidence and nature of adverse events during pediatric sedation/anesthesia with propofol for procedures outside the operating room: a report from the Pediatric Sedation Research Consortium. *Anesth Analg.* 2009;108(3):795–804.
11. Biber JL, Allareddy V, Allareddy V, et al. Prevalence and predictors of adverse events during procedural sedation anesthesia outside the operating room for esophagogastroduodenoscopy and colonoscopy in

children: age is an independent predictor of outcomes. *Pediatr Crit Care Med.* 2015;16(8):e251–e259.

12. Leroy PL, Costa LR, Emmanouil D, et al. Beyond the drugs: nonpharmacologic strategies to optimize procedural care in children. *Curr Opin Anaesthesiol.* 2016;29(Suppl 1):S1–13.
13. Jenkins K II. Needle phobia: a psychological perspective. *Br J Anaesth.* 2014;113(1):4–6.
14. Kamat PP, McCracken CE, Gillespie SE, et al, Pediatric critical care physician-administered procedural sedation using propofol: a report from the Pediatric Sedation Research Consortium Database. *Pediatr Crit Care Med.* 2015;16(1):11–20.
15. Cravero JP, Askins N, Sriswaski P, et al. Development and validation of the Pediatric Sedation State Scale. *Pediatrics.* 2017;139(5):e20162897.

Appendix

Pediatric Procedural Sedation Medications

JOHN BERKENBOSCH AND SALLY WEBB, WITH EDITORIAL ASSISTANCE BY DON WIEST

Sedatives

Midazolam (Versed©)

1. Actions
   a. Sedative
   b. Anxiolytic
   c. Anterograde Amnesia
   d. Anticonvulsant
   e. *No analgesia*
2. Mechanism and Metabolism
   a. GABA-A receptor binding
   b. Hepatic P450 system CYP34A isoform
   c. Active metabolite excreted via kidneys
   d. 97% protein bound
3. Contraindications
   a. Benzodiazepine allergy
   b. Oral midazolam is contraindicated with protease inhibitors (which inhibit cytochrome P450 CYP34A)
4. Considerations
   a. Most common agent used for sedation

   b. Combine with analgesic for painful procedure.
   c. Primary metabolite, alpha hydroxy-midazolam, is equipotent to midazolam.
   d. Elimination half-life is increased with liver disease/failure, congestive heart failure, obesity, acute renal failure
   e. Free fraction (active) increased in albumin-deficient patients
   f. WARNING: Synergistic with opioids; risk for respiratory depression. Decrease dose.
   g. Paradoxical agitation in 1–15% of children; flumazenil may be used for treatment
   h. 2017 FDA warning: long-term exposure may negatively affect brain development in children <3 years old
5. Reversal agent: flumazenil
6. Routes
   a. Intravenous (IV)
      i. Dose: 0.05–0.1 mg/kg
      ii. Recommended single max. dose: 2.5 mg
      iii. Onset of action: 1–3 minutes
      iv. Duration of effect: 20–30 minutes
   b. Intramuscular (IM)
      i. Dose: 0.1–0.15 mg/kg
      ii. Recommended single max. dose: 10 mg
      iii. Onset of action: 3–5 minutes
      iv. Duration of effect: 90–120 minutes
   c. Intranasal (IN)
      i. Dose: 0.2–0.5 mg/kg
      ii. Recommended single max. dose: 10 mg
      iii. Onset of action: 3–5 minutes
      iv. Duration of effect: 30–60 minutes
      v. Considerations
         1. Use 5-mg/mL concentration; split dose between each naris. Should not use >1.0 mL aliquots per naris to administer dose.
         2. Mucosal irritation common due to pH = 2 and benzyl alcohol. Premedicating with 0.5 mL 4% topical lidocaine IN reduces discomfort.

d. Oral (PO)
   i. Dose: 0.25–0.5 mg/kg
   ii. Recommended single max. dose: 20 mg
   iii. Onset of action: 10–20 minutes
   iv. Duration of effect: variable
   v. Considerations
      1. Unreliable clinical effect due to 1st-pass hepatic metabolism
      2. 40–50% bioavailability

Lorazepam (Ativan©)

1. Actions
   a. Sedative
   b. Anxiolytic
   c. Anterograde Amnesia
   d. Anticonvulsant
   e. *No analgesia*
2. Mechanism and Metabolism
   a. GABA receptor binding
   b. Hepatic P450 system
   c. Inactive metabolite excreted via kidneys
   d. 97% protein bound
3. Contraindications
   a. Benzodiazepine allergy
   b. Propylene glycol hypersensitivity (IV form)
4. Considerations
   a. Midazolam is generally preferred over lorazepam/diazepam because of shorter duration of activity.
   b. Elimination half-life is increased with liver disease/failure, congestive heart failure, obesity, acute renal failure.
   c. No active metabolites
   d. Readily absorbed orally
   e. WARNING: Synergistic with opioids = risk for respiratory depression; decrease dose

f. 2017 FDA warning: long-term exposure may negatively affect brain development in children <3 years old
g. Combine with analgesic (e.g., opioid) for painful procedure.

5. Reversal agent: flumazenil
6. Routes
    a. Intravenous (IV)
        i. Dose: 0.05 mg/kg
        ii. Recommended single max. dose: 2 mg
        iii. Onset of action: 2–3 minutes
        iv. Duration of effect: 6–8 hours
    b. Intramuscular (IM)
        i. Dose: 0.05–0.1 mg/kg
        ii. Recommended single max. dose: 2 mg
        iii. Onset of action: 15–30 minutes
        iv. Duration of effect: up to 17 hours
        v. Less desirable for procedural sedation due to long half-life
    c. Intranasal (IN)
        i. Dose: 0.1 mg/kg
        ii. Recommended single max. dose: 2 mg
        iii. Onset of action: <10 minutes
        iv. Duration of effect: up to 18 hours
        v. Less desirable for procedural sedation due to long half-life
    d. Oral (PO)
        i. Dose: 0.05 mg/kg
        ii. Recommended single max. dose: 4 mg
        iii. peak plasma levels: 2 hours
        iv. Duration of effect: 12 hours (adult data)
        v. 90% bioavailability

Dexmedetomidine (Precedex©)

1. Action
    a. Sedative
    b. Anxiolytic
    c. Analgesic effects

2. Mechanism and Metabolism
   a. Selective $alpha_2$-adrenoceptor agonist
   b. See peripheral $alpha_1$ activity at higher doses during induction
   c. Hepatic metabolism via glucuronidation and CYP2A6
   d. Excreted in urine
3. Contraindications
   a. Shock or heart block
   b. Use with caution if concomitant use of digoxin or beta blockers
   c. Possible or recent stroke, moyamoya disease, or intracranial arteriovenous malformation
4. Considerations
   a. Provides hypnosis, anxiolysis, and mild analgesia with minimal effect on respiratory drive
   b. Bradycardia with or without sinus arrest with rapid bolus
   c. Hypotension and bradycardia are common.
   d. Hypertension is possible, especially in children <1 year of age and with higher doses.
   e. Good option in autistic children
   f. May accumulate in hepatic failure
   g. Does not interfere with EEG results
   h. May be a neuroprotective agent when used alone or when combined with other sedative agents
   i. Use of glycopyrrolate with dexmedetomidine to treat bradycardia may cause extreme hypertension.
5. Reversal agent: none
6. Routes
   a. Intravenous (IV)
      i. Dose
         1. Load: 0.5–2 mcg/kg over 10 minutes
         2. Drip: 0.2–1 mcg/kg/hr
      ii. Recommended single max. dose: none found
      iii. Onset of action: 5–10 minutes
      iv. Duration of effect: 30–60 minutes
   b. Intramuscular (IM)
      i. Dose: 1–4 mcg/kg
      ii. Recommended single max. dose: none found

iii. Onset of action: 10–15 minutes
iv. Duration of effect: 60–120 minutes

c. Intranasal (IN)
   i. Dose: 1–4 mcg/kg (median: 2.5–3 mcg/kg)
   ii. Recommended single max. dose: none found
   iii. Onset of action: 20–30 minutes
   iv. Duration of effect: 45–60 minutes (up to 120 minutes possible)
   v. Considerations
      1. 2 mcg/kg IN dexmedetomidine has had equivalent effects to 0.5 mg/kg midazolam.
      2. Painless and odorless
      3. >90% bioavailability

d. Buccal
   i. Dose: 3–5 mcg/kg
   ii. Recommended single max. dose: 300 mcg
   iii. Onset of action: 30–45 minutes
   iv. Duration of effect: 60–120 minutes

Pentobarbital (Nembutal©)

1. Action
   a. Sedative
   b. Hypnotic
   c. Anticonvulsant
   d. *No analgesia*
2. Mechanism and Metabolism
   a. Enhances GABA activity and depresses reticular activating syndrome
   b. Hepatic metabolism; CYP2A6 and CYP34A induction
   c. Renal elimination <1%
3. Contraindications
   a. Barbiturate allergy
4. Considerations
   a. Short-acting barbiturate
   b. Terminal half-life 25–50 hours

c. No benefit with adding midazolam to pentobarbital, just more adverse events
d. 1–14% risk for paradoxical agitation during or afterwards ("pentobarb rage")
e. Longer time to sedation discharge than with dexmedetomidine
f. Prolonged recovery and risk of hypoxia, especially when combined with other sedatives
g. Injection has 40% propylene glycol.
h. 2017 FDA warning: long-term exposure may negatively affect brain development in children <3 years old.

5. Reversal agent: none
6. Routes
   a. Intravenous (IV)
      i. Dose: 1–3 mg/kg
      ii. Recommended single max. dose: 100 mg
      iii. Onset of action: 1 minute
      iv. Duration of effect: 15–45 minutes
   b. Intramuscular (IM)
      i. Dose: 2–6 mg/kg
      ii. Recommended single max. dose: 100 mg (150–200 mg in adults)
      iii. Onset of action: 10–15 minutes
      iv. Duration of effect: 2 hours
   c. Oral/Rectal (PO/PR)
      i. Dose: 3–6 mg/kg
      ii. Recommended single max. dose: 100 mg
      iii. Onset of action: 15–60 minutes
      iv. Duration of effect: 1–4 hours

Propofol (Diprivan©)

1. Action
   a. Sedative
   b. Hypnotic
   c. Anxiolytic
   d. Antiemetic

    e. Anesthesia
    f. *No analgesia*
    g. Anticonvulsant
2. Mechanism and Metabolism
    a. GABA agonist
    b. Hepatic metabolism via glucuronide and sulfation to inactive metabolites
    c. Highly lipophilic
    d. 90% renal elimination as inactive metabolites
3. Contraindications
    a. Documented anaphylaxis (not just allergy) to eggs, soybeans, or soy products
    b. Do not use in shock or if hemodynamically unstable.
    c. Avoid prolonged infusions in mitochondrial disease.
4. Considerations
    a. Ultrashort-acting sedative
    b. Be prepared for rapid loss of consciousness and deep sedation.
    c. Apnea, respiratory depression, and hypotension are possible.
    d. No analgesic effect, so an agent like ketamine or fentanyl is needed for painful procedures.
    e. Infants have higher metabolic clearance, requiring more aggressive dosing.
    f. Obese patients may have delayed emergence.
    g. Painful peripheral IV administration (less in antecubital vein) can be lessened by IV lidocaine 0.5–1 mg/kg with or without venous occlusion.
    h. Low incidence of emergence delirium and nausea/vomiting
    i. 2017 FDA warning: long-term exposure may negatively affect brain development in children <3 years old
5. Reversal agent: none
6. Route
    a. Intravenous (IV)
        i. Dose
            1. Bolus: 1–2 mg/kg
            2. Drip: 50–150 mcg/kg/min
        ii. Recommended single max. dose: none

iii. Onset of action: 30 seconds
iv. Duration of effect: 3–10 minutes

Etomidate (Amidate©)

1. Action
    a. Sedative
    b. Hypnotic
    c. Anesthesia
    d. *No analgesia*
2. Mechanism and Metabolism
    a. GABA receptor agonist
    b. Blocks adrenal stress response for 4–8 hours
    c. Hepatic metabolism via ester hydrolysis and N-dealkylation
    d. Renal (85%) and biliary (13%) excretion
3. Contraindications
    a. Do NOT use in shock or if hemodynamically unstable.
4. Considerations
    a. Ultrashort-acting hypnotic agent
    b. Accumulates in hepatic and renal failure
    c. Myoclonus common (25–45%); also associated with nausea/vomiting
    d. Painful on injection
    e. There is transient adrenal suppression from a single dose for 6–24 hours (11-B-hydroxylase inhibition). Consider exogenous corticosteroid replacement if needed.
    f. 2017 FDA warning: long-term exposure may negatively affect brain development in children <3 years old.
5. Reversal agent = none
6. Route
    a. Intravenous (IV)
        i. Dose: 0.2–0.3 mg/kg
        ii. Recommended single max. dose: none
        iii. Onset of action: 30–60 seconds
        iv. Duration of effect: 2–15 minutes (dose-dependent)

Dissociative Agent

Ketamine

1. Actions
   a. Sedative
   b. Analgesia
   c. Amnesia
   d. Anticonvulsant
2. Mechanism and Metabolism
   a. NMDA receptor antagonist and mu opioid receptor agonist
   b. Hepatic metabolism via N-dealkylation, hydroxylation, and glucuronide conjugation
   c. Metabolic product, norketamine, is also active.
   d. Terminal half-life: 2.5 hours
3. Contraindications
   a. Hypertension
   b. Aneurysms
   c. Thyrotoxicosis
   d. Psychotic disorders
4. Considerations
   a. Versatile and reliable sedative–analgesic agent
   b. Preserves cardiopulmonary stability (including heart rate, blood pressure, cardiac output) and airway reflexes
   c. May increase intracranial pressure—blunted with concomitant benzodiazepines
   d. May cause dreamlike state or hallucinations, nystagmus, and hypersalivation
   e. Nausea/vomiting common: ondansetron reduces vomiting
   f. Increasing evidence of improved sedation/analgesia when combined with propofol or dexmedetomidine
   g. May blunt cardiorespiratory events seen during solo sedation with propofol or dexmedetomidine
   h. Increased risk of respiratory depression when used with midazolam. No benefit in decreasing emergence reaction in children (as opposed to adults).

i. Causes hypersalivation but may see increased respiratory adverse events with anticholinergic use (glycopyrrolate or atropine)
j. Emergence reactions in 10–12% include hallucinations/agitation: not prevented by midazolam in children; true delirium rare (2%) when used alone

5. Reversal agent: none
6. Routes
   a. Intravenous (IV)
      i. Dose: 0.5–2 mg/kg
      ii. Recommended single max. dose: none
      iii. Onset of action: 30–60 seconds
      iv. Duration of effect: 10–15 minutes
   b. Intramuscular (IM)
      i. Dose: 2–5 mg/kg
      ii. Recommended single max. dose: none
      iii. Onset of action: 3–4 minutes
      iv. Duration of effect: 15–30 minutes
      v. Considerations
         1. Recovery with IM up to 3–4 hours possible
         2. Use 50-mg/mL concentration for IM injection.
   c. Intranasal (IN)
      i. Dose: 3–9 mg/kg
      ii. Recommended single max. dose: none
      iii. Onset of action: 5–10 minutes
      iv. Duration of effect: 30–75 minutes
      v. Use 50-mg/mL concentration for IN administration.
   d. Oral (PO)
      i. Dose: 3–10 mg/kg
      ii. Recommended single max. dose: none
      iii. Onset of action: 30 minutes
      iv. Duration of effect: 4–6 hours
      v. Considerations
         1. Unreliable clinical effect due to 1st-pass hepatic metabolism
         2. Combination with oral midazolam better in some studies

Analgesics

Fentanyl

1. Action
   a. Analgesia
   b. Euphoria
2. Mechanism and Metabolism
   a. Synthetic opioid (mu receptor) agonist
   b. Hepatic metabolism via cytochrome P450 system
   c. Renal elimination: 75% inactive, 10% active
3. Contraindications: fentanyl allergy
4. Considerations
   a. No anxiolytic or amnestic properties
   b. Potent analgesic (100 times greater than morphine) agent
   c. Chest wall rigidity with rapid, high-dose IV administration: no reports in pediatric procedural sedation
   d. Lacks histamine release—less hypotension
   e. Is a cough suppressant
   f. Respiratory depression may occur once painful procedure is finished.
   g. Infants and young children have higher clearance so more frequent dosing is required.
   h. Synergistic with midazolam and propofol
   i. Accumulates with renal failure
5. Reversal agent: naloxone
6. Routes
   a. Intravenous (IV)
      i. Dose
         1. Initial: 0.5–2 mcg/kg
         2. Subsequent: 0.5–1 mcg/kg
      ii. Recommended single max. dose: 50–100 mcg
      iii. Onset of action: 2–3 minutes
      iv. Duration of effect: 20–30 minutes
   b. Intranasal (IN)
      i. Dose: 2 mcg/kg
      ii. Recommended single max. dose: 100 mcg

iii. Onset of action: 10 minutes
iv. Duration of effect: 60–90 minutes
v. Considerations
1. Use 50-mg/mL concentration and divide the dose into each nostril with atomizer (MAD).
2. May need to repeat approx. half a dose for pain control

Morphine

1. Action
   a. Analgesia
   b. Euphoria
   c. Mild sedation
2. Mechanism and Metabolism
   a. Opioid (mu) receptor agonist at supraspinal, spinal, and peripheral levels
   b. Hepatic metabolism—glucuronide conjugation to morphine-6-glucuronide (active)
   c. Renal elimination
3. Contraindications: morphine allergy
4. Considerations
   a. Better for prolonged procedures; difficult to titrate for procedural pain
   b. Histamine release (flushing and itching), peripheral venous dilation and decreased venous return
   c. Stimulates vagal nucleus, causing bradycardia
   d. Reduce dosing when using with benzodiazepine or in opioid-naïve patients.
5. Reversal agent: naloxone
6. Routes
   a. Intravenous (IV)
      i. Dose: 0.05–2 mg/kg
      ii. Recommended single max. dose: 5 mg
      iii. Onset of action: 5–10 minutes
      iv. Duration of effect: 2–4 hours

Remifentanil (Ultiva©)

1. Action
    a. Analgesia
    b. Euphoria
2. Mechanisms and Metabolism
    a. Synthetic opioid (mu receptor) agonist
    b. Ultrashort-acting (half-life = 3–6 minutes)
    c. Hydrolysis by tissue and plasma esterases to minimally active metabolite
    d. No change in pharmacokinetics in end-stage renal disease or hepatic failure
3. Contraindications: remifentanil allergy
4. Considerations
    a. Ultrashort half-life is appealing for short procedures, especially when combined with short-acting sedative.
    b. Potent analgesic (200 times greater than morphine) agent
    c. Relatively narrower therapeutic window for apnea
    d. No accumulation due to esterase hydrolysis
    e. Chest wall rigidity may occur.
5. Reversal agent: naloxone
6. Routes
    a. Intravenous (IV)
        i. Dose:
            1. Bolus: 0.5–1 mcg/kg
            2. Drip: 0.05–0.2 mcg/kg/min
        ii. Recommended single max. dose: none
        iii. Onset of action: 2–3 minutes
        iv. Duration of effect: 8–10 minutes
        v. Dose should be based on ideal body weight in obese patients.

Acetaminophen (Tylenol©)

1. Actions: analgesia
2. Mechanisms and Metabolism
    a. Prostaglandin (central COX enzyme) inhibitor
    b. May also inhibit endogenous cannabinoid reuptake

   c. Hepatic metabolism—mainly glucuronidation and sulfation to inactive metabolite
3. Contraindications
   a. Acetaminophen allergy
   b. Liver failure
4. Considerations
   a. No published data in procedural sedation
   b. Reasonable evidence in postoperative literature that use can decrease opioid requirements
5. Reversal agent: none
6. Routes
   a. Intravenous (IV)
      i. Dose: 15 mg/kg
      ii. Recommended single max. dose: 750 mg (<50 kg); 1,000 mg (>50 kg)
      iii. Onset of action: 5–10 minutes
      iv. Duration of effect: 4–6 hours

Ketorolac (Toradol©)

1. Action
   a. Analgesia
   b. Anti-inflammatory
2. Mechanism and Metabolism
   a. Nonsteroidal anti-inflammatory (NSAID)
   b. Central and peripheral COX-1 and COX-2 inhibitor
   c. May also inhibit endogenous cannabinoid reuptake
   d. Hepatic metabolism—mainly glucuronidation to inactive metabolites
   e. Metabolites renally excreted
3. Contraindications
   a. Allergy to NSAIDs or aspirin
   b. Active peptic ulcer disease, recent gastrointestinal bleeding, or history of peptic ulcer disease or gastrointestinal bleeding
   c. Advanced renal disease
   d. Patients with high risk for bleeding

4. Considerations
    a. No published data in pediatric procedural sedation
    b. Limited (unpublished) use in Pediatric Sedation Research Consortium database (<1% of painful procedures)
    c. Some evidence of opioid-sparing effects in postoperative populations
5. Reversal agent: none
6. Routes
    a. Intravenous (IV)
        i. Dose: 0.5 mg/kg
        ii. Recommended single max. dose: 15 mg (children), 30 mg (adolescents)
        iii. Onset of action: 30 minutes
        iv. Duration of effect: 4–6 hours

Reversal Agents

Flumazenil (Romazicon©)

1. Action: benzodiazepine reversal/antidote
2. Mechanisms and Metabolism
    a. Competitively binds central benzodiazepine receptors to inhibit GABA activation
    b. Hepatic metabolism to inactive metabolites
3. Contraindications: benzodiazepine dependence or chronic use (precipitates acute withdrawal reaction)
4. Considerations
    a. Does not alter action of non-benzodiazepine GABA-based agents (e.g., ethanol, barbiturates)
    b. Reverses sedation more than respiratory depression
    c. Resedation risk, as effects may dissipate before those of parent agent
    d. Large doses are associated with precipitation of acute withdrawal reaction, including seizures.
    e. Reports of routine use in procedural sedation show more rapid awakening but not discharge time due to resedation risk.

f. Has been used to treat paradoxical midazolam reactions in children

5. Reversal agent: none
6. Routes
   a. Intravenous (IV)
      i. Dose
         1. Initial: 0.01 mg/kg every 2–3 minutes as needed, titrated to effect
         2. Subsequent: Consider infusion at 0.005–0.01 mg/kg/hr for long-acting benzodiazepine reversal
      ii. Recommended single max. dose: 0.2 mg (total dose 1 mg)
      iii. Onset of action: 1–2 minutes
      iv. Duration of effect: 30–45 minutes (depends on dose and benzodiazepine plasma level)

Naloxone (Narcan©)

1. Action: opioid reversal/antidote
2. Mechanisms and Metabolism
   a. Competitively binds mu, kappa, and sigma opioid receptors
   b. Hepatic metabolism via glucuronidation
   c. Metabolites renally excreted
3. Contraindications: chronic opioid use or dependence (precipitates acute withdrawal reaction)
4. Considerations
   a. Reverses sedation, respiratory depression, and hypotension
   b. Resedation or redevelopment of cardiorespiratory depression is a risk if reversing longer-acting opioids.
   c. For full reversal of overdose, use higher dose recommended by PALS.
5. Reversal agent: none
6. Routes
   a. Intravenous (IV)
      i. Dose to reverse respiratory depression: 0.001–0.015 mg/kg every 2–3 minutes as needed, titrated to effect
      ii. Recommended single max. dose: 0.4 mg

iii. Onset of action: 1–2 minutes
iv. Duration of effect: 30–60 minutes
v. May also give IM, SC, or ET

Anticholinergics

Atropine

1. Action
   a. Antisialogogue
   b. Antiemetic
   c. Increases heart rate
2. Mechanisms and Metabolism
   a. Inhibition muscarinic actions of acetylcholine at postganglionic cholinergic nerve sites
   b. Antiemetic effects since crosses blood–brain barrier
   c. Rapid metabolism by hepatic enzymatic hydrolysis, although up to 50% is eliminated unchanged in urine
3. Contraindications/Cautions
   a. Glaucoma
   b. Urinary retention
   c. Decreased gastrointestinal motility/obstruction
   d. Tachydysrhythmias
   e. Autonomic neuropathy
4. Considerations
   a. While hypersalivation is decreased, does not appear to decrease risk of overt laryngospasm
   b. Evidence for decreased emesis after ketamine is conflicting; balance with possible prolonged stay if tachycardia persists.
5. Reversal agent: none
6. Routes
   a. Intravenous (IV)
      i. Dose: 0.01–0.02 mg/kg
      ii. Recommended single max. dose: 0.4 mg
      iii. Onset of action: 1–2 minutes
      iv. Duration of effect: 30–60 minutes (dose-dependent)

Glycopyrrolate (Robinul©)

1. Action
   a. Antisialogogue
   b. Increases heart rate
2. Mechanisms and Metabolism
   a. Inhibits muscarinic actions of acetylcholine at postganglionic cholinergic nerve sites
   b. No antiemetic effect as does not cross blood–brain barrier
   c. 85% excreted unchanged in urine
3. Contraindications/Cautions
   a. Glaucoma
   b. Decreased gastrointestinal motility/obstruction
   c. Tachydysrhythmias
   d. Autonomic neuropathy
4. Considerations
   a. No antiemetic effects as does not cross blood–brain barrier
   b. Tachycardia more prolonged than with atropine
   c. Evidence no longer suggests benefit in decreasing laryngospasm.
   d. May actually be associated with increased risk of adverse airway events compared to atropine or no anticholinergics
5. Reversal agent: none
6. Route: intravenous (IV)
   i. Dose: 4–10 mcg/kg
   ii. Recommended single max. dose: 0.2 mg
   iii. Onset of action: 1–2 minutes
   iv. Duration of effect: 3–4 hours for tachycardia; 6–8 hours for secretions

Antiemetic

Ondansetron (Zofran©)

1. Action: antiemetic
2. Mechanism and Metabolism
   a. Selective serotonin 5-HT_3 antagonist

   b. Hepatic metabolism (primarily hydroxylation) to nonactive metabolites
3. Contraindications
   a. Long QT syndrome (dose-dependent increase in QT_c)
   b. Concomitant SSRI use (use caution)
4. Considerations
   a. Limited data on use for pediatric procedural sedation.
   b. Prophylactic use decreases emesis after ketamine sedation (number needed to treat = 13).
   c. Benefit does not appear to exist with oral ondansetron.
   d. Only published data are with use during ketamine sedation.
5. Reversal agent: none
6. Routes
   a. Intravenous (IV)
      i. Dose: 0.1–0.15 mg/kg
      ii. Recommended single max. dose: 8 mg
      iii. Onset of action: 15–30 minutes
      iv. Duration of effect: 4–6 hours
   b. Oral (PO/sublingual)
      i. Dose: 2 mg/dose (<4 years); 4 mg/dose (4–11 years); 8 mg/dose (>12 years)
      ii. Recommended single max. dose: 8 mg
      iii. Onset of action: 30 minutes
      iv. Duration of effect: 4–6 hours

Index

Page references to tables, figures, and boxes are indicated by *t's*, *f's*, *b's* respectively.